# The Christian's Guide
## to *Natural Products & Remedies*

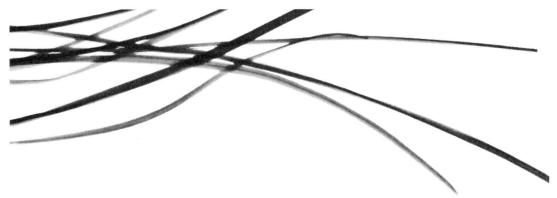

# FRANK MINIRTH, M.D.

JOHN CLAUDE KRUSZ, M.D., ALAN HOREWELL, PH.D.,
AND VIRGINIA NEAL, PH.D.

# The Christian's Guide
## to *Natural Products* & Remedies

1100 Herbs, Vitamins, Minerals, Supplements and More!

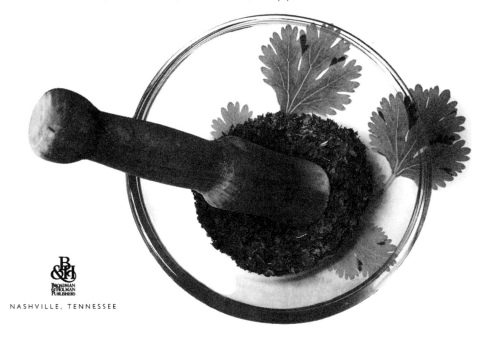

BROADMAN
&HOLMAN
PUBLISHERS

NASHVILLE, TENNESSEE

Ten-Digit ISBN: 0–8054–4082–8
Thirteen-Digit ISBN: 978–0–8054–4082–9


Published by Broadman & Holman Publishers
Nashville, Tennessee


Dewey Decimal Classification: 613.2
Subject Heading: HERBS \ NATURAL FOODS \ DIET

Unless otherwise indicated Scripture text is quoted from the New King James Version, copyright © 1979, 1980, 1982, Thomas Nelson, Inc., Publishers. Other versions are identified by acronym as follows: KJV, King James Version. NASB, the New American Standard Bible, © the Lockman Foundation, 1960, 1962, 1963, 1968, 1971, 1972, 1973, 1975, 1977; used by permission. NIV, The Holy Bible, New International Version, copyright © 1973, 1978, 1984 by International Bible Society.

1 2 3 4 5 6 7 8 9 10  10 09 08 07 06 05

# Contents

# Preface

Why should I read this book? is the first question I ask myself when considering perusal of a new book. If you, too, prefer to know the benefits of a potential read before investing your time with its content, I offer several reasons for your consideration in deciding whether to study this book carefully.

*1. Everyone is using natural products today.* Herbs and supplements are a huge business. Americans will spend over fifteen billion dollars on herbs and other supplements this year. Thirty-five percent of Americans use supplements of some kind. There are more than eight hundred dietary supplement companies. "Over the last ten years, herbal products have moved from the dusty back shelves of rarely patronized, small health food stores to prominent displays in major retail stores and pharmacies across the United States."[1] Furthermore, Christians have joined the movement with a major force.

The supplement movement cannot be ignored. Almost daily we see clients in our office who have tried herbs or other supplements. They often tell us what they have heard about herbs, seeking to understand how and whether their use will be beneficial.

Who has not had his mother put a little calamine lotion on a bug bite when he was young? Who has not had grandmother's chicken noodle soup? Who has not felt the warm, calming feeling of hot chocolate on a cold winter's day? Who has not added "a teaspoon of sugar to help the medicine go down," as Mary Poppins sang? Who has not heard Uncle George say he was trying garlic for either his high blood pressure or high cholesterol or to keep the ticks off? Who has not coughed on a long trip in the car as Cousin Billy smoked tobacco? Who has not enjoyed a good cup of coffee or a cold glass of cranberry juice? Who has not wanted a taste of Aunt Grace's blueberry pie? What about a nutritious bowl of oatmeal for breakfast? Who does not know someone using ginkgo biloba, Saint-John's-wort, ginseng, garlic, echinacea, saw palmetto, kava, grape seed extract, cranberry juice, valerian, evening primrose oil, bilberry, milk thistle, or other herbs? And finally, what does the Bible have to say about herbs?

What do all of the previous questions have in common? They all deal with natural products. Everyone uses some natural product every day, in one fashion or another. In addition, one-third of all Americans now use herbs on a more serious, routine, directed basis. Herbs and supplements are indeed big business. Yet even with the myriad of books, magazines, and Internet articles available on the subject, there seems to be a dearth of simple-to-read, easy-to-learn information. The glut of available information makes for much confusion. This book is intended to simplify the facts and provide succinct, applicable help for those wishing to reap the most benefits from herb supplements.

*2. Few books elucidate both sides of the herb and supplement story—the good and the bad.* Who would take a prescription drug without knowing some potential dangers and risks of side effects? We want to know for our safety. We anticipate the benefits of potential medications but also want to be cognizant of possible dangers. Why should natural products deserve less scrutiny? Any substance taken into the body to produce a biological response is a drug, regardless of what one calls it or whether one needs a prescription to obtain it. This book gives both sides of the story. It offers at least one salient benefit and usually one danger for a thousand different supplemental products.

Clients come in our offices every day, telling us what they have "heard" about herbs and supplements. What is daunting is what they were *not* told. The purpose of this book is to examine what is known, what is not known, the benefits, and the dangers of natural products.

Clients were often told of "wonder" herbs and other supplements for anxiety, athletic enhancement, bipolar disorder, cognitive enhancement, the common cold, diabetes, fibromyalgia, heart disease, high blood pressure, hepatitis, insomnia, headaches, obesity, obsessive-compulsive disorder, osteoarthritis, and PMS. But what are they *not* told? Are truths, half-truths, and lies all mixed together? We will try to sort this out for you.

3. *This book is worthy of consideration because it covers a legion of products.* I know of no lay book with more than a thousand natural products discussed. I know of none even close.

4. *I implore you to consider this book because of the format.* I admit the format is different after the first several chapters, but please permit me to build my case. Studying medicine requires learning a wealth of information. Medical books are often arranged with a plethora of information in a paucity of words. Here information is provided in an easy-to-learn format: a question on the left side of the page with the answer on the right. Specific chapters are allotted to herbs (chaps. 14–16), vitamins (chap. 17), minerals (chap. 18), supplements (chap. 13), hormones (chap. 20), common foods (chap. 11), spices (chap. 12), amino acids (chap. 19), beverages (chap. 10), enzymes and antioxidants (chap. 20). The format provides a quick reference and comprehension of a great deal of information. Those who want a quick reference on a specific natural product will like chapter 22, which alphabetically lists more than a thousand natural products. Use this chapter as a dictionary to look up any herb or natural product about which you have a question. Do you have a question about a specific disease? You will appreciate chapter 9 on natural products and specific diseases, again provided in alphabetical order for easy reference. Are you a medical professional? You will enjoy chapter 23.

5. *Shouldn't a book be written for Christians that addresses natural products and explores those natural products found in the Bible?* Chapter 25 deals with those products mentioned in the Bible. What does the Bible have to say about natural products? What should be the position of Christians in regard to the use of natural products? Until now Christian publishers have been both reticent and reluctant on this subject, but the Christian world is neither reluctant to use these products nor reserved to speak informally to one another about them. Isn't it time they had scientific, logical, and biblical knowledge? At the risk of seeming too confident, this book is one of the most detailed ever written in either the Christian or the secular world. The references are near legion. The appendices are in many ways analogous to a PDR (physician's desk reference) of herbal products: They describe both "what they told you" and "what they did not tell you," the good and the bad.

This book is fun and entertaining in style. Whether you are a novice in this area or a savant, you will benefit from this book. Whether you are a maverick who likes to do your own thing or a maven with great knowledge, you should benefit from this book. Do you want to know what everyone else is doing in regard to natural products? Do you want to know what is hot and what is not? Then this book is for you. Chapter 8 presents the pearls, chapter 21 the dangers, and chapter 1 the most popular herbs.

Finally, when I started to write this book a few years ago, my intent was to prove that this movement was largely specious and spurious. During the process, however, I became treatment intrigued. The more I studied, the more my preconceived concepts began to change. I began to see possibilities I had not seen before. The research began to interest me. Some of the theories seemed plausible. Pearls were unearthed. I eventually decided that the whole area of natural products could hold some fortuitous gems for us in allopathic medicine. Hopefully, the reader will find some of those gems in this book.

Frank Minirth, MD

# Authors' Note

We are neither advocates nor adversaries of today's popular movement involving the use of natural products. Instead, *1100 Natural Products* offers extensive information about vitamins, minerals, enzymes, hormones, herbs, amino acids, antioxidants, and supplements in an entertaining, easy-to-read format. You even can test your knowledge and tabulate your score at the end of the book. While much of what we explore is applicable particularly to psychiatric disorders and treatments, many other medical benefits and cautions to these natural products are discussed as well.

This book is not intended to be a specific medical guide for any individual, in any regard, for any disease. It is not intended for the purpose of diagnosing, treating, curing, or preventing any disease. Errors and inaccuracies are always possible in a book of this kind. It is not intended as a specific medical guide for those helping others. It is our belief that a personal physician is needed when making health decisions, including those related to vitamins, minerals, amino acids, antioxidants, enzymes, hormones, herbs, and supplements. We often tell our clients that almost any drug or herb can do almost anything to any organ, so to err on the prudent side is always best. It is important to consult your local doctor for any personal questions.

I wish to thank Janis Whipple, whose writing skills and input were invaluable. Many thanks are due to Megan Nichols for the tremendous help she has given in preparation of the manuscript. I want to acknowledge that I am indebted to *In Pursuit of Happiness,* published by Revell for some of the brain diagrams and associated scientific information. I am indebted to the multitude of researchers over the years. Lists of their most salient works are found in the bibliography.

## Chapter 1

# How Much Do You Know about Natural Products? An Introductory Test

How much do you know about natural products? Whether you are a tyro or a maven in natural products, you may want to check your knowledge with this introductory test. Many similar tests follow later in the book with this easy-to-learn format. Natural products have not yielded to the inexorable sands of time. They are referenced in Genesis and are increasing in popularity today. This book will test your knowledge from those nascent days to the present. The following questions deal with the most popular herbs being used today.

You may wish to hold your hand over the right side of the page for each question to see how much you already know. Each question is worth four points. There are four bonus questions.

| | QUESTION | ANSWER |
|---|---|---|
| 1. | Of all herbs with a stimulating effect, which one has been the number one in use over the past several hundred years? | Coffee |
| 2. | What herb is often not thought of as an herb but is probably the number one herb of all time? It creates a warm, calm feeling after ingested in the stomach. | Sugar |
| 3. | Name a common food and juice that is metabolized by the P450 (CYP) liver enzyme system and can interact with several drugs such as cyclosporine and valium. It is probably given more often than any other herb or food as an example of substances that interact with various medications. | Grapefruit juice |

4.  Name the best-tasting herb of all time that has a stimulating effect.

Chocolate

5.  Name the most common diet that has been tried for cancer prevention.

High fiber, low fat

6.  Of all herbs, what has contributed to the most deaths in the past few hundred years?

Tobacco

7.  What is the top-selling drug in history (over 40 billion per year), the original ingredients of which initially came from a common tree, the willow tree?

Aspirin

8.  Name one of the top-selling types of beverages of all time. One specific type of these beverages originally came from grapes and was produced in Egypt some 5,000 years ago. Over half of all automobile accidents are related to these beverages as are over half of all homicides.

Alcoholic beverages, with wine being one specific type

9.  In recent years, what has been the best-selling herb (excluding coffee, tobacco, and sugar)?

Gingko biloba

10. Of all the herbs and supplements used for depression in recent years, which one is used most often?

Saint-John's-wort

11. Of all the herbs that have been studied scientifically, which one has been studied the most?

Garlic

12. Tamiflu is one of the new prescription medications effective for the flu. Two popular herbs are said to also help with the flu. Anise is probably the number one herb in America for the flu, but it has been known to cause seizures. Name the other herb that may help with the flu but could possibly cause damage to reproductive cells in young females.

Echinacea

13. Many diets come and go with perhaps a 90 percent ineffective rate for weight loss overall. Name a high-protein diet that has been popular in recent years but has few significant or widely accepted scientific studies to back it up. In fact, with rehydration initial weight loss tends to disappear.

Atkins Diet

14. Name the most popular herb for the treatment of menopause.

Soy products

15. Pain is the most common symptom of all time. Name an herb that has been used locally for toothaches.

Clove

16. What is one of the most-used herbs to help with osteoarthritis but might make diabetes worse?

Glucosamine-chondroitin

17. Name one of the 13 top-selling natural products in the world, along with a disorder it is touted to help.

In order they are:
1.  Gingko—senility

2.  Saint-John's-wort—
    depression
3.  Ginseng—sex drive
4.  Garlic—heart disease
5.  Echinacea—the common cold
6.  Saw palmetto—benign prostatic
    hypertrophy
7.  Kava—anxiety
8.  Grape seed extract—
    antiaging
9.  Cranberry—urinary tract infection
10. Valerian—anxiety
11. Evening primrose—PMS
12. Bilberry—varicose veins
13. Milk thistle—liver disease

18. Name an interesting herb used more than any
    other for PMS, but also has been used for skin problems such
    as eczema.

    Evening primrose

19. Name an herb from Germany that outsells Prozac
    20 to 1 for depression and could be dangerous due to inter-
    actions with other modern-day medicines.

    Saint-John's-wort

20. Name perhaps the most commonly used herb for
    chronic fatigue. It can have serious side effects on the heart,
    central nervous system, and gastrointestinal tract. However,
    the biggest danger may be treating the symptoms without
    treating the cause of fatigue.

    Ginseng

21. What extremely popular herb has been used for
    weight loss and has had side effects such as anxiety, agitation,
    stroke, psychosis, and even death?

    Ephedra

22. What herb has been written about probably more
    than any other in the medical literature because of possible
    drug interactions? (Hint: It has a repulsive-sounding name.)

    Saint-John's-wort

23. Name the original herb from which digitalis came.
    This derivative (digitalis) became one of the most famous
    heart medicines of all time.

    Foxglove

24. Of all the herbal teas, which one is the best-selling?
    (Hint: It has been touted to be anti-body odor, antibacterial,
    antiseptic, antifungal, and anti-inflammatory.)

    Chamomile

25. Of all topical gels which one has been used the most
    for skin abrasions, burns, eczema, and sunburn?

    Aloe vera

26. Bonus Question:
    Perhaps 25 percent of Americans at some time suffer from
    severe headaches called migraines. Name the herb that has

    Feverfew

most often been used to help with migraines.

27.  Bonus Question:                                        Feingold Diet
     What famous diet was recommended several years ago for
     ADHD but seemed to fail to produce significant results for
     many?

28.  Bonus Question:                                        Lithium carbonate
     What has become over the past 50 years one of the most
     well-established psychopharmacologic agents for the treat-
     ment of one type of affective (depressive) disorder? It was
     initially popular in beverages in the United States in the early
     1900s. It was popularized as a mineral cure at spa resorts. It
     was also used as a salt substitute, but in 1949 reports of poi-
     soning appeared in *JAMH*.

29.  Bonus Question:                                        Willow
     Salicylic acid is in many over-the-counter preparations for
     wart removal. It is probably number one over the years in
     sales for warts. From what herb does it come?

30.  BONUS QUESTION:                                        Aloe vera
     Name the herb that may be in topical skin preparations more
     than any other.

## Grade—Chapter 1

Number correct _____ + bonus points _____ multiplied by 4 = _____ Score

*Chapter 2*

# An Overview of Herbs and Supplements

Herbs and supplements are big business! Christians in particular often seem to gravitate to natural products. Americans spent over fifteen billion dollars on herbs and other supplements in the year 2000. In 1997 Wal-Mart reported dietary supplement sales of more than 500 million dollars. The growth of the supplement industry has been phenomenal.

> 1992—$4.5 billion
> 1997—$9 billion
> 2000—$15 billion

Thirty-five percent of people use alternative treatment, most in combination with traditional treatment. Worldwide sales of Saint-John's-wort for the treatment of depression exceed expenditures on any prescription medicine. Many household magazines devote a significant amount of space to the discussion of natural products. In addition, currently there are almost one thousand dietary supplement companies.

The sheer number of available products is mind-boggling. There are over four thousand Chinese herbs alone. Although many of these herbs are applicable in psychiatry, these supplements branch into all areas of medicine. Scientific journals address herbs and supplements on a monthly basis. Multiple journal articles have appeared in well-respected medical publications during the last couple of years.

## The History of the Herb and Supplement Movement

The use of herbs dates back to antiquity. However, the late 1990s into the early 2000s have seen an unusual escalation in their use, partly as a result of several leading magazines (*Time, Newsweek, Reader's Digest,* and others) featuring lead articles on such herbs and supplements as vitamin E, melatonin, and Saint-John's-wort. In 1994 Congress passed the Dietary Supplement Health and Education Act, and in 1995 the Office of Dietary Supplements was established at the National Institute of Health. In 1998 the *Journal of the American Medical Association (JAMA)* devoted an entire issue to alternative therapies since this movement grew 47 percent during the decade. Today Americans spend over twenty billion dollars annually on herbs or supplements.

## Herbal Preparations

Herbal preparations come in a variety of forms: tablets, capsules, powder, oils, ointments, flakes, strips, teas, tinctures, fluid extracts, liniments, suppositories, granules, gum, seeds, roots, cigarettes, syrup, IV infusion, bark, and stems.

Not a day goes by in our practices without several patients bringing in examples of herbs and supplements they are taking, asking questions about safety and/or how to mix these products with their prescribed medications.

## What Are the Top-Selling Herbs and Supplements?

What are the best-selling herbs and supplements, and why are they at the top? The following data is interesting, to say the least.

In 1998 the best-selling herbs and their respective uses were:

| | Herb | Primarily Used For |
|---|---|---|
| 1. | Gingko biloba | Dementia |
| 2. | Saint-John's-wort | Depression |
| 3. | Ginseng | Aphrodisiac |
| 4. | Garlic | Heart disease, high blood pressure, and high cholesterol |
| 5. | Echinacea | Common cold |
| 6. | Saw palmetto | Benign prostate hypertrophy |
| 7. | Kava | Anxiety |
| 8. | Grape seed extract | Diabetes |
| 9. | Cranberry | Urinary tract infection |
| 10. | Valerian | Insomnia |
| 11. | Evening primrose | PMS |
| 12. | Bilberry | Circulation |
| 13. | Milk thistle | Liver damage |

Twelve additional top herbs and supplements:

| | Herb | Primarily Used For |
|---|---|---|
| 1. | Black cohosh | Menopause |
| 2. | Chromium | Diabetes, depression |
| 3. | Dong quai | Menopause |
| 4. | Ephedra | Weight loss |
| 5. | Feverfew | Migraines |
| 6. | Folic acid + B6 | Depression in females |
| 7. | Glucosamine-chrondroitin | Osteoarthritis |
| 8. | Melatonin | Insomnia |
| 9. | Omega-3 fatty acids | Bipolar disorder |
| 10. | SAMe | Depression, osteoarthritis, fibromyalgia, memory, hepatitis |
| 11. | Saw palmetto + pygeum + stinging nettle | Benign prostate hypertrophy |
| 12. | Soy | Menopause |

Other herbs and supplements of current interest are:

| Herb | Primarily Used For |
|------|-------------------|
| Acetyl L-carnitine | Age-related memory deficits |
| Acidophilus | Diarrhea |
| Aloe vera | Minor skin irritations |
| Alpha-lipoic acid | Diabetic neuropathy, heart disease |
| Amino acids | Antiaging, bodybuilding |
| Arginine and sunflower seed | Impotence |
| $B_6$ + magnesium + vitamin E and calcium | PMS |
| Calcium | PMS |
| Cayenne pepper | Heart disease |
| Chamomile | Anxiety |
| Choline | Depression |
| Coenzyme Q-10 | Heart disease |
| Cranberry juice | Urinary tract infections |
| Creatinine and androstenedine | Athletic enhancement |
| DHEA | Depression |
| Enteric-coated peppermint oil | Irritable bowel syndrome |
| Fish oil | Bipolar disorder |
| 5–HTP | Depression and anxiety |
| Flaxseed | Bipolar disorder |
| Ginger | Irritable bowel syndrome, SSRI withdrawal |
| Gymnema | Diabetes |
| Hops | Insomnia |
| Inositol | Obsessive-compulsive syndrome |
| Kava, valerian, melatonin | Insomnia |
| L-carnitine | Weight loss |
| Lemon balm | Anxiety |
| Licorice | Menopause, ulcers |
| L-tryptophane | Depression, PMS |
| Maca | Aphrodisiac, stress reduction, improve mood |
| Magnesium with B6 | Anxiety |
| Marapuama | Sexual enhancement to counteract SSRI use |
| Oat straw (avena sativa) | Insomnia |
| Passionflower | Anxiety |
| Phosphatidyl serine | Cognitive enhancement |
| Red clover | Menopause |
| Satiatrol | Weight loss |
| Selenium | Depression, weight loss |
| Vitamin E | Dementia |
| Vitex | PMS (chaste berry) |
| Zinc | Common cold |

## Why Are the Top-Selling Herbs and Supplements at the Top?

In reviewing some of the top seventy-five herbs and supplements being sold today, several questions arise. The main one: Why do they lead the pack? We suspect it is because they appeal to a broad need—menopause, depression, high blood sugar, weight loss, headache, joint problems, insomnia, mood swings, memory problems, appearing youthful, and so on. But do the herbs and supplements accomplish what they are often touted to do? On the other hand, might they hold benefits of which we never dreamed?

## Legal Restrictions

In 1994 a grassroots campaign led to congressional passage of the Dietary Supplement Health and Education Act, which restricts the authority of the US Food and Drug Administration (FDA) over any herb or supplement as long as the manufacturer makes no claim that the product is able to affect a "disease state."[1]

## Conclusion: Catching the World by Storm

Indeed herbs and supplements are big business. They have caught the world by storm. Probably everyone reading this book is either using herbs or supplements or has a friend who does. Patients daily question their doctors about the newest remedy they want to try. Every check-out lane in the grocery store carries magazines touting various herbs and supplements. What in the world is going on? Good or bad, this movement is a reality. It seems America is in desperate need of knowing "the good, the bad, and the ugly" about herbs and supplements.

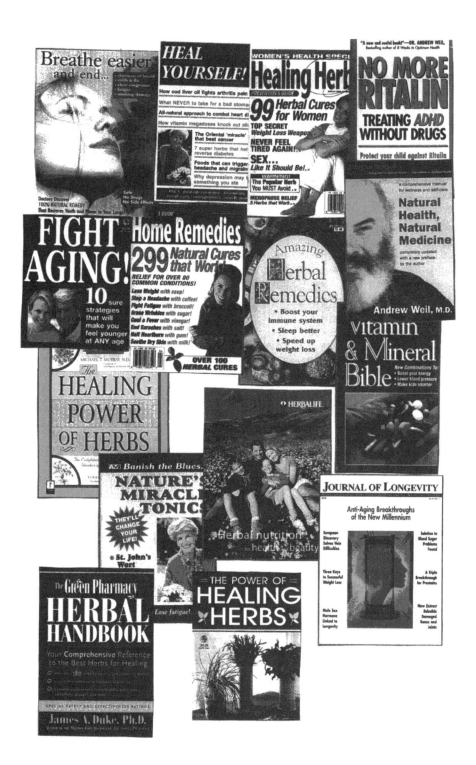

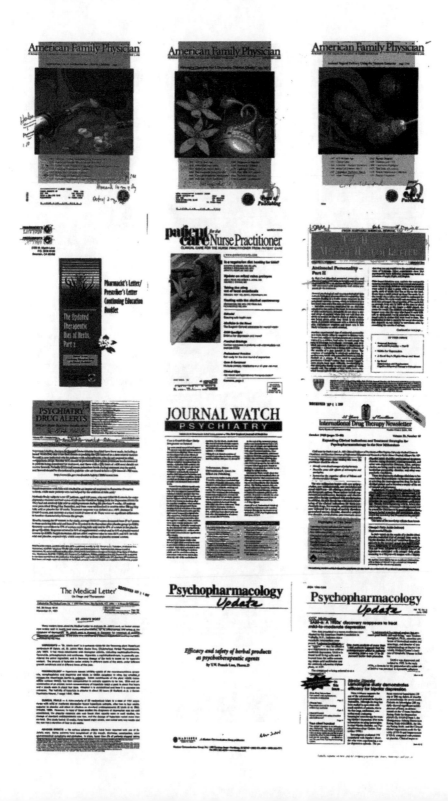

## Chapter 3

# A Deeper Look—Why Herbs and Supplements?

Interest in herbs and supplements continues to grow in the Christian world as people experience changes in insurance coverage, increased cost of prescription medications, and greater interest in what has become known as "natural" substances. A number of factors influence the use of herbs and supplements. The following are possible factors, both good and bad, involved in the plethora of new "natural" products. I trust readers will enjoy the good and be wary of the bad.

## Does the Bible Sanction Natural Products over Modern Medicine?

Many Christians believe that the Bible sanctions natural products more than prescription drugs. Is this premise true? Please consider the following thoughts.

First, any substance taken into the body to produce a biologic response is by definition a drug. Thus, herbs and prescription medicines are both drugs by definition. If one is ruled out, the other must be ruled out as well.

Second, a significant percentage of prescription medications were originally derived from herbs or natural products. Aspirin originated from the bark of the white willow tree; digitalis, used in congestive heart failure, was derived from the foxglove plant; pseudoephedrine, used in many cold remedies, came from the ephedra plant; quinine for malaria was derived from the bark of the cinchona tree; penicillin originated from a mold produced by a fungus (a primitive plant); vincristine for cancer treatment came from a periwinkle tree; and taxol, used to treat ovarian cancer, originally came from the bark of a Pacific yew tree. Therefore, if one deems modern medicine unbiblical, then one would need to rule out herbs as well.

Third, the Bible seems to give credence to both herbs (Ezek. 47:12) and the physician (Matt. 9:12). It does not give exclusivity to either.

It would seem logical that God wants his children to be as healthy as possible so that we can share Christ with others and help fellow believers grow in Christ. Both herbs and modern medicine in a sense seem minor compared with our major mission in the Great Commission. Herbs and modern medicine are only means, when necessary, to keep us healthy so we can continue to share Christ and encourage fellow believers.

## Is Natural the Best?

The influence and money of more than eight hundred dietary companies are hard to ignore. Advertisements are everywhere. One must be careful not to be caught in the fad of the moment. On the contrary one must also be careful not to assume that natural products have nothing to offer.

Our need to believe in natural aids is often deep-seated. Most can remember mother's or grandmother's admonition of chicken noodle soup "to help fight off that old cold." Numerous other old folk remedies abound from our own childhood.

Most Americans are honest, hardworking people who want to believe the best in others. Wanting to believe the best may at times lead some into gullibility. Also, most are not educated regarding the many aspects of herbs and supplements—the good, the bad, and the ugly. Many Americans are not even aware that there is no FDA (Food and Drug Administration) control over these herbs and supplements. They may believe they are safe and pure when in actuality these products have been found to contain impurities and can cause serious side effects, even death.

Many people believe that "natural is better," which is not always so. A significant percentage of prescription medicines over the years were derived from natural sources, but today we seldom use the original natural source because through scientific method and research we have developed purer medicines that are usually more effective. The key word in the previous sentence is "usually." No doubt gems still exist in the "natural," but caution is indicated. Natural is not always better. Even poisonous mushrooms are "natural."

## Beliefs about Natural Products

While something can be said for the ease of obtaining many herbs and supplements today, there is an old adage that we do well to ponder: "He who treats himself has a fool for a doctor." Many of the disorders people attempt to treat with herbs and supplements can be lethal diseases—depression, heart disease, and cancer to name a few. Is the ease of obtainment worth the risk?

Several beliefs about the use of natural products contribute to the widespread use of herbs and supplements. But each of these should be examined as to its validity when choosing to add such products to one's health-care regimen, either for preventative care or specific treatment.

### "Stigma Free" Belief

If one treats himself, no one need know. The reason for treatment may seem stigma free. But the question is—for how long? Diseases usually progress. In fact they may progress much more rapidly and with grave consequences if not treated early with the state-of-the-art medication today. Consider the dangers of undertreated hypertension and even some forms of depression that become more resistant to current medications when treated too late.

### "Cost Less" Belief

Surely herbs and supplements cost less than prescription medications. But do they? Herbs and supplements generally are not covered by insurance. And the cost of adding herbal treatments can escalate quickly. For example, an individual may spend as much as $450 per month in an attempt to lift their mood with SAMe. And this is only one product. The "cost less" belief is not always true.

### "Different Mechanism of Action" Belief

Many people believe that herbs and supplements work by different mechanisms of action than prescription medications today. It is almost as though some believe that these products miraculously and mysteriously work by natural means. Quite to the contrary, they work by the same mechanisms of action as modern psychiatric medications. True, the mechanism of action may not be as completely understood at times since herbs and supplements do not have the benefit of rigorously controlled clinical studies. Nevertheless scientists understand much more today about the mechanism of action of many herbs and supplements, and indeed they are the same as that of modern prescription medication.

Saint-John's-wort for depression works similarly in many ways to the MAO antidepressants. SAMe heightens the activity of the mood by regulating the neurotransmitters dopamine and serotonin. Valerian and kava both probably work by enhancing the activity of the neurotransmitter GABA, not dissimilar to the minor tranquilizers of today; in fact they may not be as good since they may have lurking side effects, but the mechanisms of action are similar.

## "It's Not a Drug" Belief

Herb refers to a plant used for medicinal purposes. Any time a substance is used in effect for medicinal purposes, it becomes a drug. Approximately 80 percent of the world population relies on herbs for primary health care needs. This is often the case because nothing else is available. Something unproven may be better than nothing, especially if that is all you have. Every country is not blessed with the excellent medical care available in the United States.

## "Their Effectiveness Is Based on Studies" Belief

Many people believe the effectiveness of herbs and supplements is based on studies and research. Though much more research money will undoubtedly be allocated for the study of herbs and supplements in the future, much of today's herbal medicine grew out of folklore and anecdotal reports. The scientific method of research and double-blind studies with placebo comparisons are often lacking. Modern Western medicine based on the scientific method—evidence based with randomized clinical trials—is highly successful for many classes of diseases, is dynamic and improving, and generally is reimbursable. Herb treatments are often empirical, do not meet FDA standards, may have a prominent placebo effect, may be toxic, may be of high cost, and rely on self-treatment of potentially dangerous disorders. However, the fact that they are often unproven does not mean they are not efficacious. It does mean, however, that natural products perhaps should be subjected to the same scientific method to prove if they are indeed efficacious.

## "Herbs Are Fine, but Modern Medicine Is Not" Belief

This is analogous to saying, "Model T Fords are fine, but a new Mustang is not." Herbs have been around for centuries and have been used as active constituents in many modern-day drugs (i.e., digoxin for congestive heart failure comes from foxglove; theophylline for asthma comes from thea; reserpine to lower blood pressure comes from snakeroot; and atropine for gastrointestinal uses comes from belladonna). In fact more than 25 percent of today's pharmaceutical agents have been developed by extraction and purification of crude herbs. However, just as the Model T Ford gave way to newer and better models every year, so herbs and supplements have given way to newer and better medicines that are more effective and more specific in their actions.

"The 1994 Dietary Supplement Health and Education Act permitted herbal drugs to be placed in the same category as food supplements such as vitamins. This legislation allows manufacturers to market herbal drugs without prior proof of their safety or therapeutic efficacy."[1] Thus proof of efficacy is lacking with herbs and supplements but not with modern-day medicine, which must undergo a vigorous three-step scientific method of testing. It is only fair and reasonable that natural products should undergo the same process.

## "It's Only a Vitamin, Mineral, or Amino Acid" Belief

Vitamins and minerals often can provide beneficial results. Might vitamins even act as scavengers of dangerous free radicals in the body? Certainly they are necessary for life. So how could one ever criticize the use of vitamins? They can be criticized when used in excess. Vitamins in excess have been known to cause headaches, dizziness, nausea, bone pain, anemia, liver damage, diarrhea, kidney stones, and generalized weakness. Minerals in excess have been known to cause hair loss, nausea, vomiting, irritation, and confusion. Amino acids (L-tryptophane) have been associated with death in the past.

## "Herbs Have No Side Effects" Belief

It is true that natural products overall have fewer side effects than prescription medications, but it is not true that they have no side effects. FDA psychiatric approved drugs must go through three levels of stringent tests for effectiveness and potential side effects. Herbs go through none since they are not FDA approved.

Possible side effects of natural products are especially worthy of note in pregnant females and children. Few natural products should be used by these groups.

Concerns were addressed in medical journals beginning in the mid 1990s. No consistent standards are applied to their processing or packaging, so the possibility of contamination and varying strengths must be kept in mind when evaluating them.

Because the FDA exercises no supervision, the potency and quality of products cannot be guaranteed. "*The Lancet* in 1994 analyzed ginseng from a number of sources for the percent of ginsenoisides (the active ingredients) they contained. The range varied between 2 and 9%. . . . Some ginseng products contained no ginseng, none at all."[2]

"Some herbal remedies have been found to contain lead, arsenic, and other heavy metals as well as pharmaceutical benzodiazepines."[3] After all, arsenic and strychnine are natural substances as well! From 1993 to 1998, the FDA received 2,621 reports of adverse effects linked to supplements. These complaints included reports of 101 deaths.[4]

Some of the herbs used as diet aids can have serious health risks. Aristoloclia fangchi and mutong resulted in end-stage renal disease in some patients. Other herbal preparations resulted in hepatitis with germanler, seizures and renal failure with yohimbine, and cardiovascular collapse and seizures with ephedra. Hypericum perforatum (Saint-John's-wort), gingko biloba, and echinacea purpurea have been shown to be damaging to reproductive cells in animal studies. Ephedra (ma huang), used as a stimulant, has been linked to more than thirty-eight deaths.

## Select Dangerous Herbs

1. Cannabis sativa—marijuana
2. Hallucinogenic mushrooms
3. Opium poppy—heroin addiction
4. Moldy rye (ergot)
5. Tobacco—perhaps 15 to 20 percent of all deaths are tobacco related.

## Select Potentially Dangerous Herbs

1. Chinese ephedra—psychosis, agitation, cerebral vascular accident, myocardial infarction
2. IV aloe vera—multiple deaths reported
3. Yohimbe—seizures and renal failure
4. Foxglove—the active ingredient can cause cardiac glycoside toxicity.
5. Plantain ("chanper")—same as above
6. Saint-John's-wort + UV light—sunburn
7. Rauwaulfa serpertina—the active ingredient in reserpine, thus hypotension or depression could occur.

## Select Potentially Dangerous Herb-Drug Interactions

1. Saint-John's-wort and antidepressants
2. Gingko biloba and blood thinners (ASA, Coumadin, NSAIDs, omega-3 fatty acids)
3. Echinacea plus astragalus and immunosuppressants
4. Licorice and spironolactone, digoxin, B-blockers, other diuretics
5. Herbal laxatives and digoxin, B-blockers, and diuretics
6. Passa flora, incanata, and SSRIs

7. Chromium, ginseng, bitter melon, and fenugreek—decreased blood sugar
8. Evening primrose oil plus borage oil and anticonvulsants
9. Ephedra (ma huang) and MAOIs
10. Belladonna and anticholinergics
11. Inositol and lithium
12. Omega-3 fatty acids plus garlic and blood thinners (Coumadin)
13. Saint-John's-wort, gingko, and echinacea—damage to reproductive cells
14. Saint-John's-wort and indinavir (for AIDS)
15. Saint-John's-wort and MAOIs
16. Maca and fibroids, estrogen-related cancer risks, endometriosis, or prostate cancer
17. Licorice and digoxin
18. Racemic mixtures of L-carnitine
19. Herbs that can affect bleeding time and surgery: feverfew, garlic, ginger, ginseng
20. Some herbs have potential seizure risks: eucalyptus, fennel, hyssop, rosemary, sage, savin, tansy, thuja, turpentine, and wormwood.
21. A number of anesthesiologists have reported changes in heart rates and blood pressure in patients taking Saint-John's-wort, gingko, and ginseng.

*A disclaimer is needed.* Risks, side effects, and dangers are possible. Herb manufacturers are not held to the same standards as the manufacturers of FDA-approved products. They are not required to demonstrate the safety or quality of their extracts or potions. The suppliers remain unregulated and chemical constituents can vary widely from product to product. There are wide variations in the quality of the products and the content of the active ingredients. The methods by which the plants are grown and harvested are not controlled. Most herbs and supplements do not have standardized doses or consistent strengths. Some are potentially toxic and may cause harm if mixed with other herbs and supplements or with prescription medications. Of major concern is the practice of purchasing products via the Internet that allows Americans to buy from other countries products that are banned in the United States because of their toxic danger or risk of adverse reactions. In spite of the dangers and lack of careful inspection and regulation, products continue to flood the shelves with every conceivable claim of benefit and few words of warning.

## *"They Work" Belief*

We often hear this statement regarding herbs and supplements: "But they work." Indeed these products do work at times, but what about the other times?

For a medicine to be approved, it must be significantly better than double-blind placebo controls. This placebo response is not insignificant. Dr. Minirth recalls many years ago when he used the placebo response to help a patient. The young patient was in her twenties and in the hospital for depression. She had been on every known antidepressant to no avail. Dr. Minirth felt her depression had more to do with internal conflict than a chemical depression. He decided on a plan of action and told her about a new antidepressant just out from Europe named Diatam and it was simply wonderful by all reports—highly effective and essentially free of side effects. She said, "Dr. Minirth, give me that Diatam." He said OK and called the pharmacist for a placebo. The next morning as he entered the unit, she greeted him and said, "I feel the best I have felt in years—the Diatam is a miracle drug." He then shared with the patient about the placebo response issue and how glad he was she felt better but that they needed to work on some underlying issues.

About the same time (twenty-five years ago) Dr. Minirth had another client in the hospital who was also depressed. She said that although she was very depressed she could not take antidepressants because she had bad side effects to any man-made drug. Unlike the previous patient, he believed this woman was truly medically depressed and that her response to antidepressants previously had likely been because of her fear of medication. He told her that there was a new medicine just out from Europe called Diatam and that it was practically free of side effects. She resisted the treatment, saying that any antidepressant would produce side effects. Dr. Minirth ordered it anyway. The next morning she was in bed as he entered the unit. She told him that she had had a side effect to this new medicine and had fallen during the night. He explained to her the *nocebo* response (a negative effect to a placebo drug), and they began to work on her resistance to appropriate medication.

Placebos often work, as documented in recent studies. In one example, the pooled population of 2,045 patients was treated with (1) a placebo, (2) an SSRI medication, and (3) Effexor XR. Twenty-five percent of the patients in the study had a "placebo response." A placebo response occurs when a patient has improvement without benefit of the medication. Usually this takes the form of ingesting a sugar pill or capsule instead of medication. We now know that the placebo effect involves an endogenous opiate release, which occurs when the person thinks he or she has taken medication to relieve the symptoms. If one hundred depressed people were given a placebo but told that it was a new antidepressant that showed great promise, perhaps as many as 30 percent would have a significant lifting of mood. The usual placebo response is around 30 percent. The problem arises in knowing whether the positive responses are due to the herb or supplement. An additional problem is not knowing what else the herb might do that is not necessarily helpful.

A recent and groundbreaking study at UCLA revealed ongoing beneficial changes, documented by PET scans, in the frontal lobes in 25 percent of those taking placebo alone. In general, however, many herbs are lacking in double-blind, placebo-controlled studies to determine their efficacy, side effects, and contaminations. Dangerous combinations can occur, and perhaps the biggest danger is the self-treatment of potentially dangerous and truly life-threatening disorders. Herbs and supplements that do help often produce only mild results, are not covered by insurance, and can be very expensive preparations. They are a mixed bag. Some help, some do not, and some even harm.

To be fair, we as clinicians know that prescription medications can also have side effects. The difference is that these side effects are known. The drug is prescribed and supervised by a physician. The drugs are researched through three stages of extensive double-blind, placebo-controlled studies. Significant benefits must be demonstrated and side effects documented for herbs and other supplements.

### "The Mysterious, Magical Fountain of Youth" Belief

The search for the mysterious, magical fountain of youth lurks in almost all of us. Surely some supplement or herb will mysteriously and almost magically cure whatever ails us, we think. Men died in such search years ago because the appeal was so strong. The allure still beckons today. Perhaps three things draw us into this belief. First, mystery is interesting. It seems to appeal to something within us. Knowledge seems to remove some of the allure. Second, the magical draw seems to fit into our need for hope. Finally, the search itself for the fountain of youth is compelling. It offers not only hope for a cure but a chase that is fun and intriguing. The search will surely continue.

## The Good, the Bad, and the Ugly

Though the "good" certainly exists regarding herbs and supplements and can benefit us in many ways, we must heed the rest of the story. We've already begun to explore the "bad," and sometimes it becomes the "ugly."

The use of some herbs really provides great benefit. Sometimes prescription medications are limited in certain disease-ridden states. In some countries prescription medications are limited, so herbs have filled the void. Some people even fear using a prescription medication and are more likely to try an herb; thus they may receive help they would otherwise not receive.

As wonderful as natural products have proven to be over the years, however, there is a dark side. Honest people seeking help over the centuries were deceived by others who took advantage of them. A quick historical sketch uncovers some terms that are applicable to our search for the truth about "natural products" today.

During the Middle Ages, Italians often did their banking on benches in the streets. Jugglers, singers, and clowns often added to the atmosphere. Deceptions were prevalent in this setting. Since the workers sat around benches, they were called *montimbancos* or *mountebanks*. Today, *mountebank* refers to a charlatan who sells quack medicine from a public place. A person today who tricks or misleads others with spurious statements about natural products would be a mountebank.

In the 1600s the Great Plague ravaged Europe. Quacks took advantage of this situation, too, and made their own secret remedies. Their mixtures were known as *nostrum,* meaning "our own remedy." No one knew exactly what was in these remedies or why they supposedly just worked, but people in need took nostrums. Today, *nostrum* means quack medicine.

In the sixteenth century, charlatans selling useless remedies were so prevalent that they sounded like the quacks of ducks; they were called "quack-salvers." Today, *quack* means any ignorant pretender to medical skills, one who misleads with some truth adulterated with error. A quack overstates and misleads for selfish purposes.

*Qui vive* is a term from France that also has application to the world of natural products. It means "to be on the alert." The herb and supplement industry contains both truth and error, both the scrupulous and the unscrupulous, both honest exponents and charlatans. Because of a lack of FDA accountability with natural products, the buyer should be on the *qui vive.*

*Specious* is another interesting word with application to our topic. It means "appearing to be true but actually being deceptive." *Specious* indicates something that is superficially reasonable but not so in reality. While many claims regarding natural products are true, others are specious.

In the fifth century BC, a pernicious term entered the language. *Sophists* were itinerant Greek teachers paid to teach the children of the upper class. They had great rhetorical skills. In fact their exceptional articulation skills sometimes led to deceptions in their teachings. Today *sophistry* means "a superficially plausible statement filled with deception." Thus, misleading and overstated advertisements regarding natural products is sophistry.

*Surreptitious* is another word worthy of note. It means "characterized by secrecy and done in a secret, sly manner in order to avoid notice." Some natural products are salubrious, health giving; others are promoted in a sly manner to avoid notice of their false claims.

*Panacea* contains the prefix *pan* from Greek. *Panacea* means "a remedy for all diseases." Charlatans claim to have panaceas. When a person claims that his product has many wonderful and varied benefits, one does well to be on the *qui vive.*

*Beguile* periodically has application to the world of natural products. It means "to deceive and mislead." In Genesis 3:13, Eve said, "The serpent beguiled me" (KJV). The prefix *be* means "completely." The word *guile* means "deceit and treacherous teaching." With the upsurge of interest in natural products, the buyer does well not to be beguiled by the many claims.

*Subterfuge* is an underhanded scheme. Subterfuge refers to any secret plan with a concealed motive. Because of the popularity of natural products and the potential wealth available from the sale of these products by overzealous promoters, one does well to be on the alert for subterfuges.

Finally, *caveat emptor* means "let the buyer beware," because the seller might be trying to sell inferior merchandise. In the world of natural products, sometimes vendors overstate the benefits of their products.

In summary, natural products have undoubtedly done a lot more good than harm over the years, but honest people can be deceived by sophistry, so be cognizant of the limitations of any natural product and be aware of potential dangers.

## Conclusion

Indeed, a number of factors influence the use of herbs and supplements. None of us are immune to these factors. We need to do our best to ask if we are being objective.

To be fair, herbs and other supplements can have significant benefits. Dangers are also possible. In other words, there are many unknowns. These products always should be used under a knowledgeable medical doctor's supervision, realizing the potential dangers.

One of the most important dangers is the self-treating of potentially lethal conditions (i.e., major depressive disorder, mania, congestive heart failure) with an herb or supplement as the primary or only form of treatment. Heart disease kills over half a million people each year. Major depressive disorders result in over thirty thousand suicides annually. Twenty percent of those with bipolar disorder commit suicide. Cancer is the second-leading killer each year. Such serious diseases need state-of-the-art medications as the primary treatment.

## Chapter 4

# Looking into Images of the Mind

Can we now actually see the emotions of the mind, and can supplements help when needed? If we could concretely see emotional disorders, might Christians be more amenable to treatment?

Many of the disorders we treat in psychiatry include a significant neurophysiological or biochemical imbalance. This component can now be observed by the sophisticated technological advancements of nuclear medicine. Supercomputerized images provide photos of mental processes and thus aid in diagnosis and subsequent treatment. Many mental problems are not disorders in the anatomy of the brain but problems in how the brain works at the chemical level. In some cases, however, if the physiological malady is more acute—as in schizophrenia, Alzheimer's dementia, severe major medical depression, and posttraumatic stress disorder—anatomical deficits in the brain can actually be seen.

SPECT (single proton emission computerized tomography) and PET (positron emission tomography) scans can directly observe the blood flow and metabolism of brain cells. Scientists have now been able to identify certain patterns of brain activity that correlate with psychiatric problems. Several of these psychiatric disorders are revealed by the following computerized images, or PET scans (see fig. 1).[1] From a review of these PET scans, clearly some disorders—such as major depression, attention-deficit/hyperactivity disorder (ADHD), obsessive-compulsive disorder (OCD), schizophrenia, and others—have a major neurophysiological component, and state-of-the-art medications and medical treatment may be needed.

But what about supplements? Are natural products usually effective enough, specific enough, selective enough, and scientifically proven enough to deal with the extremely complex cascade of biochemical events occurring in serious emotional issues? Could it be that at times supplements may be helpful adjuncts? Can we learn from what they have to offer?

Observing the brain of an individual with major depressive disorder (see fig. 1), we find that deep structures of the brain are involved, along with the temporal lobes, frontal lobes, parietal areas, and occipital regions. Depression affects multiple areas of the brain and frequently results in a "don't care" attitude, low energy, little willpower, hopelessness, and sleep and appetite changes. Note the difference in the *control* image representing a brain that is not depressed. Pay special attention to the *recovered* brain, following medical treatment for depression. Also, please note the areas of increased glucose uptake in the manic high as opposed to the decreased uptake in depression low of the bipolar brain.

In the brain of an individual with ADHD, the frontal parts of the brain are less active, as revealed by "cooler" shades of color on the scan. The frontal areas of the brain are responsible for supervising, guiding, focusing, and directing the individual's behavior. They are responsible for self-control and for planning ahead. Decreased activity in the frontal area of the brain as revealed by less activity ("cooler" shades) results in short attention span, distractibility, poor impulse control, short-term memory difficulty, and random unfocused activity.

Now observe the brain of an individual with schizophrenia and other psychotic disorders, which affect a person's ability to determine reality from fantasy. Often the individual will present hallucinations (hearing voices), delusions, and distorted thinking (misunderstanding others' communication or motives). A dramatic, computerized photo of brain activity in a patient with schizophrenia and one without the disorder is shown.

In an individual with OCD, obsessive-compulsive patterns are commonly seen in the form of inflexibility, having to do things a certain way, becoming upset if plans are changed, counting, checking, excessive washing, overconcern about germs, and recurrent disturbing thought patterns. Areas of the brain associated with this disorder include the frontal lobes and the cingulate gyrus. After effective treatment, follow-up studies will show less activity in the area of the frontal lobe and cingulate gyrus along with less worrying, more flexibility, fewer obsessions, and greater cooperation.

An individual with Alzheimer's disease has a tragic, progressive form of dementia more commonly present in the elderly. Individuals suffering from this disorder become forgetful, may get lost in familiar places, and cannot do tasks they once knew how to do. It takes a heavy toll on the lives of its victims and their families. These Alzheimer's scans show a shrinking of the brain, represented by the shadows around the edges and in the middle sections of the brain.

Despite the overwhelming nature of these mental disorders, some herbs and supplements have been found helpful in treatment if patients are also provided with state-of-the-art medications and other modern treatments as well. Although these products may be useful in certain conditions and situations, it is important that patients be protected from the known dangers and serious side effects of some herbs and supplements and that precious time is not lost when they could be benefitting from more modern approaches.

The following PET scans allow us to look into the image of the mind, to see how stress and genetic factors work. The complexity of this knowledge, however, raises the question of whether herbs and supplements are able to produce the desired effect. Yet even if they prove not always or totally to be up to the task, might we still benefit from what natural products have to offer?

## THE BRAIN UNDER STRESS

### NEUROIMAGING OF PSYCHIATRIC DISORDERS

Through PET (Positron Emission Tomography) scans, glucose metabolism and thus, cerebral functioning can be seen in the brain. PET scans allow us to actually see the damaging effects of stress and genetic factors. Here are some common patterns simulated below.

**BIPOLAR DISORDER:**

**DEPRESSION:**

**ADHD:**

**SCHIZOPHRENIA:**

**ALZHEIMER'S DISEASE:**

**OCD:**

© 2002 Frank Minirth, M.D.
Illustrations by Felix Flores

## Chapter 5

# The Brain and Emotions, Natural Products, and Psychiatric Medications

The use of natural products and psychiatric medications for emotional well-being speaks to a tremendous need in the Christian world. Similarities exist between the two remedies: both can be helpful; both can carry danger; both may have similar mechanisms of action. However, they also have significant differences. One of the major differences exists in the area of knowledge. As complete as we attempted to be in this book, the knowledge in general regarding herbs pales in comparison to the knowledge of psychiatric medication. A second area in which they differ is effectiveness. While natural products may help some significantly, overall they are far less effective. The following is a discussion of the brain and its chemistry, the effects of stress, the possible benefits of natural products and psychiatric medications, and how both natural products and psychiatric medications work.

## The Brain—the Last Frontier

The study of the brain may be the last and most exciting biological frontier. More than 50 percent of the human genome is dedicated to the central nervous system. The 1990s were declared the decade of the brain. Current research is intense, and the findings are highly encouraging to the understanding of depression, anxiety, panic, obsessive worries, weight issues, inattention problems, pain, headaches, memory, anger, energy, sleeplessness, logic, motivation, association, drug abuse, and sexual issues, to name just a few.

### Neurotransmitters and Emotions

Neurotransmitters exist between nerves in the space called the synapse. With perhaps upward of one hundred billion nerve cells in the brain, each having more than one hundred thousand synapses, the total number of synapses in one brain is unimaginable. Thus the power of these synapses and their neurotransmitters is awesome. We now know that these neurotransmitters can be altered by psychiatric medication to relieve mental disorders. Mental issues are very complex and biochemical in causation. Helping individuals with such issues involves not only altering neurotransmitters but also receptive sites, secondary messenger systems, brain-derived neurotrophic factors of brain cell nourishment, ion transport, and even the DNA within the nucleus of the nerve cell. Antidepressant medications often block the reuptake and therefore the metabolism of serotonin at the presynaptic nerve terminal. If serotonin (or norepinephrine and/or dopamine) is not taken up and metabolized, then it increases in the synapse, the mood lifts, and anger and worry may go down. Today we not only know which neurotransmitters alter certain emotions, we even know about neurotransmitter subsystems. For example, there are at least thirty-two subtypes of serotonin receptors alone. Medications today can affect not only specific neurotransmitters but also specific subsystems. The biochemistry of emotions has become a science in and of itself.

Incidentally, while neurotransmitters and amino acids are important, one cannot simply take amino acids and overcome depression. The brain is complex and this theory is antiquated.

## The Brain and Emotions

Several parts of the brain are extremely important in emotions. For example, the midbrain (with the raphe nucleus [serotonin production], locus ceruleus [norepinephrine production], and the substantia nigra [dopamine production]) is very important. The limbic system (with the hippocampus [important in memory], the amygdala [important in anger], the nucleus accumbens [important in addictions and motivation/reward], and the hypothalamus [important in eating and endocrine regulation issues]) also play significant roles. The frontal lobes of the brain are the centers for executive function, planning, impulse control, motivation, actions, and volition. Finally, the autonomic nervous system can affect all organ systems in the body.

The brain has many known neurotransmitters and often many different functions for one neurotransmitter. Here are some oversimplified but nonetheless helpful points. Serotonin may play a role in depression, anxiety, sleep, sexual issues, headaches, eating symptoms, pain perception, obsessive worry, panic disorders, aggression, and PMS. Norepinephrine may play a role in bipolar disorders, depressions, and attention problems. Dopamine may play a role in a loss of touch with reality, attention deficit issues, drug addictions, and mood. GABA may play a strong role in anxiety and some addiction issues. Acetylcholine plays a role in memory. Histamine may play a role in sleep and weight gain. Thus medications that can alter the above neurotransmitters have incredible potential benefits. The following studies are interesting.

Functional imaging techniques have revealed detailed correlations between localized brain activity and emotional states such as happiness and sadness. Happiness has been associated with increased activity in the ventral frontal cortex; sadness has been associated with increased activity in the anterior insular cortex.

From PET scans of the brain, we also know that many mental issues show anatomical changes in specific parts of the brain. In OCD positron emission tomography (PET) studies have shown elevated metabolic rates in the cingulate region and the heads of the caudate nuclei and orbital gyri. In schizophrenia important PET scan findings include reduced prefrontal metabolism and an increased density of $D_2$ receptors in schizophrenia. In bipolar disorder the main findings shown with MRI are that they tend to have what are called subcortical hyperintensities.

In Alzheimer's dementia, single photon emission computer tomography (SPECT) perfusion studies have demonstrated that the presence of apathy is also associated with frontal cortex changes. The strongest correlations with apathy are with reduced perfusion in the anterior cingulate region, and then to a lesser extent in orbital-frontal and anterior temporal regions. The cholinergic deficits from neuronal destruction that are implicated in the cognitive impairment of Alzheimer's disease may also contribute to behavioral disturbances. The atrophy of the small nucleus at the base of the brain, the nucleus basalis, occurs early in the disease process. Choline acetyltransferase is synthesized at this site, and its decreased production as the site atrophies leads to decreased production of acetylcholine. The nucleus basalis is poised between limbic and paralimbic afferents and cortical efferents. This site is positioned, then, to influence environment. Diseases such as Alzheimer's disease affecting nucleus basalis disrupt the integration of limbic-neocortical interactions that mediate cognitive and emotional functions.

# The Parts of the Brain and Emotions

The following specific discussion of the parts of the brain and the role each play in emotions may help clarify this complex organ and how it is interconnected with emotional and mental disorders.

## *Cerebrum*

1. Cerebral cortex—Center for reasoning, planning, volition, impulse control, motivation, and action are located in the cerebrum. The orbital cortex in the front part of the brain is where thought and emotions combine. It is a warning system in the brain and works overtime in OCD. The orbital cortex mixes thoughts with emotions and then allows choices to be made.

The brain consists of five lobes:
- *Frontal lobe*—intellectual functions, communication, personality, voluntary movement of skeletal muscle.
- *Parietal lobe*—speech center, sensations from skin and muscles, facial recognition, motor control of movements.
- *Temporal lobe*—interpretation of sound, auditory and visual memory, moods.
- *Occipital lobe*—visual images.
- *Insular*—memory, integration of other cerebral lobes.

2. Limbic system—The limbic brain is diffuse. It consists of the following parts:
- *Cingulate gyrus*—This structure is located deep in the center of the hemisphere of the brain. It helps one shift attention from one thought or behavior to another. If it malfunctions, one becomes stuck on certain behaviors or thoughts, as in OCD. It is also the part of the brain that signals danger.
- *Hippocampus*—This structure controls emotional memory. With prolonged stress cortisol remains high, and the hippocampus is suppressed in activity and eventually seems to atrophy. Thus memory distortions may occur, and painful memories will not dissipate, as in posttraumatic stress disorder.
- *Amygdala*—The amygdala is involved in memory just as the hippocampus, but it has to do more with memory of emotionally charged events. If physical damage occurs to the amygdala or is induced, as in laboratory animals, then rage can result. When in danger, the amygdala signals an alarm to the hypothalamus. The hypothalamus will then signal the sympathetic nervous system, which in turn activates the adrenal gland to release epinephrine and norepinephrine for fight or flight. The hypothalamus also signals the release of corticotropin-releasing hormone (CRH), which signals the pituitary to release adrenocorticotropic hormone (ACTH), which then signals the adrenal gland to release cortisol, which continues until the danger signal is halted. In those with PTSD, however, the alarm signal is not halted because the hippocampus is damaged. In any event the amygdala signals the initial alarm.
- *Nucleus acumbens*—The nucleus acumbens is involved with the sensations of pain and pleasure and therefore is important in addictions. It receives messages, in part, from the hippocampus, the amygdala, the septum, the hypothalamus, and the frontal lobes of the cerebral cortex. Dopamine is the neurotransmitter important in addictions.
- *Other areas of the limbic system* include septal nuclei, mammillary bodies of the hypothalamus, the anterior nucleus of the thalamus, the olfactory bulb, and interconnecting pathways of the various components of the limbic system.

The limbic system is the emotional brain—pain, pleasure, anger, depression, affection, and sexuality all originate in the limbic brain. Stimulation of the amygdala in animals results in rage; stimulation of the nucleus acumbens results in pleasure. Malfunction of the cingulate gyrus results in obsessive worry; malfunction of the hippocampus results in painful memories that will not go away.

3. Basal ganglia—The basal ganglia consists of several groups of nuclei located deep in the cerebral hemisphere. It is wrapped around by limbic structures and lies just above the midbrain. It consists of the corpus striatum, caudate nucleus, lenticular nucleus, putamen, and globus pallidus. The caudate nucleus in particular is interesting because it is the gate for unwanted intrusive thoughts. For example, after an untreated streptococcal sore throat, some with a disorder may have a swelling of the caudate nucleus and then begin to have obsessive worries.

## Diencephalon

1. Thalamus—The thalamus is that part of the brain called diencephalons, which relays all sensory input to the cerebral cortex except smell. If it malfunctions, one can become hyperaware of sensory input. It also functions in emotions, memory, cognition, and awareness. It is located near the midbrain and flanks the limbic system.

2. Hypothalamus—The hypothalamus controls the autonomic nervous system, which affects all internal organs of the body, smooth muscles, and visceral responses to stress. With stress one is ready for fight or flight as organs and hormones are affected by the autonomic nervous system. The autonomic nervous system also affects sexual arousal and orgasm. In short, the hypothalamus controls the visceral activities of the body: cardiovascular, temperature, gastrointestinal, sex, electrolytes, endocrine, and blood pressure.

3. Pituitary gland—The pituitary gland controls multiple endocrine functions and thus has broad implications concerning emotions, pain, and headaches. It serves as the interface between emotions and the endocrine system.

4. Pineal gland—The pineal gland secretes melatonin, which controls the onset of puberty and also plays a role in sleep.

## Midbrain and Neurotransmitters

The midbrain serves as a relay station for both motor and sensory impulses. But what is so important emotionally is that it is the home to the production of some of the most important neurotransmitters in the brain—serotonin, dopamine, and norepinephrine. Neurotransmitters transmit electrical impulses from one nerve cell to the next. In one sense they control emotions. Every emotion results from biochemical reactions in the brain. Today we know a lot about which neurotransmitters are important in various emotions. For example, low serotonin plays a role in depression, obsessive worry, and anger. And overly high dopamine plays a role in psychosis. Low dopamine can play a role in low energy, low motivation, and movement disorders. Low norepinephrine may be a factor in depression.

Within the midbrain the raphe nucleus produces serotonin, the locus ceruleus produces norepinephrine, and the substantia nigra produces dopamine. Thus the midbrain indeed is important in regard to emotions.

## Medulla Oblongata

The medulla is part of the brain stem, along with the pons and midbrain. It contains at least part of the reticular formation (along with the pons, midbrain, and diencephalon), which functions in arousal and consciousness. The reticular formation runs throughout the entire brain stem.

## Cerebellum

The cerebellum plays a major role in the timing of motor activity. However, it also may play a role in emotions.

# Testing for the Chemistry of Emotions

In the near future, in all probability a single blood test will determine whether one has significant chemical depression, anxiety, OCD, ADHD, schizophrenia, and so on. Even now, dramatic advances are being made with PET scans and other research tools. To some degree even now we can track the chemistry of emotions.

In the recent past, blood tests (DST/dexamethasone suppression test; TRH/thyroid releasing hormone test) were used for depression, along with sleep studies—rapid eye movement (REM) and reflected disturbances in the onset of REM sleep. However, these tests needed more specificity and reliability.

Other tests are also being used and providing exciting results. These include EEG/electroencephalography, PET/positron emission tomography, MRI/magnetic resonance spectroscopy, CT/computerized axial tomography, MRS/magnetic resonance spectroscopy, Functional MRI, SPECT/single photon emission computed tomography, and EEG/EP topographical mapping.

## How Stress and Genetic Factors Affect the Brain

The brain is affected by stress and genetic factors, just like organs. Sometimes genetic factors are more important, as in bipolar disorder. While in general we do not inherit mental disorders, we do inherit a level of neurotransmitters, which play a role in all emotions. Sometimes stress factors are more important, as in adjustment disorders. Often both genetic and stress factors interact to produce emotional problems. The same is often true for other medical problems, such as heart disease.

The effects of stress can be temporary, or the changes can be permanent and never corrected. Too much stress for too long may cause permanent alterations in brain chemistry and structure. This again is similar to heart disease. In heart disease there comes a time when the stress has gone on too long, and the damage to the heart or vessels becomes permanent.

The illustration at the end of this chapter shows the effects of stress and genetics on the brain as well as the complexity of the amount of knowledge we have about the brain and its connection to emotions. The question is, Are herbs and supplements up to the task of treating emotional and mental disorders? At times they certainly do help some individuals, but we have found them not nearly as effective as modern psychiatric medications. The study of the brain is the last frontier. It is the most important organ of the body. Should we trust our brain, our very self, to herbs and supplements? Are herbs and supplements up to the task? You decide!

## Where Psychiatric Medications and Natural Products Work

To further aid in our quest to determine the effectiveness and appropriateness of natural products versus psychiatric medications for mental/emotional disorders, we must consider how these products affect the brain biochemically. Though this information again is presented in scientific terms, its detailed analysis helps us see inside the brain to where these products actually cause a positive or negative effect for those suffering with such disorders. It can help us determine what methods are most helpful to those who need help on a daily basis.

As we have seen, to be most effective, prescription medications and/or herbs and supplements work on neurotransmitters, and they can do so at a number of different sites.

### Site 1

Some psychiatric medications and natural products work on postreceptor sites by being an agonist at a specific serotonin site (5HT1), as with the antianxiety medication Buspar. Other medications work as antagonists at the postreceptor site, as does the antidepressant Serzone, which works as an antagonist at the serotonin postreceptor site, 5HT2, and by doing so may lift mood. In addition, it may also decrease anxiety by antagonizing the 5HT2 site in the frontal cortex. Furthermore, by antagonizing 5HT2 receptor sites in the spinal cord, it may lead to less sexual dysfunction.

Antipsychotics such as Haldol, Thorazine, Stelazine, and Prolixin largely work on the postreceptor of dopamine (DA). Some antipsychotics have not only DA antagonism on the postregular site but also block 5HT2, which could have a mood-lifting effect and might decrease the negative symptoms of schizophrenia, such as flat-affect alogia and social withdrawal. Some antipsychotics work at DA antagonism on the postregular site but also work at site 3 (described below) to block the reuptake of serotonin and norepinephrine.

An antianxiety agent such as Xanex, Serax, and Ativan essentially works as an agonist for the neurotransmitter GABA on the postreceptor site.

Certain herbs such as valerian and possibly kava work as GABA agonists against evoking GABA and therefore have calming effects. Side effects and impurities, however, have limited their use.

## Site 2

Some psychiatric medications work by stimulating the release of neurotransmitters at the prereceptor site, as Adderall does for ADHD by causing the release of more dopamine and norepinephrine, which increase attention span. It also works at site 3 (described below) by blocking the reuptake of dopamine and norepinephrine.

Some psychiatric medications work by causing the release of neurotransmitters at the prereceptor site. Psychostimulants like Adderall work in this manner by causing the release of dopamine, which increases the ability to pay attention. In contrast, a similar natural product, ephedra, probably works by a nonselective alpha and beta receptor agonist.

## Site 3

Antidepressants such as tricyclics (Tofranil, Sinequan, Elvil), tetracyclics (Ludiomil), selective serotonin reuptake inhibitors (Prozac, Paxil, Zoloft, Luvox, and Celexa), Effexor, Serzone, to some degree, and Wellbutrin all work at site 3. They work by blocking the reuptake of different neurotransmitters. Selective serotonin reuptake inhibitors (SSRIs) block the reuptake and degradation of serotonin, so mood lifts, anger decreases, and obsessions decrease. Wellbutrin blocks the reuptake and degradation of dopamine so mood lifts and energy and motivation increase. Tricyclics and tetracyclics block the reuptake of many neurotransmitters, and yet they may have many side effects. Effexor blocks the reuptake of neurotransmitters (serotonin, norepinephrine, and dopamine). Saint-John's-wort works at least partially at this site.

## Site 4

Psychiatric medications also work by decreasing or increasing the number of receptor sites at the postreceptor site. There is not enough research to know if Saint-John's-wort works here.

## Site 5

Some psychiatric medications, possibly lithium, may effect changes through a second messenger system. In fact, many psychiatric medications may ultimately work through secondary messenger systems.

## Site 6

Some psychiatric medications (MAO inhibitors) alter the metabolism of neurotransmitters and thus increase the amount available for release at the prereceptor site. Saint-John's-wort may work at least partially at this site.

## Site 7

The amount of neurotransmitter available could theoretically be altered by providing more or less of the precursor ingredients. For example, L-tryptophane, a naturally occurring amino acid, is a precursor of serotonin and was used to help relieve depression more in the past than it is today. However, problems arose. First, the response usually seemed mild at best, and then, possibly due to impurities, several deaths caused by eosinophilia occurred in those using L-tryptophane.

Consider the natural synthesis of some monoamines (tyrosine→hydroxylation→DOPH→decarboxylation→ dopamine→hydroxylation→norepinephrine→methylation→epinephrine). Tyrosine has been tried in depression but usually has poor results.

Controlled studies are lacking for these precursors. Digestive juices may weaken effects. The blood-brain barrier may weaken effects. A happy mood may also be a very complex chemical reaction, and one precursor simply will not be effective.

The same question could be asked about 5HTP (5–hydroxytryptophane). As with giving L-tryptophane directly, the benefit usually seems mild and dangers such as eosinophilia always harm.

Giving the neurotransmitter directly could be considered, as with GABA, which is sold as a supplement. The possible dangers and ineffectiveness, for the reasons mentioned above, argue for caution.

## Selectivity

Not only do psychiatric medications affect certain neurotransmitters and subneurotransmitters, in some cases they also may work selectively in specific brain regions. For example, the new neuroleptics, such as Risperdol, Seroquel, Zyprexa, and Geodon, are antagonists on the postreceptor side of dopamine 2 (DA2) and serotonin 2 (5HT2), but they selectively work in the limbic brain to produce the desired effects and do not work as much in the basal ganglia of the brain. Consequently, fewer undesirable side effects, such as parkinsonism, are produced. The antidepressant Serzone not only blocks the prereceptor serotonin reuptake, which might cause sexual side effects, but also is an antagonist at the postreceptor site of serotonin 2 (5HT2), and this selective action in the spinal cord could block the sexual side effects as serotonin increases.

The new neuroleptic Abilify (aripipezole) is especially interesting because it works as an antagonist of DA2 in the limbic brain, and as a result, hallucinations go away. It also may work as an agonist at DA2 in the basal ganglia, so movement disorders are often avoided.

## Isomers in Psychiatric Medications and Natural Products

What are known as single isomer drugs will take a prominent role in psychiatry in the future. Already Lexapro (escitalopram), one of the isomers of Celexa (citalopram), is big news, as is Focalin, one of the isomers of methylphenidate (Ritalin). In natural products L-carnitine, an amino acid, has made news because the racemic mixture (a mixture of the two isomers) is toxic.

Isomers are mirror-image molecules but are not always superimposable on each other and may have dramatically different biologic effects. Thus in the future the more effective isomer of a drug will be isolated and used. This will no doubt result in lower dosages, fewer side effects, and fewer drug interactions. Single isomer drugs are an important step forward in psychiatry.

## Summary

In reality, mental issues are biochemically complex in causation; therefore, helping individuals biochemically involves not only altering neurotransmitters but also receptor sites, ion transport, secondary messenger systems, brain-derived neurotropic factors of brain cell nourishment, and even the DNA within the nucleus of the nerve cell. In general, natural products are not as effective, specific, or selective as modern allopathic medicines.

# THE BRAIN UNDER STRESS

## AN OVERVIEW

Under stress the brain changes. The specific parts of the brain affected by stress are illustrated. The diagram below is for educational purposes and is not drawn to scale.

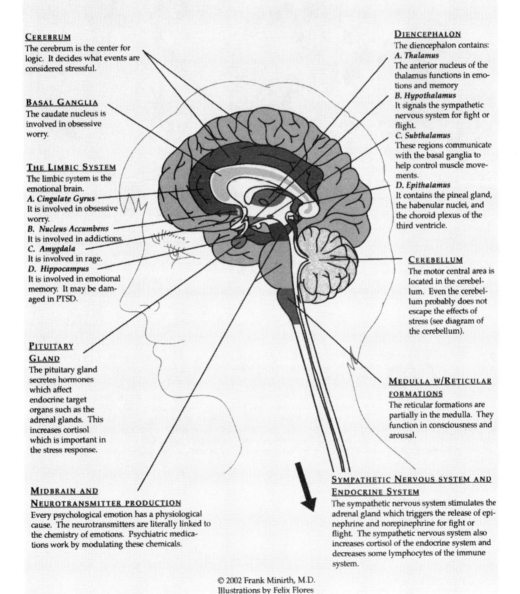

**CEREBRUM**
The cerebrum is the center for logic. It decides what events are considered stressful.

**BASAL GANGLIA**
The caudate nucleus is involved in obsessive worry.

**THE LIMBIC SYSTEM**
The limbic system is the emotional brain.
*A. Cingulate Gyrus*
It is involved in obsessive worry.
*B. Nucleus Accumbens*
It is involved in addictions.
*C. Amygdala*
It is involved in rage.
*D. Hippocampus*
It is involved in emotional memory. It may be damaged in PTSD.

**PITUITARY GLAND**
The pituitary gland secretes hormones which affect endocrine target organs such as the adrenal glands. This increases cortisol which is important in the stress response.

**MIDBRAIN AND NEUROTRANSMITTER PRODUCTION**
Every psychological emotion has a physiological cause. The neurotransmitters are literally linked to the chemistry of emotions. Psychiatric medications work by modulating these chemicals.

**DIENCEPHALON**
The diencephalon contains:
*A. Thalamus*
The anterior nucleus of the thalamus functions in emotions and memory
*B. Hypothalamus*
It signals the sympathetic nervous system for fight or flight.
*C. Subthalamus*
These regions communicate with the basal ganglia to help control muscle movements.
*D. Epithalamus*
It contains the pineal gland, the habenular nuclei, and the choroid plexus of the third ventricle.

**CEREBELLUM**
The motor central area is located in the cerebellum. Even the cerebellum probably does not escape the effects of stress (see diagram of the cerebellum).

**MEDULLA W/RETICULAR FORMATIONS**
The reticular formations are partially in the medulla. They function in consciousness and arousal.

**SYMPATHETIC NERVOUS SYSTEM AND ENDOCRINE SYSTEM**
The sympathetic nervous system stimulates the adrenal gland which triggers the release of epinephrine and norepinephrine for fight or flight. The sympathetic nervous system also increases cortisol of the endocrine system and decreases some lymphocytes of the immune system.

© 2002 Frank Minirth, M.D.
Illustrations by Felix Flores

## THE BRAIN UNDER STRESS

### THE SYNAPSE, NEUROTRANSMITTERS, AND CHEMICALS WITHIN THE NERVE CELL

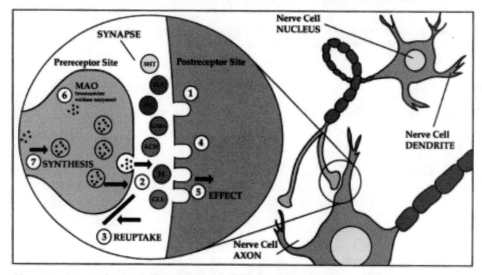

Neurotransmitters are chemicals (made from amino acids) that transmit nerve impulses from one cell to the next. There are perhaps 200 of these and many more if one considers several kinds of even one neurotransmitter receptor such as serotonin. Every psychological emotion has a physiological component and certainly neurotransmitters are a part of that component. Neuropeptides (endorphines, enkephalins, dynorphins) are also neurotransmitters and they are the body's natural painkillers. Important issues regarding neurotransmitters are:

1. Neurotransmitters are extremely important in brain functioning. We could not think or feel without neurotransmitters.

2. Neurotransmitters are very important in emotions. Every psychological emotion had a physiological cause and neurotransmitters are part of the cause.

3. Psychiatric medications often begin to work by initially altering neurotransmitters which result in changes at post receptor sites, ion transport, secondary messenger systems, brain derived neurotrophic factor, and eventually the DNA within the nucleus of the cell.

For example, antidepressants that prevent the reuptake of serotonin (5HT) may result in improved mood in depressed individuals, less worry in obsessive-compulsive individuals and less anger. Also increasing norepinephrine (NE) and dopamine (DA) may lift mood. Dopamine also plays a role in sexual activity. Acetylcholine (ACH) plays a role in memory. GABA plays a role in calmness. Blocking histamine receptors could help sleep but increase weight. Glutamate, an excitatory neurotransmitter, may play a role in degenerative disease, Alzheimer's dementia, and schizophrenia. Herbs also alter neurotransmitters but usually with a much less dramatic, selective, and specific effect than psychiatric medications.

(5HT) = Serotonin = Important in mood, worry, and anger
(DA) = Dopamine = Important in energy and motivation
(NE) = Norepinephrine = Important in mood and energy
(ACH) = Acetylcholine = Important in memory
(GABA) = Gamma-aminobutyric acid
(H) = Histamine
(GLU) = Glutamate

*Chapter 6*

# Positive and Negative Effects on Emotions

As we have seen, the science of treating mental disorders is complex. The brain is an intricate and multifaceted organ and deeply connected to our very selves. Dealing with diseases related to the brain requires results at this complex level of understanding. Yet though our emotions are triggered biochemically, other factors are crucial to understand—factors that cause our brain's mechanisms to set our emotional reactions in motion.

## Factors That Alter Neurotransmitters and Emotions

Several issues can alter neurotransmitters for the worse and have potentially profound influences on the emotions. They are:

### 1. Stress

Stress certainly can alter the brain with profound influence on the emotions and body. Stress can be defined as emotional tension. It can come from present issues such as relationship conflicts, financial worries, and job stress, or from past issues such as abuse, abandonment, and self-image. It is determined by one's perception (what is stress to one is not to another). In addition, one's general physical health can be a factor in stress. During stress the body is poised for either fight or flight. In fight-or-flight mode, chemical changes occur, which may have far-reaching implications. With stress can come corresponding behavioral changes: angry verbal responses, being ready to run, exercising, drinking, smoking, binge eating, and so on. The autonomic nervous system balance is altered and blood pressure increases (which, in some individuals, may trigger a heart attack), along with other physiological parameters. Blood pressure may not go back down totally and may result in hypertension and acceleration of atherosclerosis.

The hypothalamus is also affected during stress, which in turn affects the pituitary gland, which in turn affects the adrenal medulla (with the resulting release of adrenaline) and the adrenal cortex (with the resulting release of cortisol), which eventually results in accelerated aging, decreased bone mineral density, alterations in immune system response, and possible permanent alterations in the functioning of the brain through effects on the hippocampus, amino acids, and neurotransmitters. Because stress may alter the hippocampus, which controls memory, continued stress may result

31

in an inability to access the information necessary to decide that a situation is no longer a threat. Thus stress begets stress. In fact, magnetic resonance imaging has shown that stress-related disorders such as post-traumatic stress disorder and recurrent major depression are associated with atrophy of the hippocampus. Furthermore, ongoing stress may result in a disregulation of the hypothalamus-pituitary-adrenal axis, resulting in cognitive impairment. Finally, stress alters the neurotransmitters of the brain that control mood, logic, disposition, sleep, attention, weight, and pain perception.

## 2. Genetic Factors

Genetic factors can affect the brain as well. For example, 90 percent of individuals with bipolar disorder also have a first-degree relative with bipolar disorder; 50 percent of individuals with a major depression have a first-degree relative with the same disorder; 40 percent of individuals with obsessive compulsive disorders have a first-degree relative with the same or related disorder; 35 percent of individuals with attention-deficit disorders have a first-degree relative with the same disorder. Furthermore, if one identical twin has schizophrenia, the other twin has a high probability (80 to 90 percent) of developing it as well; if one identical twin has bipolar disorder, there is a 60 percent chance the other twin will have the disorder. These probabilities drop significantly in nonidentical twins or other siblings as compared to identical twins.

Research is perhaps the most interesting in the area of identical twins. Even personality traits to some degree are inherited. Identical twins reared apart from birth show behavioral similarities; many laugh alike and show similar nervous mannerisms.

For example, "Joy" and "Jan," identical twins, were separated at birth. Thus, they had no common environmental factors except in utero. Both named their children identical names; both wore identical jewelry including seven rings on their fingers. Then there is the story of "Joe" and "Jim," identical twins, also separated at birth. Both loved carpentry; both built circular benches around trees in their yards. Furthermore, the story of identical twins, "Al" and "Ike," is striking. They too were separated at birth, raised in separate countries, and did not meet until they were in their fifties when they showed up at the same time for a job interview. Both wore blue shirts with epaulets; both wore aviator glasses; both wore rubber bands on their wrists; both flushed the toilet before and after use; both liked to startle people in elevators by sneezing. Finally, the story of identical twins separated at birth, "Bill" and "Bob," is interesting. They had grown up only forty-five miles apart but never met until they were adults and learned the following. Both drove a blue Chevrolet; both had a dog named Toy; both chain-smoked Salems; both chewed their fingernails; both vacationed in the same neighborhood in Florida; both tested almost identical in personality traits.

## 3. Illegal and Addictive Drugs

Illegal drugs can be dangerous because they permanently alter the brain chemistry, functioning, and emotions. Marijuana is of special concern because it actually becomes part of the brain structure. Its changes are so insidious because it produces "amotivational syndrome."

## 4. Medical Disease

Medical diseases can produce many emotions. For example, possible causes for depression are pernicious anemia, mononucleosis, hypothyroidism, Cushing's syndrome, Addison's disease, cancer of the pancreas, multiple sclerosis, various drugs, and perhaps to some degree even upper respiratory infection. Possible causes for anxiety include mitral valve prolapse, hyperthyroidism, hypoglycemia, pheochromocytoma, and drugs such as caffeine and nicotine. In a loss of touch with reality, possible causes include porphyria, prescription drugs, brain tumors, endocrine abnormalities, Wilson's disease, alcohol, bromide-containing compounds, LSD, PCP, marijuana, and cocaine. Personality changes may be caused by Alzheimer's disease, dementia, various illegal drugs such as marijuana ("amotivational syndrome"), vascular disorders, viral infections of the central nervous system, Parkinson's disease, disease of the central nervous system, lupus, multiple sclerosis, and temporal lobe epilepsy. To some degree even violence may be related to such disorders as temporal lobe epilepsy, various illegal drugs, alcohol, and so on. Medical causes of insomnia include sleep apnea, myoclonic jerks, and caffeine. Obsessive-compulsive disorder in some cases may be precipitated by an untreated strep throat. Paniclike feelings can come from mitral value prolapse and hyperthyroidism.

## Positive Influences on Brain Chemistry and Emotions

Positive factors can alter neurotransmitters for the better and potentially have a profound influence on the emotions. They are:

### 1. Behavioral-Cognitive Techniques

From PET scans of the brain, we know that simple, repeated, behavioral, cognitive techniques can actually alter the metabolism of the brain for the better.

### 2. Volition

We have powerful chemicals in our brains that, to some degree I believe, are released through our own volition. For example, even placebos work to some degree, perhaps 30 percent of the time.

### 3. Laughter

Laughter probably releases endorphins and enkephalins, which help lift mood and decrease pain.

### 4. Herbs and Vitamins

This is an area of much debate and the discussion of this book. The use of herbs and vitamins has a pro and a con. The pro side is that in some circumstances they work. The con side is that sometimes they do not work, and just because they are "natural" does not mean they are safe (strychnine and cyanide are also "natural"). Remember, there is no FDA control over safety or dosage, and in some cases herbs and supplements could have dangerous interactions with medicines. The claims are interesting to ponder but worthy of great caution.

### 5. Sex

Powerful chemicals are released during sex. These chemicals have a relaxing and calming effect and are so strong that when used inappropriately they seem to be potentially addicting. For example, a new medication that has gained great media attention is Viagra (sildenafil citrate), used to treat erectile dysfunction in men. Sexual emotions throughout history have often overruled sound logic. However, used appropriately in marriage, they are a gift blessed by God himself.

### 6. Exercise

Exercise releases adrenaline (epinephrine) and endorphins, which are natural stimulants and mood enhancers.

### 7. Medication

Mediations can do wonderful things today. Moods can be lifted and stability can be returned. Attention can be focused. Pain can be released. Worries can be abated. Energy can be increased. Anxiety can be mitigated. Sex drive can be increased (or decreased). Anger can be lessened. Hallucinations can be eliminated. And the ability to relate can be enhanced.

## *8. Scripture Memory*

What we take in through the eye affects the frontal lobes and other areas of the brain involved in memory. Secondary-messenger systems are altered, and memory is stored. We become what we take into the brain. We can become Christlike by taking in the Word of God.

## Summary

Understanding the effectiveness of natural products and prescription medications for those suffering with emotionally charged disorders can help us determine how to help them fight disease and have a more productive life. Although much of what offers help does occur biochemically, we can affect other factors that can either cause or worsen such disorders. By decreasing any external factors over which we have control, and by utilizing these positive factors, we can provide much-needed relief to people who need assistance in dealing with mental and even some physical disorders.

# THE BRAIN UNDER STRESS

## THE LIMBIC SYSTEM

The limbic brain is the emotional brain. Pain, pleasure, anger, depression, affection, and sexuality all originate in the limbic brain. Stimulation in animals of the amygdala results in rage. Stimulation of the nucleus accumbens results in pleasure. Malfunction of the cingulate gyrus results in obsessive worry. Malfunction of the hippocampus results in painful memories that will not go away.

### NUCLEUS ACCUMBENS

The nucleus accumbens has to do with pain and pleasure. It is important in addictions. It receives input from the hippocampus, the amygdala, the septum, the hypothalamus, and the frontal lobes of the cerebral cortex. Dopamine is the neurotransmitter important here in addictions.

Under stress, unfortunately some individuals turn to drugs of abuse that have a major effect here.

### AMYGDALA

The amygdala is involved in memory just as the hippocampus is, but the amygdala has to do more with memory and emotionally charged events. If physical damage occurs to the amygdala or it is induced in laboratory animals, then rage can result. When in danger, it is the amygdala that signals the alarm to the hypothalamus. The hypothalamus will then signal the sympathetic nervous system, which in turn activates the adrenal medulla to release epinephrine and norepinephrine for fight or flight. The hypothalamus also signals the release of corticotrophin releasing hormone (CRH) which signals the pituitary gland to release adrenocorticotropic hormone (ACTH) which then signals to the adrenal cortex to release cortisol which continues until the danger signal is halted (but with PTSD the alarm signal is not halted because the hippocampus is damaged.) It is the amygdala that signaled the initial alarm.

Under stress anger may result and play a role here.

### CINGULATE GYRUS

This structure is located deep in the center of the cerebral hemisphere of the brain. The cingulate gyrus helps one shift attention from one thought or behavior to another. If it malfunctions one becomes stuck on certain thoughts as in OCD. It is also the part of the brain that signals danger.

Under stress some individuals may obsessively worry because of damage here. Their activity here is similar to a biochemical seizure that can often be quelled with psychiatric medication.

### HIPPOCAMPUS

The hippocampus controls emotional memory. With prolonged stress cortisol remains high and the hippocampus is suppressed in activity and eventually seems to atrophy. Thus, memory distortions may occur and painful memories will not go away as in post-traumatic stress disorder.

Under severe stress (PTSD) the memories of the event continue to occur because of damage here.

# THE  BRAIN  UNDER  STRESS

## THE LIMBIC SYSTEM

The limbic brain is the emotional brain.  Pain, pleasure, anger, depression, affection, and sexuality all originate in the limbic brain.  Stimulation in animals of the amygdala results in rage.  Stimulation of the nucleus accumbens results in pleasure.  Malfunction of the cingulate gyrus results in obsessive worry.  Malfunction of the hippocampus results in painful memories that will not go away.

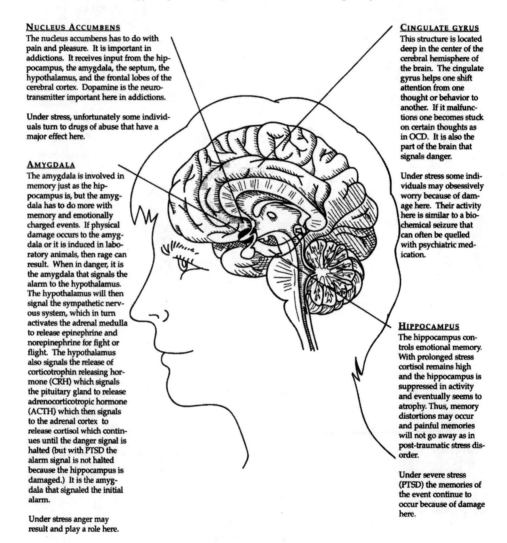

### NUCLEUS ACCUMBENS

The nucleus accumbens has to do with pain and pleasure.  It is important in addictions.  It receives input from the hippocampus, the amygdala, the septum, the hypothalamus, and the frontal lobes of the cerebral cortex.  Dopamine is the neurotransmitter important here in addictions.

Under stress, unfortunately some individuals turn to drugs of abuse that have a major effect here.

### AMYGDALA

The amygdala is involved in memory just as the hippocampus is, but the amygdala has to do more with memory and emotionally charged events.  If physical damage occurs to the amygdala or it is induced in laboratory animals, then rage can result.  When in danger, it is the amygdala that signals the alarm to the hypothalamus.  The hypothalamus will then signal the sympathetic nervous system, which in turn activates the adrenal medulla to release epinephrine and norepinephrine for fight or flight.  The hypothalamus also signals the release of corticotrophin releasing hormone (CRH) which signals the pituitary gland to release adrenocorticotropic hormone (ACTH) which then signals to the adrenal cortex to release cortisol which continues until the danger signal is halted (but with PTSD the alarm signal is not halted because the hippocampus is damaged.)  It is the amygdala that signaled the initial alarm.

Under stress anger may result and play a role here.

### CINGULATE GYRUS

This structure is located deep in the center of the cerebral hemisphere of the brain.  The cingulate gyrus helps one shift attention from one thought or behavior to another.  If it malfunctions one becomes stuck on certain thoughts as in OCD.  It is also the part of the brain that signals danger.

Under stress some individuals may obsessively worry because of damage here.  Their activity here is similar to a biochemical seizure that can often be quelled with psychiatric medication.

### HIPPOCAMPUS

The hippocampus controls emotional memory.  With prolonged stress cortisol remains high and the hippocampus is suppressed in activity and eventually seems to atrophy.  Thus, memory distortions may occur and painful memories will not go away as in post-traumatic stress disorder.

Under severe stress (PTSD) the memories of the event continue to occur because of damage here.

# THE BRAIN UNDER STRESS

## THE ENDOCRINE SYSTEM

The endocrine system consists of endocrine glands that secrete specific chemicals called hormones into the blood or surrounding interstitial fluid. The endocrine system functions closely with the nervous system in regulating and integrating body processes. In general, the action of hormones is relatively slow and the effects are prolonged, whereas the action of nerve impulses is fast and the effects are of short duration. Hormones regulate metabolic functions. They exert profound effects on their target organs (see below). They are controlled by three factors: hormonal, humoral, and neural.

### HORMONAL
Hormones control themselves by a feedback system. The hypothalamus hormones such as TRH, CRH, GHRH, GnRH, and PIF regulate pituitary hormones and the pituitary hormones such as GH, TSH, ACTH, FSH, LH, PRL, oxytocin, and ADH regulate the hormonal release at the final target organs (as thyroid and adrenal glands).

### HUMORAL
Certain ions and nutrients stimulate hormonal release. For example, PTH are decreased by decreasing blood calcium levels. Then PTH reverses the decline of blood calcium.

### NEURONAL
The nervous system can stimulate the release of hormones. For example, stress stimulates the sympathetic nervous system which then stimulates the adrenal gland to release the catecholamines norepinephrine and epinephrine.

The nervous system can even override the endocrine controls. For example, under stress blood sugar may rise dramatically.

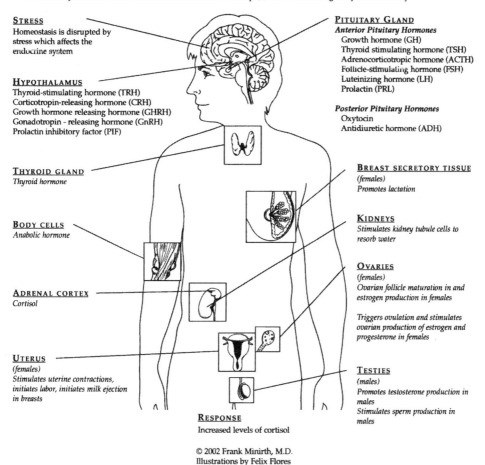

**STRESS**
Homeostasis is disrupted by stress which affects the endocrine system

**HYPOTHALAMUS**
Thyroid-stimulating hormone (TRH)
Corticotropin-releasing hormone (CRH)
Growth hormone releasing hormone (GHRH)
Gonadotropin - releasing hormone (GnRH)
Prolactin inhibitory factor (PIF)

**THYROID GLAND**
*Thyroid hormone*

**BODY CELLS**
*Anabolic hormone*

**ADRENAL CORTEX**
*Cortisol*

**UTERUS**
*(females)*
*Stimulates uterine contractions, initiates labor, initiates milk ejection in breasts*

**PITUITARY GLAND**
*Anterior Pituitary Hormones*
Growth hormone (GH)
Thyroid stimulating hormone (TSH)
Adrenocorticotropic hormone (ACTH)
Follicle-stimulating hormone (FSH)
Luteinizing hormone (LH)
Prolactin (PRL)

*Posterior Pituitary Hormones*
Oxytocin
Antidiuretic hormone (ADH)

**BREAST SECRETORY TISSUE**
*(females)*
*Promotes lactation*

**KIDNEYS**
*Stimulates kidney tubule cells to resorb water*

**OVARIES**
*(females)*
*Ovarian follicle maturation in and estrogen production in females*

*Triggers ovulation and stimulates ovarian production of estrogen and progesterone in females*

**TESTIES**
*(males)*
*Promotes testosterone production in males*
*Stimulates sperm production in males*

**RESPONSE**
Increased levels of cortisol

© 2002 Frank Minirth, M.D.
Illustrations by Felix Flores

## THE  BRAIN  UNDER  STRESS

### THE DIENCEPHALON (HYPOTHALAMUS), THE SYMPATHETIC NERVOUS SYSTEM, THE PITUITARY GLAND, THE ENDOCRINE SYSTEM, AND THE IMMUNE SYSTEM

The Sympathetic Nervous System prepares the body for emergency situations. It is primarily concerned with processes involving the expenditure of energy. When the body is in homeostasis, the main function of the sympathetic division is to counteract the parasympathetic effects just enough to carry out normal processes requiring energy. During physical or emotional stress, however, the sympathetic dominates the parasympathetic. Physical exertion stimulates the sympathetic division as do a variety of emotions such as fear, embarrassment, or rage. Emergency, excitement, exercise, embarrassment will set off sympathetic responses. Activation of the sympathetic division and release of hormones by the adrenal medulla set in motion a series of physiological responses collectively called the alarm reaction or fight-or-flight response. When in danger, it is the amygdala that signals the alarm to the hypothalamus. The hypothalamus will then signal the sympathetic nervous system, which in turn activates the adrenal medulla to release epinephrine and norepinephrine for fight or flight. The hypothalamus also signals the release of corticotrophin releasing hormone (CRH) which signals the pituitary gland to release adrenocorticotropic hormone (ACTH) which then signals to the adrenal cortex to release cortisol which continues until the danger signal is halted (but with PTSD the alarm signal is not halted because the hippocampus is damaged).

Cortisol results in more glucose and more fatty acids for energy needs. Cortisol also enhances epinephrine's vasoconstrictive effects to deliver nutrients quickly. With continued stress the sympathetic nervous system overrides the normal inhibiting feedback system of high cortisol and the cortisol remains high. Sustained high cortisol can lead to hyperglycemia, hypertension, osteoporosis, bruising, poor wound healing, and a continued state of high alert. Under the high cortisol and continued stress a gene for brain derived neurotrophic factor (BDNF), a chemical that sustains the brain neurons, is repressed leading to atrophy of the neurons in the hippocampus. Thus, individuals under prolonged stress may have trouble realizing that the stress is over even when the stressor is gone because the emotional memory cells are atrophied. Furthermore, in mature animals intense stimulation of the amygdala even one-time can produce lasting changes in neuronal excitability in the direction of either fight or flight. In other words, prolonged stress is not good to say the least. Under stress the sympathetic nervous system is affected and can result in traumatic memories that continue to occur. Finally, since hormones such as cortisol and epinephrine provide chemical links between the endocrine and immune system, under stress T lymphocytes are depressed, increasing the susceptibility to physical disease (perhaps even cancer).

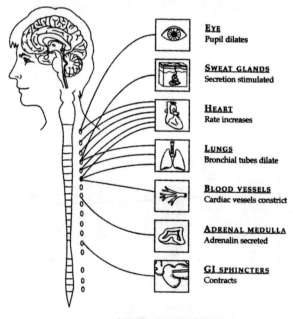

**EYE**
Pupil dilates

**SWEAT GLANDS**
Secretion stimulated

**HEART**
Rate increases

**LUNGS**
Bronchial tubes dilate

**BLOOD VESSELS**
Cardiac vessels constrict

**ADRENAL MEDULLA**
Adrenalin secreted

**GI SPHINCTERS**
Contracts

© 2002 Frank Minirth, M.D.
Illustrations by Felix Flores

# THE BRAIN UNDER STRESS

### THE MIDBRAIN

The midbrain serves as a relay station for both motor and sensory impulses. But what is so important emotionally is that it is the home to the production of some of the most important neurotransmitters in the brain (serotonin, dopamine, and norepinephrine).

Neurotransmitters transmit electrical impulses from one nerve cell to the next. They are throughout the central and peripheral nervous system. They play an important role in emotions. Every emotion results from biochemical reactions in the brain. Today we often know which neurotransmitters (and even sub-neurotransmitters) are important in various emotions.

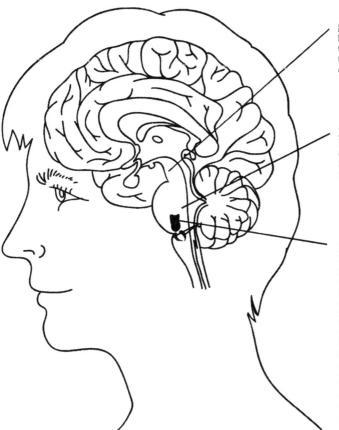

**SUBSTANTIA NIGRA**
Dopamine production occurs in this nucleus. Dopamine is important in energy, motivation, mood and attention.

**LOCUS CERULOUS**
Norepinephrine production occurs in this nucleus which is also important in energy, motivation, mood, and attention.

**RAPHE NUCLEUS**
Serotonin or 5-hydroxytrypto-phan (5HT) is concentrated in the neurons in a part of the brain stem called the raphe nucleus. Axons projecting from the raphe nucleus terminate in the hypo-thalamus, thalamus, and other parts of the brain and spinal cord. Serotonin is thought to be involved in inducing sleep, sensory perception, temperature regulation, and control of mood. The antidepressant drugs (Prozac, Paxil, Zoloft, Luvox, Celexa, and Lexapro) are selective inhibitors of serotonin reuptake (SSRI's). SSRI's thus make more serotonin available in the synapse cleft and eventually result in lifting of mood.

# THE BRAIN UNDER STRESS

## THE BRAIN STEM

The brain stem consists of the midbrain, the pons, and medulla. All are important in emotions. Psychiatric medications initially work by altering these neurotransmitters which then alter postsynaptic neurotransmitter receptors, ion transport, secondary messengers and chemicals such as brain-derived neurotrophic factor (BDNF) that nourish and sustain brain cells.

Under stress chemical changes take place within the nerve cell.

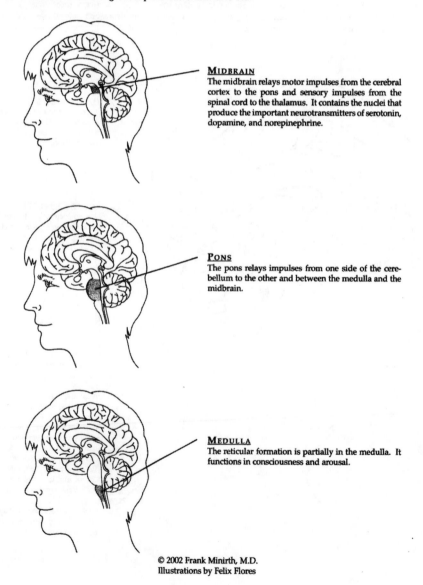

**MIDBRAIN**
The midbrain relays motor impulses from the cerebral cortex to the pons and sensory impulses from the spinal cord to the thalamus. It contains the nuclei that produce the important neurotransmitters of serotonin, dopamine, and norepinephrine.

**PONS**
The pons relays impulses from one side of the cerebellum to the other and between the medulla and the midbrain.

**MEDULLA**
The reticular formation is partially in the medulla. It functions in consciousness and arousal.

© 2002 Frank Minirth, M.D.
Illustrations by Felix Flores

# THE   BRAIN   UNDER   STRESS

## CEREBELLUM

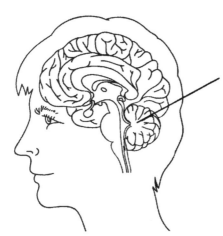

### CEREBELLUM

The cerebellum compares intended movements with what is actually happening to smooth and coordinate complex skilled movements. It regulates posture and balance. It too probably has to do with emotions. Babies who are not rocked and cuddled (functions of the cerebellum) may have more emotional difficulty. Stress early in life can even potentially affect the cerebellum.

*Chapter 7*

# Selected Natural Products in Psychiatry

Though we are skeptical that natural products used in psychiatry hold forth the potential found in other areas of medicine, they are, nonetheless, of great interest and worth more research. Christians might want to study the following herbs and supplements.

## Saint-John's-Wort

Saint-John's-wort is by far the most popular herb in psychiatry. In Germany it outsells Prozac twenty to one. It may help some with more mild depressive disorders. However, its use is complicated by many potentially dangerous drug interactions and by the treatment of a potentially lethal condition (major depressive disorder, which can lead to suicide) with mild benefits.

## Omega-3 Fatty Acids

The best natural product in psychiatry may prove to be omega-3 fatty acids for mood stabilization, but the proof is far from conclusive.

## L-Tryptophane, 5HTP, and Tyrosine

Precursors of various neurotransmitters that are important for mood have become more popular in recent years. L-tryptophane, a precursor of serotonin, has been used to treat insomnia and depression and appears to help to a mild degree in some, but contaminants have limited its use. Another precursor of serotonin, 5HTP, also might help some with depression but leads to the fear of eosinophilia. Tyrosine, a precursor of dopamine, has been used for improving alertness following sleep deprivation and it appears to help some.

# GABA

Neurotransmitters themselves are now being sold over the counter. GABA, the primary inhibitory neurotransmitter, is touted to calm anxiety and lift mood. Effectiveness is not proven.

# Lithium

By far the most effective natural product for a major mental disorder over the last fifty years has been a mineral—lithium carbonate. It remains the gold standard for treating bipolar disorder.

# Gingko

Medications such as Reminyl with galantamine (originally derived from daffodils) are of great benefit in Alzheimer's dementia. Gingko biloba is highly touted among all natural products for helping decrease dementia, yet it may offer only limited benefits for some and also carries many possible adverse reactions and drug interactions.

# Inositol

Inositol, a B vitamin, has been tried in panic disorders and OCD (obsessive-compulsive disorder). More research is needed, and while it may help some, we doubt it will be a major benefit for most.

# Coffee

One of the number-one herbs of all time, coffee is a mild stimulant, and even with all of its drawbacks and potential drug interactions, it likely helps many people, to a mild degree, with mental alertness.

# Kava, Valerian, and Melatonin

Concerning anxiety and insomnia, an herb with GABA agonist effects, kava, may prove to be dangerous to the liver and to have dangerous interactions with benzodiazepine and alcohol. Valerian is another herb with a GABA-like agonist effect similar to benzodiazepine, but it could potentially produce tolerance. Overall valerian is probably safer than kava and does seem to help some with anxiety and insomnia. Melatonin, a hormone, has been used for insomnia more than any other natural product; however, it is probably only helpful in circadian-rhythm disturbance insomnia. Melatonin use in tardive dyskinesia is an interesting possibility.

# SAMe

SAMe, a naturally occurring substance found in all body tissue, may be of help for some who suffer with depression.

## Folic Acid and B$_6$

Folic acid and B$_6$, when added to SSRI antidepressant medications, seem to help some women with resistant depression.

## L-Arginine

L-arginine has been touted to help in female sexual dysfunction, but research is lacking, and side effects (such as decreased platelet count and increased serum creatinine) are possible.

## Vitamin E

Vitamin E, like melatonin, might help in some cases of tardive dyskinesia. It has been used for neuroprotective effects in Alzheimer's dementia with equivocal results.

## Feverfew

Feverfew helps some people with the mental anguish of migraine headaches. It may help in prevention and probably helps more when headaches are infrequent and not severe.

## Wild Yam

Wild yam, a "natural alternative" for estrogen replacement, was the precursor of all the commercial preparations of hormones. Its effectiveness is not known.

## Evening Primrose Oil

While evening primrose oil is the number one herbal treatment of all time for PMS, it is probably not truly effective for most women.

## MACA and Maragamma

MACA, an herb used by Native Americans, and maragamma, an Amazonian herb, have been touted for sexual enhancement, but again, research into effectiveness is lacking.

## DHEA

DHEA is a popular hormone that can be bought over the counter. It has been touted for fighting depression and erectile dysfunction. It probably helps some, but it can be dangerous with many potential side effects, which have limited its use.

*Chapter 8*

# Pearls for the Taking: My Top Twenty-Three Picks of Natural Products

Are there natural products that are pearls of wisdom for the taking? Of course there are. Twenty-five percent of current medicines come from natural products. In medical school we were always looking for pearls from the professors. Here are my top twenty-five pearls from natural products. I must caution that pearls of today do not always hold true for the future, so these are given with a degree of caution concerning the unknown. Please give yourself four points for each correct answer.

| QUESTION | ANSWER |
|---|---|
| 1. Of all the natural products for *mental health,* one seems to stand out above the rest. It might help to calm a bipolar. It might help to lift depression. In addition, it might even lower cholesterol. What is it? | Omega-3 fatty acids in fish oil |
| 2. Of all the products to *lower cholesterol,* one seems to be a real pearl. After all, heart disease is the number one killer, and high cholesterol is often a factor in heart disease. It might even help in weight loss. It might cause gastrointestinal upset and fatigue in some, but it seems very safe usually. What is it? | CLA (conjugated linoleic acid) |
| 3. This drug proved to be an unbelievable pearl. Its original ingredient, salicylic acid, comes from the willow tree. It helps in *angina.* It can decrease the number of heart attacks, the number one killer in America. It is an analgesic. It is the number one drug of all time. Thirteen billion are sold per year. What is it? | Aspirin |

4.  *Migraines* affect perhaps one in every four people                  Feverfew
    in America. The pain is excruciating. There is a natural prod-
    uct that many claim often really helps. What is it?

5.  A simple diet and lifestyle can really help                          High-fiber, low-fat diet,
    decrease the likelihood of some forms of *cancer*.                   nicotine free
    It is a wonderful pearl. What is it?

6.  *Diabetics* can suffer from horrible pain and                        Alpha lipoic acid
    discomfort from neuropathy. If anything could ever help to
    reverse this, it would be a wonderful pearl. What might help
    in some cases?

7.  When the heart begins to fail, fear sets in.                         Coenzyme Q10
    There are great treatments for *congestive heart failure* today.
    In fact, digoxin originally came from the foxglove plant. There
    may be another pearl for some as an adjunctive help in CHF.
    It is generally well tolerated. What is it?

8.  Venous insufficiency is a big problem for many                       Grape seed extract
    people with *varicose veins*. Wouldn't it be a pearl if a natural
    substance might help, especially if it seemed very safe for
    most? This herb is also rich as a scavenger of free radicals. It
    might even improve night vision. What is it?

9.  Free—Give yourself four points.

10. *Hepatitis* is a horrible disease. It is often                       Milk thistle
    chronic and can be deadly. Until recent years there was little
    we could do medically. Now there is more hope with drugs
    such as interferon. There also exists an herb that might help
    nourish the liver. It might even decrease insulin resistance in
    some. It is usually well tolerated in most. It is a pearl for
    some. What is it?

11. The words *Alzheimer's dementia* strike fear in the                  Reminyl
    hearts of the elderly. In recent years, from daffodils came a
    wonderful drug for Alzheimer's dementia and possibly other
    forms of dementia. What is the drug? It has proved to be a
    real pearl.

12. Repeated *urinary tract infections* are a hassle for                 Cranberry juice
    many elderly females. Of course, there are great medical
    treatments today. In addition, people benefit by a wonderful
    natural herb from a berry. It might help in the prevention of
    UTI for some, and it is usually well tolerated. What is this
    pearl?

13. This has been one of the pearl finds of the                         Coffee
    last several centuries, although some would debate its being a

pearl. It is true it can have side effects in some: insomnia, anxiety, gastric irritation, rapid heartbeat, headache, arrhythmias, fibrocystic disease in women possibly, increased osteoporosis possibly, habituation, and many drug interactions. However, many would agree that it is a pearl, and most people probably do not have major side effects. Benefits include *increased mental alertness,* pain relief, and possible delay in Parkinson's disease in some. It is America's beverage to help people awaken in the morning. It is a social custom. Most would say it is a real pearl, the pearl of the last several centuries. What is it?

14. *PMS* has plagued women since the beginning of time. We now know it is usually physiological and not psychological. One herb has become the number one over-the-counter help for PMS. Multiple small studies have demonstrated possible benefits for PMS, but significant research for significant effectiveness is lacking. It is usually well tolerated. Overall, many women consider it a pearl. What is it?

Evening primrose oil

15. This natural substance probably does not improve sleep for most people (except it might very well help in circadian rhythm sleep disturbance). It probably does not help in depression. However, it still might be a pearl because of other possible benefits in some: in tardive dyskinesia, thrombocytopemia, some forms of tumor regression when added to conventional chemotherapy, and benzodiazepine withdrawl. It can cause daytime drowsiness, depression, and headaches in some. It is currently under investigation by the FDA for various complications, so I would not list it as an absolute pearl yet.

Melatonin

16. *BPH* (benign prostatic hyperplasia) is a problem for many men as they grow older. There are excellent drugs for this today. However, there is an herb that many men have turned to for help. It is usually safe and well tolerated. What is it?

Saw palmetto

17. *Diabetics* often worry about developing retinopathy of the eyes. There is an herb that might improve retinal lesions from diabetic or hypertensive retinopathy. It might even help circulatory problems. It is usually safe and well tolerated. What is it?

Bilberry

18. *Diabetes mellitus* afflicts millions of Americans. Various natural products have been touted to decrease blood sugar (gymnema, fenugreek, etc.). However, there is one that is usually very safe, very nutritious, might even lower cholesterol, and probably does lower blood sugar after a meal in some, even though it is a complex carbohydrate. What is this pearl?

Oat bran

19.   *Osteoarthritis* is a common problem as people grow                    Glucosamine
      older. In recent years a natural product has been used by
      many to help in osteoarthritis. It is often used in combination
      with another natural product, chondroitin. It has also been
      used in TMJ.

      I debated whether to include this as a pearl because of its
      possible side effects (elevated blood glucose, drowsiness,
      headaches, mild gastrointestinal problems, etc.). Nevertheless,
      many would claim it is truly a pearl. What is it?

20.   Of all the minerals there is one I would pick as a                     Zinc
      pearl. It is not vanadyl, which has been used in diabetes and
      has been associated with some deaths. It is not selenium,
      which might reduce total cancer mortality but can also cause
      a toxicity similar to that of arsenic. It is not even magnesium,
      which might help in preventing migraines, increasing bone
      density in osteoporosis, and helping to prevent hearing loss in
      individuals exposed to loud noise.

      This mineral might help in the common cold, improve
      depressive symptoms, increase weight gain in anorexia ner-
      vosa, and help prevent peptic ulcers. Topically, one form of it,
      calamine lotion, helps with *poison ivy*. Topically, it might
      decrease acne. It is used in mouthwashes to decrease plaque
      formation. It is used topically for herpes simplex infections.
      High doses do carry risks (ex: sideroblastic anemia, possible
      increased BPH, copper deficiencies, kidney damage, flu-like
      symptoms, and impaired immune function). Nevertheless,
      overall this mineral has been a pearl for some. What is it?

21.   There is an herbal product that is a would-be                          Stevia
      pearl. It would be a pearl (lowers blood sugar, lowers blood
      pressure, bacterialicidal against E. coli, one hundred times
      sweeter than sugar) if it were not for significant safety con-
      cerns (mutagenic in vitro, reduced sperm production and
      testisweight in rats). What is this product that is one hundred
      times sweeter than sugar with no calories? We have not done
      well in sweeteners: sugar contributes to obesity, a major
      killer; saccharin is a known carcinogen; and aspartame might
      cause agitation in some.

22.   This is a natural product that is a potential pearl.                   Deer velvet
      It is only a potential pearl because there is insufficient
      research at this time. It contains fifty amino acids, chon-
      droitin, vitamin A, the sex hormones estrone and estradiol
      that stimulate sexual function in females, growth hormone,
      and gargliosides and sphingomyelins, which are involved in cell
      metabolism and growth. It seems to speed wound healing,
      reduce fatigue, increase muscular strength, and improve

health. In short, it seems to have some *antiaging effects*. Few adverse reactions have been reported so far. Let's hope some of the above prove true. Then it might be a pearl. What is it?

23.    What is the all-time number one topical                    Aloe vera gel
       product used for various *skin conditions*? It is certainly a pearl.

24.    Name a possible pearl used for *anxiety*.                   GABA
       Pearls in natural products for anxiety and depression are
       indeed rare. There is one that is a main inhibitory neuro-
       transmitter in the entire brain. Anecdotal reports claiming
       that it does calm anxiety and gives a sense of well-being
       seem impressive. Thus far, adverse reactions that have been
       reported seem few. However, significant research is lacking, so
       it is only a possible pearl. Name it.

25.    Free—Give yourself four points.

## Grade—Chapter 8

Number correct _____ + bonus points _____ multiplied by 4 = _____ Score

*Chapter 9*

# Questions and Answers about Specific Diseases and Herbs Used to Treat Them

T he following questions relate to specific diseases. You may want to cover the right side of the page as you answer each of the questions to see how much you really know. Give yourself one point for each correct answer.

| QUESTION | ANSWER |
|---|---|
| 1. Various vitamins and minerals have been touted to help in *acne*. Name some of these vitamins and minerals. | Vitamin C, Vitamin A, and Zinc |
| 2. _____ pansy helps topically with *acne*. | Wild |
| 3. Many herbs have unsuccessfully been tried for *ADHD*. Which one is not often touted?<br>A. Omega-3 fatty acids<br>B. SAMe<br>C. Feingold diet<br>D. Coffee<br>E. Kola nut<br>F. Gingko<br>G. Valerian<br>H. Ephedra<br>I. Guarana<br>J. Green tea<br>K. Red dye<br>L. Beta carotene | K. Red dye is not often touted. In fact, a few years ago the Feingold diet recommended the intake of no red dye. Incidentally, restricting red dye never proved helpful for most children with ADHD. Furthermore no natural product has been found to significantly help people with ADHD. |
| 4. Many herbs and natural products are touted for *allergies*. Which one of the following is not? | E. Pollen aggravates allergies. |

A. Garlic
B. Gingko
C. Stinging nettle
D. Horseradish
E. Pollen
F. Vitamin C
G. Anise
H. Ginger
I. Peppermint

5.  Many herbs or supplements have been tried for either cognitive enhancement in normal people or dementia in the elderly. Only one has been developed into a scientifically proven substance that does help in *Alzheimer's disease*. Name it.
    A. Gingko biloba
    B. Vitamin E
    C. L-carnitine
    D. Choline
    E. Lecithin
    F. "Smart drugs" (Piracetam, Aniracetam, Praminacetam)
    G. Phosphatidylserine
    H. Galantamine
    I. Ginseng
    J. SAMe
    K. DHEA
    L. Melatonin
    M. Hyperzia serata
    N. Omega-3 fatty acids
    O. Vitamin C
    P. Coenzyme Q10
    Q. Vitamin B complex

H. Galantamine is marketed as the prescription drug Reminyl, which is for Alzheimer's dementia.

6.  Several natural products have been touted to help in *anemia* at times. Which one of the following is not usually touted?
    A. Vitamin C
    B. Iron in small amounts
    C. Yellow dock
    D. Seaweed
    E. Burdock
    F. Mint
    G. Linden
    H. Any product that causes chronic bleeding

H is false. The most common cause of anemia is excessive blood loss.

7.  Herbs touted for *angina* include all of the following except which one?
    A. Willow bark
    B. Garlic
    C. Ginger

H. Ergot could have a constricting effect on blood vessels and, thus, would not be good for angina. Most in the list are blood thinners and might, in

D. Bilberry
E. Hawthorn
F. Angelica
G. Evening primrose oil
H. Moldy rye (ergot)
I. Khella
J. Kudzu
K. Cereus

some cases, allow blood to flow through constricted heart vessels more easily and with less pain (angina). Aspirin, which has been used so much in angina, is from willow bark.

8.  Several herbs have been touted for *anxiety*.
    Which of the following is not touted to calm anxiety?
    A. Kava
    B. Valerian
    C. Magnesium
    D. Passionflower
    E. Lemon balm
    F. Chamomile
    G. Green tea
    H. GABA
    I. Calcium
    J. B complex
    K. Thiamin

G. Green tea is high in caffeine, which can produce anxiety.

9.  *Arrhythmias* are irregular rhythms of the heart.
    Certainly a doctor should be consulted for arrhythmias of the heart. Though not usually adequate, various natural products have been touted through the centuries. Which one of those listed below is not often touted?
    A. Magnesium and potassium
    B. Hawthorn
    C. Coenzyme Q10
    D. Ephedra
    E. Cactus grandiflorus
    F. The amino acids of taurine and carnitine

D. Ephedra is known for producing heart palpitations.

10. Folklore touts which of the following for *arthritis*?
    A. Stinging nettle
    B. Red pepper—topically
    C. Pineapple with bromelaine
    D. Ginger
    E. SAMe
    F. Glucosamine-chondroitin
    G. Boswellia to reduce inflammation
    H. Sea cucumber to reduce pain
    I. CLA
    J. MSM
    K. All of the above

K. All of the above

11. Many athletes have tried various herbs and

C. GHB

supplements for *athletic enhancement.* Which one of the following was originally sold as a nutritional supplement but then banned in 1990 after reports of addiction?
A. Aldrostenedione
B. Creatine
C. GHB
D. ATP
E. Vitamins

12. *Athlete's foot* is caused by a fungus, tinea pedis. Name a natural product that is reputed by some to help when used topically.

Tea tree oil

13. _____ used topically seems to help your *athlete's foot* problem, which is totally out of control.

Lavender

14. *Bad breath* has been curtailed with all of the following herbs except which one?
A. Spearmint and peppermint
B. Cinnamon
C. Garlic
D. Fennel
E. Basil
F. Lavender
G. Cardamom
H. Ginger
I. Nutmeg
J. Turmeric
K. Hyssop
L. Eucalyptus

C. All of these herbs have been used for bad breath. They all have a good fragrance except garlic, which is notorious for bad odor. Several of the others are common ingredients in food preparation, soaps, cosmetics, and commercial breath mints.

15. Natural products have been tried in *benign prostatic hypertrophy* (BPH). All of the following have been suggested except which one?
A. Saw palmetto
B. Pygeum
C. Stinging nettle
D. Flaxseed oil
E. Zinc
F. All of the above

F. All of those listed have been touted. BPH is a risk factor for prostate cancer. A simple blood test, PSA, that a local doctor can do, can help to rule this out.

16. Which of the following herbs has been touted to help with *bipolar disorder,* while it also might make it worse by precipitating manic episodes in some individuals?
A. Omega-3 fatty acids
B. Flaxseed
C. Fish oil
D. All of the above
E. None of the above

D. Omega-3 fatty acids, flaxseed, and fish oil may all cause manic episodes.

17.  Topically several herbs have been used for *body odor.* Which one is not on the usual list?
     A.  Vinegar
     B.  Baking soda
     C.  Turnip juice
     D.  Zinc

D. While zinc has been used orally by some in an attempt to decrease body odor, it is not used topically for that purpose.

18.  Several herbs have been touted to promote *breast enlargement.* Which one of the following is not on the list?
     A.  Fenugreek
     B.  Fennel
     C.  Ephedra
     D.  Wild yams
     E.  Cumin

C is not usually on the list. Most of the others have estrogen-like activity and have been touted to promote breast enlargement.

19.  *Bronchitis* with its irritating cough has supposedly been helped in some by all of the following except which one?
     A.  ACE inhibitors
     B.  Echinacea
     C.  Astragalus
     D.  NAC (N-acetylsteine) that reportedly thins mucus secretions
     E.  Horehound tea that reportedly thins mucus
     F.  Slippery elm with soothing qualities
     G.  Marshmallow

A. ACE inhibitors are prescription medications for high blood pressure that induce a cough in 40 percent of some populations.

20.  Assume you are lost on an island that has many fruits and plants. Although you are in good health you seem to be bruising. You find a book on herbs, and it touts all of the following for *bruises* except which one?
     A.  Raw potato—topically
     B.  Pineapple
     C.  Grapes
     D.  Bilberry
     E.  Ginger

E. Ginger is not on the list. It would, if anything, tend to increase bleeding and could theoretically cause a person to bruise more easily.

21.  Natural products have been used over the years for *burns.* All of the following have been touted except which one?
     A.  Cool water
     B.  Topical aloe vera gel
     C.  Topical chamomile tea
     D.  Topical lavender
     E.  Topical calendula
     F.  Repeated cayenne topically
     G.  Goldenseal cream
     H.  Echinacea

F. Repeated cayenne use has been implicated in possible skin cancer.

I.  Gotu kola
J.  Vitamins C and E
K.  Zinc

22. Several herbs and diets have been touted for *cancer* or cancer prevention. Which of the following seems to hold the most promise?
    A.  Red clover
    B.  Pineapples
    C.  Carrots
    D.  Cucumber
    E.  High-fiber, low-fat diet
    F.  Celery
    G.  Nuts
    H.  Onions
    I.  Tomatoes
    J.  Olives
    K.  Lemons
    L.  DHEA
    M.  Grape seeds
    N.  Antioxidants such as vitamin E and the mineral selenium
    O.  Green tea
    P.  Soy that has genistein

E. A high-fiber, low-fat diet holds the most promise. However, several of the ones listed seem fairly innocuous for most people. Other natural products less often included in the list are MSO, maitake, shark cartilage, and melatonin.

23. *Canker sores* can be a problem when eating, talking, and kissing. All of the following have been touted to help except which one?
    A.  Acidic, spicy, and salty foods
    B.  Vitamin C and B complex
    C.  The amino acid lysine
    D.  Echinacea
    E.  Topical goldenseal
    F.  Topical licorice
    G.  Topical lemon balm tea
    H.  Selenium

A. Acidic, spicy, and salty foods may be one factor in precipitating canker sores.

24. Several natural products and actions have been touted for help in *carpal tunnel syndrome*. Which one of the following is usually not touted?
    A.  Vitamin B$_6$
    B.  Bromelain
    C.  Turmeric
    D.  Prolonged, repeated movements of the injured hand and fingers

D. Carpal tunnel syndrome is often a stress injury that can be caused by prolonged, repeated physical stress.

25. Which of the following is not usually touted for *cataract* prevention?
    A.  Vitamins C and E
    B.  Bilberry

D. Prolonged UV light may be a factor in the causation of cataracts.

C. Rosemary
D. A good healthy dose of sun
E. Carrot
F. Selenium

26. Natural products have been used to decrease *cholesterol* and triglycerides. Several are reputed to have such effects. Which one in the list below is usually not included?
   A. CLA
   B. Fish oil
   C. Red yeast rice
   D. Guggulipid
   E. Niacin
   F. Vitamins C and E
   G. New York sirloin
   H. Garlic

G. New York sirloin increases cholesterol. The others have been tried by many in attempting to decrease cholesterol.

27. For *chronic fatigue* several herbs have been touted, but sometimes side effects have developed. Which of the ones below do not match up?
   A. Ginseng—hypertension
   B. Ginger—bleeding
   C. Caffeine—anxiety
   D. SAMe—formaldehyde in blood
   E. Spinach—seizures
   F. Goldenseal—respiratory failure
   G. Lemon Balm—thyroid medication interference
   H. Echinacea—reproductive problems
   I. Licorice—kidney damage

E. Spinach is high in vitamins. It is usually very safe and is not known for causing seizures.

28. The most common two natural products in *commercial preparations* are _____ and

_____

Aloe and Vitamin E

29. A search continues for a cure for *the common cold*. This search by individuals over the years has included all but which of the following?
   A. Echinacea
   B. Zinc
   C. Goldenseal
   D. Rhinovirus
   E. Boneset
   F. Catnip
   G. Elderberry
   H. Eucalyptus
   I. Vitamin C

D. Rhinovirus is one of the viruses that causes the common cold. It is a cause, not a cure.

30. *Conjunctivitis* is an inflammation of the eye. Natural products touted to help at times include all of the following except which one?

B. Smoke is an irritant and as such may be a factor in the causation of some conjunctivi-

A. Vitamins A and C
B. Smoke
C. Fresh eyebright

tis. Other causes include
bacteria and viruses, and thus, a
medical doctor is needed.

31. Many commercial products used for *constipation*
contain an herb or supplement. Which one of
these is not usually on the list?
A. Rhubarb
B. Prunes
C. Psyllium
D. Fiber
E. Tea
F. Ground flaxseed
G. Anthroquinone herbs (senna, cascara,
blackthorn, aloe, fragula)
H. Fenugreek
I. Castor oil
J. Magnesium
K. Ground fenugreek

E. Tea has been touted for
diarrhea but not for
constipation.

32. Many herbs and other products have been tried
topically for *dandruff* (calendine, comfrey, burdock,
ginger, sage, rosemary, vinegar). They are usually
safe, but name a problem that does arise at times
when they are used.

Allergic skin reactions or
contact dermatitis

33. Twenty million people in America are medically
*depressed*. The majority do not avail themselves
of psychiatric medication. The search in the herb
and supplement world is strong. Unfortunately, side
effects are possible. Which of the following does
not match up?
A. Saint-John's-wort—interactions with other drugs
B. L-tryptophane—eosinophilia
C. SAMe—formaldehyde in the blood
D. DHEA—prostate cancer
E. Selenium—low platelet count (thromboeytupenice)
F. Ginseng—bleeding issues
G. Folic Acid + $B_6$—neural tube defects
H. Choline—fish smell
I. L-Carnitine—confusion
J. Chromium—cancer
K. Omega-3 fatty acids—mania

G does not match. Folic acid is
used in pregnant females to
prevent neural tube defects. It
does not cause them. Folic acid
plus $B_6$ has resulted in added
antidepressant effects when
added to Prozac in females.

34. Several herbs and supplements have been touted
for *diabetes mellitus*. Which one is not usually
on the list?
A. Fenugreek
B. Gymnema
C. Chromium

G. Bee pollen is made by bees
just as honey is, and it too will
raise blood sugar rather than
lower it.

D.  Grape seed extract
E.  Ginseng
F.  Bitter melon
G.  Bee pollen
H.  Alpha-lipoic acid
I.  Garlic
J.  Coenzyme Q10
K.  Oats
L.  Cinnamon
M.  Billberry

35.  You have some *diabetic neuropathy* with pain and locate _____ for it.

Evening primrose oil

36.  *Diarrhea* can have a significant medical cause, but sometimes it does not. Various herbs have been tried for diarrhea. Which one of the following has not?
A.  Berries—bilberry, blackberry, raspberry, blueberry
B.  Carrots
C.  Rhubarb pie, senna, and cascara
D.  Oats
E.  Acidophilus for diarrhea related to antibiotic use

C. Rhubarb pie, senna, and cascara are used for constipation, not diarrhea.

37.  *Diverticulitis* has been supposedly helped in some by all of the following except which one?
A.  Psyllium
B.  Peppermint
C.  Ground flaxseeds
D.  All of the above have been reputed to help

D. All of the above have been reputed to help.

38.  *Eczema* has been touted to be helped by all of the following except which one?
A.  Flaxseed oil
B.  Zinc, short term
C.  Animal fur

C. Animal fur may trigger the red, scaly skin of eczema in some.

39.  _____ and gotu kola help topically with *eczema*.

Avocado

40.  For *female sexual dysfunction* and female sexual enhancement, several herbs and supplements have been touted. Which of the following has not been touted?
A.  Viacreme
B.  Rose root
C.  Deer velvet
D.  L-arginine
E.  Yohimbe
F.  L-tryptophane

F. L-tryptophane is a precursor of serotonin, and increased serotonin in the frontal cortex and spinal cord could theoretically decrease sex drive and function.

41.  Which herbs have been tried over the years

F. All of these herbs have been

for *fever?*
A. Willow Bark
B. Meadowsweet
C. Red Pepper
D. Cinnamon and peppermint
E. Ginger
F. All have been tried
G. None of the above have been tried

tried over the years for fever.

42. *Fibromyalgia* is an interesting disease characterized
by aches and pain and fatigue. The following herbs
have been tried. Fill in the blank on B.
A. SAMe
B. Coenzyme _____
C. Magnesium plus malic acid
D. Vitamin E
E. Lecithin
F. Black walnut and boswellia
G. Astragalus

Q10

43. Many herbs have been sought for a *fountain of
youth* experience. All of the following herbs
except one are touted for antiaging. Name it.
A. Amino acids
B. DHEA
C. Coenzyme Q10
D. Omega-3 fatty acids
E. L-phenylalanine
F. Human growth hormone
G. Tobacco

G. Although no fountain of
youth has been found, tobacco
is the herb known to accelerate
aging.

44. Natural products have been touted to sometimes
help in *gallstones*. Ones often listed include all
of the following except which one?
A. Flaxseed oil
B. Milk thistle
C. Inositol
D. Fatty food
E. Choline
F. Methionine

D. Fatty food is certainly not
needed in gallstones.

45. Herbs tried for *gas* relief include all of the following
except one. Pick the one not suggested.
A. Ginger
B. Cinnamon, peppermint, and cornmint
C. Nutmeg
D. Basil
E. Fava beans
F. Lemon
G. Fennel, sage, and cloves

E. Fava beans. Some feel that
cooking fava beans, which are
known for producing gas pain,
with wormwood, wormseed,
and carrots will decrease the
problem.

    H.  Thyme and savory
    I.  Allspice
    J.  Rosemary
    K.  Oregano
    L.  Bergamot
    M.  Lavender
    N.  Onion
    O.  Marjoram
    P.  Tarragon
    Q.  Chamomile

46.   Which of the following herbs have been tried for *gout*?       O. All of the above
    A.  Cherry
    B.  Celery
    C.  Chiso
    D.  Avocado
    E.  Procumbers
    F.  Oats
    G.  Olives
    H.  Bromelain
    I.  Licorice
    J.  Turmeric
    K.  Avocado
    L.  Cat's claw
    M.  Willow
    N.  Nettle
    O.  All of the above
    P.  All of the above except A and B
    Q.  None of the above
    R.  All of the above except D

47.   Herbal remedies for *hair loss* have not faired too well.    B. Selenium
    In fact, one of the supplements below can end up
    causing hair loss in mega doses. Which one is it?
    A.  Saw palmetto
    B.  Selenium
    C.  Silicon
    D.  Rosemary
    E.  Sage
    F.  Horsetail
    G.  Sesame
    H.  Stinging nettle

48.   Several herbs have been touted for *headaches*.    A and B. Feverfew has been
    Which two of those listed below have been    tried the most for migraines.
    tried the most?    Since the original ingredient
    A.  Feverfew    came from willow, and since
    B.  Willow bark    aspirin is the number one drug
    C.  Evening primrose oil    of all time (over forty billion
    D.  Garlic    sold per year), indirectly, willow

E.  Ginger
F.  Gingko
G.  Red pepper
H.  Lemon balm
I.  Magnesium
J.  Peppermint

49.  Herbs touted for *heartburn* include the following.
     Which one generally has acute, dangerous side
     effects in some people?
     A.  Licorice
     B.  Angelica
     C.  Chamomile

is number one.

A. Licorice is probably the most
likely to be dangerous at times,
causing hypertension, nausea,
vomiting, and dangerous drug
interactions. However, all herb
use should be monitored. Chamomile
can cause spontaneous abortions in
pregnant females. It can also cause
bleeding and increase the effects of alcohol. Even angelica can have estrogen-like
effects, which might be good or bad, and
it can cause a rash if the user spends
time In the sun.

50.  Different medications have been tried for different
     aspects of *heart disease*. Which of the following
     are true?
     A.  Coenzyme Q10—CHF—modest help at best.
     B.  Hawthorn—CHF—interferes with other heart
         medicine. Research looks promisingly possible.
     C.  Garlic—high cholesterol—mild effect at best.
     D.  Soy—high cholesterol—diets that are low in
         saturated fats and include 75 grams of soy
         protein may reduce the risk of heart disease.
     E.  Cholestine—high cholesterol—This is a statin
         similar to several prescription medications. It
         is dangerous to treat the number-one killer
         without a doctor.
     F.  Guggal gum—high cholesterol—The preliminary
         data is promising. More data is needed.
     G.  All of the above are true.
     H.  None of the above are true.

G. All are true statements.

51.  Natural products have been used for *hemorrhoids*.
     All of the following have been tried except
     which one?
     A.  Psyllium seed
     B.  Flaxseed
     C.  Topical Saint-John's-wort
     D.  Comfrey paste
     E.  Goldenseal topically
     F.  Mullein topically
     G.  Tannins topically

J. Constipation is often a factor
in hemorrhoids.

H.  Menthol topically
I.  Camphor topically
J.  Constipating foods

52.  Interferon is now often helpful in *hepatitis C.*
     However, in the past, little was available. Herbs
     were tried. Which one of the following was tried
     the most?
     A.  SAMe
     B.  Milk thistle
     C.  Shusaikotu
     D.  Dandelion
     E.  Goldenseal
     F.  Colostrum

B. Milk thistle has probably been
used the most. It can have these
side effects: nausea, vomiting,
diarrhea, menstrual changes.

53.  Of all the herb and supplement suggestions, few
     seem to help with *high blood pressure.* One of the
     suggestions below has been given most often to
     encourage the decreasing of blood pressure. Name it.
     A.  More garlic
     B.  More celery
     C.  Less sodium
     D.  Hawthorn
     E.  Onion, broccoli, and carrot soup
     F.  Kudzu
     G.  Saffron

C. Less sodium chloride, or less
table salt, might help to
decrease blood pressure.

54.  Assume you are itching and have *hives.* If you can
     avoid an unlikely allergic reaction, you might try
     topical applications of _____, ginger, stinging nettle,
     chamomile, oregano, clove, caraway, lemon balm, and
     peppermint.

Jewelweed

55.  Natural products have been touted to help at
     times in *impotence.* All of the following have
     been tried except which one?
     A.  Gingko biloba
     B.  Flaxseed oil
     C.  Vitamin C
     D.  Testosterone derivatives
     E.  Beta blockers

E. Beta blockers are prescription medications that decrease
sympathetic response and cause
impotence in some.

56.  Fill in the blank in this paragraph about
     *insomnia* herbs:
     You are stressed from flying all night to a land far, far away.
     You can't sleep. A friend is with you, and she is big into herbs.
     She offers you several different herbs. You do not want her
     kava, because you heard of some cases of liver failure. You
     don't want her valerian because you heard it might be addict-
     ing. You don't want hops because it might decrease your sex
     drive. Your cat is with you, so you don't want catnip. You can't

Melatonin

wait several weeks for oat straw to work. You are allergic to the daisy family and can't take chamomile. You are on thyrotropin and can't take California poppy. Your wife is pregnant, and you don't want her to accidentally get lemon balm, passionflower, or skullcap. You tried wild lettuce, but your insomnia got worse. Thus, you try a low dose of _____ for a few nights to help with your circadian rhythm sleep disturbance.

57. You have been in Mexico for a couple days now on vacation. Your *irritable bowel syndrome* is much worse. From which of these herb categories might you consider picking an herb?
    A. Peppermint, ginger, cinnamon, valerian, colostrum, onion
    B. Castor oil, blackthorn, cascara
    C. Prunes

A. Peppermint, ginger, cinnamon, valerian, colostrum, onion

58. Natural products have been touted to help some with systemic *lupus* erythematosis (SLE) with its wide array of symptoms on various organs. All but one of the items below are often listed. Which one is usually not listed?
    A. Flaxseed oil
    B. Zinc
    C. Vitamins C, E, B complex
    D. Sunlight

D. Sunlight may trigger an attack in some.

59. You go back in time to different places in the world. You are female, you are beginning to go through *menopause,* and you need help. Only herbs are available. Which of the following has information that does not match?
    A. America—deep South, 1900s—soybeans
    B. America—Ohio River area, 1900s—black cohosh
    C. Europe—Dark Ages—red clover
    D. China—ancient times—licorice
    E. The Mediterranean—1800s—chasteberry
    F. England—1800s—hops
    G. Mars—vitex

G. Mars—vitex

60. Natural products have been touted for *migraines.* Which one is not often listed to help in migraines?
    A. Feverfew
    B. Melatonin
    C. MSG

C. MSG (monosodium glutamate) in oriental food is known for triggering migraines in some people.

61. If a person taking modern medicine for *multiple sclerosis* (MS) wanted to add herbs for nourishment and knew the possible side effects of the herbs, he might choose which of the following?
    A. Pineapple

F. All of the above

B.  Blueberry
C.  Stinging nettle
D.  Black currant
E.  Evening primrose oil
F.  All of the above
G.  None of the above

62.  Name a natural product that has been used in *muscle strain.*

Rosemary oil compresses

63.  You have been eating too fast and feel *nauseated.* You already take daily aspirin for your heart, and your heart rate is rapid. You are almost hyperventilating because you are so nervous. You have heard that ginger, peppermint, and cinnamon have all been used for nausea. Of these three, which one would you choose?

You would probably choose peppermint. Ginger thins the blood, as does aspirin. The risk of bleeding might be too great. Cinnamon can cause a rapid pulse and respirations, and your heart rate is already high.

64.  *Obesity* is a major problem in America, with perhaps one in three to one in four Americans being obese. Naturally, many people turn to herbs and supplements for help. This area of herbs and supplements seems especially dangerous at times. Which does not match up as a possible side effect?
A.  Ephedra—CVA, MI, arrhythmias, seizures, psychosis, and death are possible.
B.  L-carnitine—The Racemix mixture is toxic.
C.  Selenium—Chronic toxicity can resemble arsenic poisoning.
D.  Gaurana—Anxiety is possible.
E.  All of the above.

E. All of the above

65.  What B vitamin has been touted for *OCD?*

Inositol

66.  Fill in the blank:
SAMe, bromelain, MSM, and CLA have been touted for *osteoarthritis.* However, _____ is probably the most popular herb combination touted for osteoarthritis.

Glucosamine-chondroitin

67.  You are growing older and have *osteoarthritis.* You are on Actonel, a modern medication for osteoporosis, but you also want to be wise in how you eat. You are in a cafeteria, and before you are beans, black pepper, cabbage, dandelion, avocado, pigweed, horsetail, and parsley. You are a bit of a hypochondriac. Which might you choose, given that you have heard all of these have been touted for nourishment in MS?

Beans, cabbage, and black pepper are usually benign in side effects, so you would probably choose them. You would not choose dandelion since it could interact with several medications you are on at the time. You would not choose horsetail because it has nicotine, and you are already nervous. Plus, you don't like the name. It also interacts with many medications. You might choose a little avocado and just a tad of parsley for bad breath. Finally, the idea of pig-weed is just too much. Oh yes, you might be looking for stinging nettle as you pass through the line.

68.  *Osteoporosis* is characterized by a decrease in bone mass. When this occurs in the vertebral column, pain can occur. All of the following natural products have been touted for use in osteoporosis except which one?
    A.  Cannabis sativa
    B.  Calcium, magnesium, and vitamin C
    C.  Bromelain
    D.  Glucosamine
    E.  Flaxseed oil

A. Cannabis sativa is marijuana and is not touted for osteo-porosis. In fact, its dangers are often insidious but significant.

69.  _____ and _____ taken orally seem to help your general aches and *pains,* as does _____, with its menthol effects.

Willow bark and ginger; peppermint

70.  Your wife is named Rosemary, and she is partial to _____ for her *pain.*

Rosemary

71.  Chewing a few _____ seeds seems to help. The *pain* lessens a little, perhaps because of the phenylalanine effects.

Sunflower

72.  Fill in the blank:
*Parkinsonism* is a difficult disease. It is relatively common. It is characterized by rigidity, tremors, slow movements, postural instability, a lack of facial expression, and a shuffling gait. However, the degree varies tremendously, and various combinations of symptoms may or may not be present. It is due to a dopamine depletion in the nigrostriatal area of the brain. It can be caused by recreational use of MPTP. It can come on postencephalitic. Toxins (_____, dust, carbon disulfide) can cause it. The old neuroleptic medications frequently caused it in the past.

Manganese

Treatment today is directed at addressing an imbalance of neurotransmitters in the brain. For example, anticholinergic drugs block the effects of acetylcholine, and Levadopa, a precursor of dopamine, augments dopamine in the brain.
_____ is a vitamin that has been touted for nutritional help in Parkinsonism. Foods that are encouraged by some for those with Parkinsonism include _____ beans

Vitamin E

Fava

and _____ beans. Herbs that are
touted include _____ _____ oil
and _____ flower. Other natural products
that have been touted for Parkinsonism include
vitamins $B_6$, C, E; flaxseed oil; gingko biloba;
phosphatidylserine; coenzyme Q10; and NADH.

Velvet
Evening primrose
Passion

73. Several herbs have been touted for *PMS*, such as
dong quai, vitex, and Saint-John's-wort. Several
minerals have been touted, such as magnesium
and calcium. An amino acid, L-tryptophane, has been
touted. But number one in sales by far is _____
except in Europe, where _____ is number one.

Evening primrose oil
Chasteberry

74. I was once on a mountain vacation when I
developed a rash from *poison ivy*. My wife suggested an
herb. I said, "But I am a medical doctor; I will try a topical
corticosteroid." And I did, but the rash grew worse. Then I
said to myself, "Well I will try a topical antibiotic ointment.
Maybe it had become infected." The rash almost seemed to
eat this ointment and spit it out. I then tried benadryl
cream but to no avail. The rash intensified. My wife said,
"Why don't you just try _____ lotion?" I went into a
small country store and humbly asked if they had any of the
lotion. The attendant said, "Sure." I applied it that night, and
my rash began to disappear.

Calamine

75. _____ seems to help *rheumatoid arthritis* a little.

Turmeric

76. *Schizophrenia* is a serious mental disorder often
characterized by hallucinations and delusions. _____ natural product has been proven to be of significant benefit.
Ones that have been touted include evening primrose, fo-ti,
gotu-kola, omega-3 fatty acids, and glycine.

No

77. Many herbs have been tried for *sexual enhancement*,
but side effects have been a problem for many of the
herbs tried. Which of the following does not match?
A. Yohimbe—high blood pressure and hallucinations
B. Ginseng—mania, headaches, estrogen-like effects
C. Gingko—bleeding
D. MACA—possible increased cancer risk
E. Fava beans—priapism in extremely large doses
F. Cardamom, cinnamon, anise, velvet bean, muira,
puama, wolfberry, ashwaganda, guarana,
countrymallow, saw palmetto—no side effects

F is the wrong match. Almost
any herb can have side effects.
(See the individual herb
section.)

78. Natural products have been touted for *sinusitis*.
All of the following except one are often touted.
Which one is usually not listed?
A. Ragweed

A. Ragweed may trigger
sinusitis.

B. Echinacea
C. Astragulus
D. Cat's claw
E. Maitake mushrooms
F. Vitamin C

79. Other herbs used topically for *skin irritations*
include all of the following except which one?
A. Walnut
B. Purslane
C. Calendula
D. Poison oak
E. Cucumber
F. Hamamelis
G. Carrot
H. Ivy
I. English plantation
J. Marshmallow
K. Camphor
L. Menthol

D. Poison oak

80. Vitamin E and _____ _____ oil have been taken
orally to improve *skin quality.*

Evening primrose

81. Several herbs have been tried topically through
the years for *sunburn* (e.g., calendula, cucumber,
tea, plantain, eggplant), but which one has been
tried the most?

Aloe vera

82. Natural products have been touted for *tinnitus.*
Name two.

Inositol
Zinc, short-term

83. Name the number one herb tried topically
for *toothaches.*

Clove

84. A *toothache* is terrible, so you find some _____
to soothe it locally.

Clove

85. Natural products have been touted to help some
with *ulcers.* Although these are certainly inadequate
for an ulcer, some commonly listed are all of the
following except which one?
A. Glutamine, an amino acid
B. Marshmallow
C. Cabbage juice
D. Alcohol, coffee, caffeinated soda, acid fruit juice,
nonsteroid anti-inflammatory drugs

D. These are the substances to
avoid in ulcers.

86. Name the number-one herb tried over the years
for *urinary tract infections?*

Cranberry juice

87.  Many herbs have been tried for *varicose veins* (e.g.,                     Horse chestnut
     violet, witch hazel, butcher's broom, lemon, onion,
     bilberry, gingko, and gotu kola), but which one does
     the famous Commission E in Germany endorse? It
     should be pointed out that the FDA in America
     does not endorse this herb for varicose veins.

88.  Several herbs have been touted to help when                     Willow, with its salicylic acid
     topically applied for *warts* (e.g., dandelion,
     pineapple, soybean, basil, castor, celandine, fig,
     milkweed, yellow cedar), but which one has been
     tried the most over the years in an attempt to
     remove warts?

89.  Many topical herbal applications are touted                     Horse chestnut
     to decrease *wrinkles* (e.g., carrot, witch hazel,
     cocoa, cucumber, purslane, rosemary, sage, almond,
     aloe, avocado, castor oil, grape, olive oil, and
     pineapple). If you were in Japan, which herb
     might be number one?

90.  _____ helps topically with *wrinkles*.                       Pineapple

91.  _____ helps topically with *yeast infections*.               Chamomile

92.  100 Bonus Points

# Grade—Chapter 9

Number correct _____ + bonus points _____ = _____ Score

# Chapter 10

# Questions and Answers about Beverages and Natural Products

The following questions relate to beverages. You may want to cover the right side of the page as you answer each of the questions to see how much you really know. Give yourself three points for each correct answer.

| QUESTION | ANSWER |
|---|---|
| 1. What percent of Americans use caffeine? | 80 percent |
| 2. What is the average consumption of caffeine per day among the 80 percent of Americans who use caffeine? | 200 milligrams (mg) per day |
| 3. How much caffeine is in a cup of coffee? | 100 mg |
| 4. How much caffeine is in a cup of tea? | 50 mg |
| 5. How much caffeine is in a chocolate bar? | 25 mg |
| 6. How much caffeine does one have to consume to become intoxicated? | 200–500 mg |
| 7. What are the effects from caffeine that people like? | Caffeine to a mild degree may increase energy, increase alertness, and elevate mood. |
| 8. What are the symptoms of caffeine intoxication? | Symptoms of caffeine intoxication include anxiety, agitation, tremors, rapid heartbeat, elevated blood pressure, restlessness, insomnia, apprehension, and headaches. |
| 9. What are the symptoms of caffeine withdrawal? | Symptoms of caffeine withdrawal include anxiety, agitation, fatigue, depression, and |

poor concentration.

10    How long does it take for tolerance to develop to the consumption of 500 mg or more per day of caffeine?

2 weeks

11.   When an individual recurrently consumes caffeine to the point of intoxication and in spite of social or occupational complications, the individual suffers from what?

Caffeine abuse

12.   Name three diseases made worse by caffeine.

1.  Peptic ulcer disease
2.  Fibrocystic disease
3.  Gastroesophageal reflux disease

13.   Name four psychiatric and/or medical conditions that must be distinguished from caffeine abuse.

1.  Panic disorder
2.  Generalized anxiety disorder
3.  Hyperthyroidism
4.  Akathesia from neuroleptic medications

14.   Name a common breakfast drink that is cardioprotective or healthy for the heart.

Red grape juice

15.   Name a common breakfast drink that can interact with many of the 100 top-selling prescription drugs.

Grapefruit juice

16.   Does black tea or green tea have more caffeine?

Black tea

17.   This tea has recently become popular in America. It has been popular in China for many years. Although there is no significant research to back up its claim of helping in the case of cancer, this claim along with the stimulating effect from the caffeine present are reasons for its popularity.

Green tea

18.   This tea has been touted as a "blood purifier" but can cause hallucinations, hypertension, liver cancer, and death. Name it.

Sassafras tea

19.   Energy drinks often contain which three herbs?

1.  Caffeine
2.  Guarana
3.  Ginseng

20.   Weight-loss drinks often contain which stimulating herb that can be dangerous?

Ephedra

21.   Drinks that may reverse weight loss in some people often contain what kind of protein?

Whey protein

22.   What kind of milk has been touted for menopausal symptoms, high lipids, and osteoporosis prevention?

Soy milk

23.   High protein drinks often contain which natural products?

1.  Soy protein
2.  Amino acids

3.   Vitamins
4.   Minerals

24.   Drinks touted to be high in antioxidants often
      contain which natural products?

1.   Beta carotene
2.   Green tea
3.   Vitamins (A, C, and E)
4.   Minerals (selenium, zinc, calcium, iron)

25.   Drinks promoting the micronutrients of vitamins,
      minerals, proteins, fats, and carbohydrates often contain what
      algae?

Spirulina chlorella

26.   Name a plant made into a drink that mothers
      have long touted for eye health.

Carrot

27.   Name some fruits often touted for their
      nutritional benefits although they contain high
      fructose, a close cousin to glucose.

1.   Orange juice
2.   Apple juice
3.   Pineapple juice
4.   Grapefruit juice

28.   Name a fruit drink that has been used for
      urinary tract infections.

Cranberry juice

29.   For various medical diseases extra nutrition is
      often needed in drinks. Drinks providing extra nutrition are
      often high in what?

Vitamins and minerals

30.   What percentage of Americans drink alcohol?

65 percent

31.   What percentage of Americans have a lifetime
      prevalence of alcohol dependency?

14 percent

32.   What popular soft drink today contained
      cocaine in the early 1900s?

Coca-Cola

33.   This drink is often consumed on cold winter
      nights. It is touted for weight loss; however,
      long-term use in excess could possibly cause potassium loss
      and even osteoporosis.

Apple cider vinegar

# Grade—Chapter 10

Number correct _____ + bonus points _____ multiplied by 3 = _____ Score

*Chapter 11*

# Questions and Answers about Common Foods

The following review questions cover common foods. You may want to cover the right side of the page as you answer each of the questions to see how much you really know. Give yourself two points for each correct answer. There are five bonus questions.

| QUESTION | ANSWER |
|---|---|
| 1. What is another name for seaweed? It has been used as a *laxative*. It does have high thyroid content. It should not be used by those on thyroid medication. | Agar |
| 2. This legume is usually cultivated as feed for cattle and horses, but some people also eat this food. It has been touted to help in *menopause*, but it might trigger a recurrence of systemic lupus erythematosous in some individuals. | Alfalfa |
| 3. This vegetable when pickled or cooked is touted to help with *indigestion*. What is it? | Artichoke |
| 4. This vegetable probably has a diuretic effect and increases urine output. It has been touted to help prevent *kidney stones*. What is it? | Asparagus |
| 5. This food is often found in salads at Mexican restaurants. It has been touted to *decrease cholesterol*. What is it? | Avocado |
| 6. This food has been touted for *nausea* related to car sickness. What is it? | Barley |
| 7. These beans have been touted as one of the best | Fava bean |

sources of *L-dopa,* a natural precursor of dopamine in the brain. Since it has high levels of L-dopa, some believe that it is helpful for those with Parkinson's disease. What is it?

8. This food is red and has been touted to help with *liver disease,* but significant research is lacking. What is it? — Beets

9. Of all the nuts, which one contains a high amount of unsaturated fats, which might *lower cholesterol?* It is also one of the best sources of vitamin E. It also contains calcium, magnesium, and the B vitamins niacin and riboflavin. — Almonds

10. Which walnut has been touted for *Montezuma's Revenge* after traveling to Mexico? — Black walnut

11. What bran has been touted to lower cholesterol and possibly to *lower postprandial blood sugar* in some diabetics? — Oat bran

12. Which fruit contains *quercetin,* a phytochemical that scavenges free radicals and contains fiber that aids in digestion and lowers cholesterol? — Apple

13. Which fruit has been touted to help with *arthritis?* — Pineapple

14. What kinds of pancakes are touted to help with *varicose veins* and hemorrhoids? — Buckwheat pancakes

15. Name a vegetable that is often served with sausage and is touted to help with *gastritis.* — Cabbage

16. Which pepper comes in different colors (green, yellow, orange, red), boosts the immune system, and contains large amounts of vitamin C and *beta carotene?* It should be noted that natural beta carotene as in this red pepper is healthy but in supplements might not be. — Bell peppers

17. The Hershey Company became famous from this food that is touted to have a *stimulating* effect. Name it. — Chocolate

18. What berry is especially high in vitamin E and *lycopene,* which may help prevent cell damage? — Blackberry

19. Give another name for *chili pepper.* Topically, it has been used for pain. It is also known as cayenne pepper. — Capsaicin

20. Name a nut that is high in vitamin E and *selenium,* a mineral that scavenges free radicals. — Brazil nuts

21. Sticks of this herb are often served at parties. It has been touted to *lower blood pressure,* but since it might lower circulating neurotransmitters such as dopamine, norepinephrine, and epinephrine, it could conceivably also decrease — Celery

mood. What is it?

22. This delicious fruit has been touted to help in
    *colds and gout.* What is it?

    Cherry

23. Name a vegetable rich in phytochemicals that
    might decrease the risk of *cancer* in some. It is also rich in
    lutein, an antioxidant that might offer some vision protection.

    Broccoli

24. This berry has been touted to help in *urinary
    tract infections.* What is it?

    Cranberry

25. This food is what pickles are made from. It is
    touted to have a *diuretic effect.* Name it.

    Cucumber

26. What has been touted as a *perfect complex
    carbohydrate?* It contains fiber, magnesium, phosphorus, sele-
    nium, zinc, and B vitamins; and it is not as allergenic as wheat.

    Brown rice

27. The current trend in America is to eat more
    cereals for breakfast. Which ones of these are known to be
    high in *fiber?*

    Whole-grain cereals

28. Those who eat beans several times a week
    might decrease their risk of *heart disease.* Name one that is
    especially rich in vitamin C and iron. It also contains calcium,
    magnesium, and potassium.

    Chickpeas

29. Name an underground stem (rhizome) that
    decreases *nausea* and motion sickness.

    Ginger

30. Name a tea that is lightly steamed rather
    than fermented, as black tea is, allowing its *free radical con-
    stituents* of phytochemicals and polyphenols, to be better pre-
    served.

    Green tea

31. This cabbage vegetable may offer more *antioxidants*
    than any other vegetable. It contains vitamin C, vitamin E, beta
    carotene, folate, calcium, magnesium, and lutein. Name the veg-
    etable.

    Kale

32. What type of fish is known to be especially high
    in *omega-3 fatty acids,* which are thought to be healthy for the
    heart?

    Salmon

33. This fruit may be the best source of *carotenoids,*
    which are touted to help prevent cancer. It is also high in
    vitamins C and E. Name the fruit.

    Mangos

34. Asians ate this fungus, believing that it increased
    *longevity.* It also contains eritadenine, a substance that might
    lower cholesterol. Name the fungus.

    Mushroom

35. Name a vegetable oil that might help some
    have a more healthy heart. It is high in *monounsaturated fat.*

    Olive oil

36. This fruit *decreases absorption* of many common
    prescription drugs. What is it?

    Grapefruit

37. This food is often consumed with prime rib
    although some hate its taste. It has been used to clear the
    *sinuses* and help with upper respiratory infections. What is it?

    Horseradish

38. Name a tropical fruit that is full of *beta carotene
    and vitamin C.* It is touted to improve immune function, lower
    cholesterol, aid digestion, and mitigate inflammations.

    Papaya

39. Name a type of grape that is steeped with
    polyphenols, antioxidants touted to help the heart. It also
    contains tartaric acid, which is touted to help decrease the
    risk of *colon cancer.*

    Red grape

40. What food is well known for its seasoning
    ability and has been touted by some to help with the *common
    cold?*

    Onion

41. Pioneers would often go through the woods
    gathering this plant to make salads. They used it as a *laxative,*
    but it could also cause significant gastrointestinal upset.

    Pokeweed

42. The consumption of which fish in particular is
    touted to help produce a *healthy heart,* decrease the symp-
    toms of rheumatoid arthritis, decrease the risk of some can-
    cers, have antidepressant actions, and have mood stabilizing
    effects in those with depression?

    Salmon

43. Name two seeds that might lower *cholesterol.*

    Sesame seeds, Flaxseeds

44. Name a health food from the Orient touted
    to increase *metabolism* and lower cholesterol.

    Tofu

45. This vegetable is known to be extremely high in
    complex carbohydrates that cause weight gain. However,
    extract of it has been tried for possible *weight loss.* What is
    it?

    Potato

46. This food is very popular in pies at Thanksgiving.
    It has been touted to help in *benign prostatic hypertrophy.*
    What is it?

    Pumpkin

47. *Lycopene* is touted to help in the prevention of
    heart disease and cancer. Name a fruit, often thought to be a
    vegetable, that is high in lycopene.

    Tomato

48. What kind of bread may be the most healthy
    since it contains fiber, protein, and B vitamins? The main ingre-

    Whole wheat bread

dient in this bread is touted to decrease the risk of *heart disease.*

49. This tasty fruit has been touted for *menstrual cramps,* but because it can possibly cause uterine contractions, it should not be used during pregnancy. What is it?          Raspberry

50. This food has been touted for *stimulating growth* in children since it contains several vitamins and minerals. What is it?          Spinach

51. Bonus Question          Strawberry
    This berry looks good, tastes good, and is touted to have a *diuretic effect.* What is it?

52. Bonus Question          Yogurt
    This food contains a *live bacteria* that might help the gastrointestinal tract. It might also decrease yeast infections and lower cholesterol.

53. Bonus Question          Sweet potato
    Wild yams come from this potato. It has been touted for various *menstrual disorders* although significant research is lacking. Name the potato.

54. Bonus Question          Orange
    This fruit, which is orange in color, prevented *scurvy* in the early voyagers coming to America. Name it.

55. Bonus Question          Garlic
    Name a spice that is touted to *promote circulation,* lower cholesterol, decrease the risk of cancer, and keep ticks off.

# Grade—Chapter 11

Number correct _____ + bonus points _____ multiplied by 2 = _____ Score

## Chapter 12

# Questions and Answers about Spices

The following questions relate to spices. You may want to cover the right side of the page as you answer each of the questions to see how much you really know. Give yourself five points for each correct answer.

| QUESTION | ANSWER |
|---|---|
| 1. Name a spice that is commonly found in pasta sauces and has been touted topically for *wart removal.* | Basil |
| 2. This spice is found in Tabasco sauce in many restaurants. It has been touted topically for *pain relief* and orally as a digestion aid. Name it. | Capsicum |
| 3. This spice is commonly found on rye bread. It has been used to *reduce gas* since ancient times. Name it. | Caraway |
| 4. This spice is a common flavoring agent in foods and has been touted to rid infected individuals of *worms.* Name it. | Chives |
| 5. This spice is very popular. It has been used for gastrointestinal problems and for its reported *antiseptic* qualities. Name it. | Cinnamon |
| 6. This is a popular spice. It is even found in many mouthwashes. It has been used for centuries for its ability to *dull pain,* as in toothache. Name it. | Clove |
| 7. This spice is often used in small amounts as a flavoring in foods. It probably does help with loss of appetite and *upset stomach,* for which it is touted. It belongs to the carrot family. Name the spice. | Coriander |

77

8. This spice is found in certain kinds of pickles. It has been used for *gastrointestinal problems*. Name it.

Dill

9. This herb is popular with chefs. It was listed in the *U.S. Pharmacopoeia* until 1970. It has largely been used to relieve gas and help *digestion*. Name it.

Fennel

10. This spice has a strong odor and has been touted for *reducing high blood pressure*. Name it.

Garlic

11. This spice is used as a condiment on hamburgers and hotdogs. It has been touted to help in upper *respiratory infections* and flatulence. Name it.

Mustard

12. This spice is used in custard pies. It has also been used for bad breath and indigestion. It is touted to help *anti-inflammatory actions*. However, if taken in excess, dangerous reactions are possible including seizures, confusion, and even death. Name it.

Nutmeg

13. This spice was used as far back as the ancient Greeks for *bad breath*. It has long been used as a flavoring agent in soups and sauces. It is often used with various servings of meats in restaurants. Name it.

Parsley

14. This spice has been touted to help bad breath and indigestion. It has been touted to help with *perspiration* in menopause. While it is safe for most people, excessive use of this could result in convulsions and rapid heartbeat. Name it.

Sage

15. This spice has been used for flavoring and as an ingredient in *antacid* preparations. It is touted for motion sickness. Name it.

Ginger

16. This spice is a cousin to ginger. It is a major ingredient in curry powder. It has been touted to have *anti-inflammatory* effects. Name it.

Turmeric

17. This spice has been used as a flavoring agent in some alcoholic beverages. It has been touted for indigestion. Topically it has been used for *insect bites*. Excessive amounts can result in confusion, hallucinations, seizures, and even death. Name it.

Wormwood

18. True or False:
Indium is a spice.

False. Indium is a trace element that has been touted to help with anti-aging effects, but research is lacking and toxicity is possible in excessive amounts.

19. True or False:
Riboflavin is considered a spice.

False. Riboflavin is a vitamin. It is $B_2$.

20. True or False:

False. Arginine is an amino acid

Arginine is a common spice.

that is popular and is sold as a natural product today.

## Grade—Chapter 12

Number correct _____ + bonus points _____ multiplied by 5 = _____ Score

# Chapter 13

# Questions and Answers about Supplements

How much do you know about supplements? You may want to cover the right side of the page as you answer each of the questions to see how much you really know. Give yourself one point for each correct answer. There is one bonus question.

| QUESTION | ANSWER |
|---|---|
| 1. What are usually derived from natural foods, are touted to have various health benefits, and are popular today? | Supplements |
| 2. In biochemistry and neurophysiology this component is often discussed as a source of energy for cells. It can be bought over-the-counter and is touted to increase energy and build muscle. Name it. | ATP (Adenosine Triphosphate) |
| 3. Name a supplement that is known for its abundance of minerals. | Alfalfa |
| 4. Name a popular supplement that is found in many skin care products and is used for all kinds of skin irritations. | Aloe vera |
| 5. Name a supplement that is touted to help in pancreatitis and has many amino acids. | Barley |
| 6. Name a supplement touted to have antibacterial effects. Its cousin, bee pollen, has been touted for fatigue and depression. | Bee propolis |
| 7. This supplement is touted for many bacterial, | Beta-1, 3-Glucan |

viral, and fungal infections. It has also been touted for benefits
with cancer and is said to be antiaging. Name it.

8.   This supplement is touted to help in liver disease,            Bifidobacterium bifidum
     yeast infections, and digestion. Name it.

9.   This supplement, like its cousin shark cartilage,             Bovine cartilage
     has been touted for arthritis, ulcerative colitis, and psoriasis.

10.  Because of its long name, this supplement is                  Cerasomal-Cis-9-
     often just referred to as CMO. It is touted                   Cetylmyristoleate
     to help with arthritis. Name it.

11.  This alga is a complete food. It has been                     Chlorella
     touted to protect against ultraviolet radiation. Name it.

12.  This supplement is a connective tissue found                  Chondroitin sulfate
     in joints. It is often marketed with glucosamine and is touted
     to help in osteoarthritis.

13.  Name a supplement that is found in a number                   Citrin
     of preparations touted for weight loss.

14.  Which is more beneficial, this supplement or                  Coenzyme A
     coenzyme Q10? This is touted to help with energy and the
     immune system.

15.  This coenzyme is touted to help the heart.                    Coenzyme Q10

16.  Name a supplement used topically for                          Colloidal silver
     fungal infections.

17.  Name a supplement high in zinc.                               Corn germ

18.  Name a supplement that has been touted                        Creatine
     for athletic enhancement, but in excess it could be danger-
     ous.

19.  This supplement is a derivative of the amino                  DMG (Dimethylglycine)
     acid glycine and is touted to increase energy and mental
     functioning. It is also said to lower blood pressure and blood
     glucose. Name it.

20.  What supplement is similar to the amino acid                  DMAE
     choline and is touted to increase mental capacity?

21.  This supplement comes from wood and has been                  DMSO (Dimethylsulfoxide)
     used topically for all kinds of injuries to decrease pain. Name
     it.

22.  Which supplement is composed of the omega-3                   EFAs (essential fatty acids)
     and omega-6 fatty acids? This supplement has been touted to
     decrease cholesterol, decrease blood pressure, and help in

bipolar disorder. It is the polyunsaturated fatty acids. They are found in fish and flaxseed.

23. What supplement has been used topically for hemorrhoids, insect bites, and wrinkles?

Emu oil

24. What is the most common commercial fish oil on the market?

Cod liver oil

25. What supplement of seeds is high in omega-3 fatty acids that have been touted to lower cholesterol, help in arthritis, and stabilize mood in bipolar disorder?

Flaxseed

26. What supplement of seeds has a nutty flavor, is high in linoleic acid, has no cholesterol, and has no sodium?

Grape seed oil

27. What popular supplement for PMS should not be used by those with breast or cervical cancers since it results in more estrogen?

Evening primrose oil

28. Taking this supplement one hour before meals absorbs water and thereby decreases appetite and has been touted for diabetes and weight loss. Name it.

Glucomannan

29. This gum supplement has been touted for diabetics, for decreasing the appetite, and for lowering cholesterol. Name it.

Guar gum

30. These supplement brans have been used to lower cholesterol. Name them.

Oat bran and rice bran

31. What supplement is found in fruits and vegetables and is touted to be helpful in colitis, constipation, varicose veins, hemorrhoids, and colon cancer prevention?

Cellulose

32. This supplement is touted to be helpful in preventing gallstones. It is touted also to be good for diabetics and in colon cancer prevention. Name it.

Lignin

33. This supplement slows the absorption of food and is found in apples. Name it.

Pectin

34. Name a supplement that contains tryptophane and is currently popular and touted for depression.

5-HTP (5-hydroxyl L-tryptophane)

35. What supplement is often sold in preparations with chondroitin and is touted for osteoarthritis? It can make diabetes worse since it comes from glucose.

Glucosamine

36. What groups of "drinks" are made from plants and are touted as blood cleansers?

"Green drinks"

37. What supplement is high in vitamins, minerals, and enzymes, and is touted to help in digestion?     Papaya

38. This great-tasting food is high in carbohydrates, protein, amino acids, vitamins, and minerals. It is sweeter than sugar. It is not only eaten as a food, but it is applied topically for wounds. Name it.     Honey

39. This supplement has been touted by weight lifters. It is involved in ATP production.     Inosine

40. This supplement is a type of seaweed that contains many vitamins, minerals, and iodine. It is touted to be good nutrition for the brain.     Kelp

41. This supplement is a bacteria that has been touted for digestion, to decrease cholesterol, and to help in yeast infections.     Lactobacillus acidophilus

42. Name a supplement touted to improve the immune system. It is a protein found in human bile, tears, and milk.     Lactoferrin

43. This supplement was experimented with in the past for Alzheimer's dementia, but it was not found to be effective. The logic was that it consists mostly of choline, and the neurotransmitter acetylcholine is low in Alzheimer's dementia. It has been touted for improving brain functioning, decreasing atherosclerosis, increasing energy, and helping the liver. Soybeans are high in this substance. Name it.     Lecithin

44. This supplement is a mushroom that has been touted to inhibit the growth of cancer and viruses (HIV). It has also been touted for fatigue, diabetes, hepatitis, high blood pressure, and obesity.     Maitake

45. What supplement is a naturally occurring hormone that decreases at puberty and is used to help in insomnia?     Melatonin

46. What popular supplement is a derivative of DMSO and is touted for arthritis and pain?     MSM (Methylsulfonylmethane)

47. What supplement is a form of niacin, increases the levels of dopamine, and is thus touted for Parkinsonism?     NADH (Nicotinamide Adenine Dinucleotide)

48. Octacosanol comes from a supplement that has long been touted for many ailments: neuromuscular disorders, low endurance, and muscle pain. It is high in vitamin E. Name it.     Wheat germ

49. Extracts from this plant leaf are touted to be     Olive

antiviral, antibacterial, and antifungal. A topical oil has been used for various skin irritations. Name it.

50. Oil from this supplement is high in omega-3 fatty acids. It is touted to increase cognitive ability. Name it.

Perilla oil

51. This supplement is touted for dementia, depression, and ASHD (atherosclerotic heart disease). Name it.

Phyophatidyl choline

52. What supplement is currently popular and is touted for enhancing cognitive ability?

Phosphatidyl serine

53. What supplement is a precursor of several hormones (DHEA, progesterone, testosterone, and estrogen) and thus could potentially carry the danger of these hormones?

Pregnenolone

54. What supplement is a group of bacteria such as acidophilus and bifidobacterium bifidum, which are important in digestion?

Probiotics

55. What hormonal cream has been touted for menopausal symptoms?

Progesterone cream

56. What food supplement contains statins that are found in several cholesterol-lowering prescription medications?

Red yeast rice

57. What supplement from bees contains the only natural source of acetylcholine, along with many vitamins, minerals, amino acids, and hormones? It is touted to be antibacterial.

Royal jelly

58. What supplement has been touted for depression, arthritis, and fibromyalgia? A few people taking it become manic.

SAMe

59. What marine animal has been used for all kinds of arthritis? Hint: it sounds like a cucumber.

Sea cucumber

60. What shellfish has been touted for arthritis and the healing of wounds?

Sea mussel

61. What mushroom supplement may be number one in China and is touted to have antiaging effects?

Reishi

62. What mushroom supplement is touted to help in cancer by increasing T cells?

Shiitake

63. What algae supplement is high in protein and is touted to help the immune system?

Spirulina

64. This thin grass supplement has been touted in cancer and anemia. Name it.

Wheat grass

65. This protein supplement has been touted for muscle building and for those with cancer. It comes from cheese.

Whey protein

66. This organism is consumed for energy. It is touted to boost the immune system. It is used in beer production.

Yeast

While almost any supplement could be unsafe at times, some are especially dangerous when used in certain conditions. In questions 67–83, please indicate which of the following combinations are potentially dangerous. Answer "true" if the combinations are dangerous and "false" if they are not.

**QUESTION**

**ANSWER**

67. Candidiasis and yeast

True

68. Excessive sleepiness and melatonin

True

69. Infant and honey

True—The infant's immune system is immature. A botulin toxin can develop.

70. Diabetes mellitus and glucosamine

True—Glucosamine is a derivative of glucose.

71. High eosinophil count and 5-HTP

True

72. Breast cancer and evening primrose oil

True

73. Aggression and DHEA

True

74. Diabetes mellitus and bee pollen

True

75. Obesity and sugar

True—Obesity is probably the number one cause of death. It contributes to heart disease, high blood pressure, some cancers, and many of the top causes of death in America.

76. Skin irritations and topical aloe vera

False—While contact dermatitis is possible with almost any substance, aloe vera has an extremely long history of use in various commercial preparations for skin irritations.

77. High cholesterol and omega-3 fatty acids

False—While omega-3 fatty acids are not for everyone (some diabetics), they do have a long history of being used in high cholesterol.

78. Blood thinners and the "G" supplements

True—"G" supplements thin

(garlic, gingko, ginseng, ginger)

the blood also and therefore can be dangerous with other blood-thinning medications such as aspirin.

79.    Psychosis and ginseng

True—Ginseng has been known to produce a psychosis in some.

80.    OCD and Inositol

False—Inositol probably has helped a minority of individuals with OCD. However, it has also induced mania in a few.

81.    Emaciated individual and kelp

False—Kelp is rich in vitamins and minerals. It can be a good food source for some.

82.    Emaciated individual and shiitake, reishi, and monitake mushrooms

False—These mushrooms have long been used in China as a food source touted to have many health benefits including nutrition.

83.    Diarrhea due to antibiotics and acidophilus

False—Acidophilus has long been used to return normal bowel functioning disturbed by antibiotics.

84.    The most-studied supplement of all time is probably _____.

Gingko

85.    The most-used supplement of all time, which has a distinct odor, is _____.

Garlic

86.    Probably the most-used supplement of all time touted to enhance sexual functioning is _____.

Ginseng

87.    The supplement that has probably been studied more than any other for possible benefits in bipolar disorder is _____.

Omega-3 fatty acids

88.    The supplement that actually has statins present, as do modern cholesterol-lowering drugs, is _____.

Red yeast rice

89.    Which of the following do not match?
   A. Marine animals—sea cucumber
   B. Bees—royal jelly
   C. Sharks—shark cartilage
   D. Shellfish—sea mussel
   E. All of the above match.
   F. None of the above match.

E. All of the above match.

90.    Which of the following do not match?
   A. Bees—bee pollen

H does not match. A sea cucumber is not a cucumber plant at all;

B. Algae—spirulina
C. Single-celled organism—yeast
D. Bacteria—bifidobacterium bifidum
E. Bacteria—lactobacillus acidophilus
F. Plant component—chlorophyll
G. Fish—omega 3-fatty acids
H. Cucumber—sea cucumber
I. Bacteria—probiotics

it is a marine animal.

91. Name a cooking substance that has been used topically for athlete's foot and to get rid of *ticks and chiggers*.

Vinegar

92. Name one of several common substances that has been used topically for *body odor*.

1. Vinegar
2. Baking soda
3. Turnip juice

93. What nutritional supplement is known to have exceptional *nutritional power*, with many trace elements and vitamins?

Kelp

94. Of all the supplements and/or herbs that have been tried for *bipolar disorder*, which one has been used the most by the general population?

Omega-3 fatty acids

95. What popular supplement has probably been used the most in *fibromyalgia*?

SAMe

96. Name a supplement that is the same as the first substance from the mother's breast after the birth of a baby. It is touted for many ailments including *irritable bowel syndrome*.

Colostrum

97. _____ Plus is a popular supplement that is often described as a wellness product that helps with *weight loss*. The theory behind it is a bit simplistic, and significant scientific studies are lacking.

Collagen

98. What current herb supplement is derived from L-tryptophane and has been used in the treatment of *depression*?

5HTP

99. What coenzyme is widely used today in an attempt to decrease free radicals and thus is touted to decrease the probability of *cancer*? It has also been touted to help heart functioning.

Coenzyme Q10

100. Many *diets* come and go with perhaps a 90 percent ineffective rate for weight loss overall. Name a high-protein diet that has been popular in recent years but has few rigorous and widely accepted scientific studies to back it up. In fact, with rehydration the initial weight loss

Atkins diet

tends to disappear.

101.  Bonus Question                                                            Honey
      This food tastes great and has a good smell. It has been used
      topically for *minor skin irritations*. It is made by a bee. Native
      Americans love it. Name it.

## Grade—Chapter 13

Number correct _____ + bonus points _____ = _____ Score

## Chapter 14

# Questions and Answers about Herbs

How much do you know about herbs? Here are more than one hundred herbs used for medicinal purposes. You may want to cover the right side of the page as you answer each of the questions to see how much you really know. Give yourself one point for each correct answer. There is one bonus question.

| QUESTION | ANSWER |
|---|---|
| 1. Name a Chinese herb that has been touted for just about everything, although significant human research is either totally absent or severely lacking at best. | Bupleurum |
| 2. Name an herb in Europe that is found in many food preparations and is touted to have (but is far from proven in humans) antibacterial and antitumor effects. As with many claims of many herbs, this one's claim for *anorexia nervosa* is not substantiated. | Burdock |
| 3. Name an herb that has long been used as *a cough suppressant* in spite of the fact that it can damage the liver and its flower bud may be carcinogenic. Hint: Its name is the same as the foot of a young horse. | Coltsfoot |
| 4. Name a fungus from China that is touted for but unproven for *anxiety*. It is often sold in Asian pharmacies under the name reiski. It is often in alcohol extracts. | Ganoderma |
| 5. Gentian and gentiana are related. One of them could be especially dangerous since it grows next to hellebore, which is highly toxic. Which one is it? | Gentian |
| 6. This herb is in many mouthwashes used for *plaque*. Name it. (Hint: It sounds like something for the movie *Dracula*.) | Bloodroot |

7.  Ginseng comes in different types: American                    Siberian ginseng
    (panax quinquefolices), Asian (panax ginseng), and Siberian
    (eleutherococcles), to name a few. All three of the above are
    touted for *fatigue, depression, to boost the immune system, and
    for sexual issues.* Any of them can have potentially dangerous
    side effects, but one produces less anxiety and insomnia.
    Which one?

8.  Name a Chinese herb that has been used for                    Magnolia flower
    *nasal congestion*; animal research suggests antibacterial, anti-
    fungal, antiviral effects; and so far serious reported side
    effects seem few.

9.  Name a wonderful wild herb from Europe that                   Marshmallow
    tastes great and *soothes irritations* of the mouth, throat, and
    stomach. Although one would think that it would raise blood
    sugar, in the wild form it is touted to lower blood sugar. Hint:
    A similarly named treat is often added to hot chocolate and
    is also often eaten around a campfire.

10. Name an herb commonly known as panax                          Notoginseng root
    pseudoginseng that is touted to stop *nosebleed.*

11. Name a Chinese herb touted by some to                         Polygonum (Fo-Ti)
    even treat *schizophrenia* but certainly is not up to the task.

12. Name a tree common throughout the world that                  Birch
    contains salicylate, the chemical from which aspirin was
    made. Hint: The willow tree also has salicylate. Name another
    tree.

13. Name an herb that bears the name orange that                  Tangerine peel
    is touted for *belching* and other digestive disorders.       (mandarin orange)

14. Lozenges are made from a group of algae and                   Usnea
    fungi in the Northern Hemisphere and are sometimes used
    to treat a mild sore throat. Name the herb.

15. Name an ancient herb used topically to treat                  Yarrow
    wounds. Orally it might have a calming effect. Because of its
    diuretic effect, it has been used in high blood pressure. Hint:
    It rhymes with narrow.

16. Name an herb that is touted to lower blood                    Fenugreek
    sugar in diabetes types I and II and smells like maple syrup.

17. Name an herb that has been used for impotence                 Nux vomica
    but contains strychnine and can kill. It is analogous to the
    legend of the men who found the Amazon tribe of women.

18. Name an herb that, although it is not used                    Belladona

much in medicine today because of its side effects, was one
of the forerunners in the treatment of asthma.

19. What hot-tasting fruit taken orally for | Capsicum (also known as
gastric problems and applied to the skin | cayenne, red pepper, chili
to relieve pain has historically been described | pepper, Tobasco, and
as the plant that bites back? | paprika)

20. Name an herb that resembles a cucumber, | Burnet
has been used in salads, and is touted for uterine bleeding,
but its effectiveness is not known.

21. Name an herb that questionably has been | Bugle
touted for both hypothyroidism and hyperthyroidism.

22. The American flag has three colors. This herb is | Blue flag
more commonly used as a laxative, has one of those colors in
its name, and is called _____. It can be toxic.

23. Native American females used this herb | Black haw
for menstrual cramps. It has a rather grim-sounding name.

24. Name an herb used by Native American | Blue cohosh
females to induce menstruation. Hint: It has a blue color. It
could be dangerous, and self-medication with this one should
not be done.

25. Name an herb often found in potpourri in | Borage
bathrooms, often found in salads, and often found in various
drinks. It is touted to help in PMS, arthritis, and colds but
may prove to be somewhat of a bore.

26. Name an herb that acts similar to quinidine, | Broom
the heart-stabilizing medication. Just as quinidine could be
dangerous, so can this herb. Hint: The plant from which this
herb comes has been used as a broom.

27. Name a seed found on rye bread used for | Caraway
flatulence.

28. Name an herb that is touted strongly by | Carob
herbalists for indigestion and is touted as a chocolate substitute.

29. This herb can interact with innumerable | Cola
medications. It can have many side effects although it often
does not. It was made famous by a soda.

30. Name a common South American beverage | Maté
of this herb that is stimulating, and long-term use has been
associated with many different cancers.

31. Name an herb used to make pancakes that | Buckwheat

might help *varicose veins* and hemorrhoids.

32. Although unproven and not known for
degree of safety, various herbs are touted to
*slow heart rate* and seem safe for many (there are always
exceptions such as pregnant females, etc.). Name one.

1. Motherwort
2. Chicory

33. Name an herb that is interesting, to say the
least. It might help indigestion. It contains insulin that might
boost the immune system. It contains a digitalis-like compound that might slow the heart rate. It seems to have some
anti-inflammatory and bacteriostatic activity. Its lactucopicrin
gives it a little sedative effect, and thus it is often added to
canned brands of coffee. It might even lower cholesterol and
blood sugar a little according to some. It seems safe for most
and with low drug interactions.

Chicory

34. Although not proven in effectiveness or
safety scientifically, it seems safe in that few adverse side
effects have been reported. It has been used in the Amazon
jungle for many years.

Muira puama

35. Name an herb used by Native Americans
for *menstrual cramps*.

Partridge berry

36. This herb contains the famous cancer-
fighting substance, vincristine, which has helped so many but
can damage kidneys, liver, and bone marrow. It is a common
decorative flower that is usually blue.

Periwinkle

37. Name the herb from which the well-known
laxative psyllium comes.

Plantain

38. Although potentially dangerous, what was
pleurisy root used for by Native Americans?

Pleurisy

39. Name an herb that has been given for *high
blood pressure*, but it is possible that in some the drop in
blood pressure is due to toxicity.

Prickly ash

40. Name a pie popular in the fall of the year. The
seed of the herb might help to a mild degree to relieve the
discomfort of BPH (benign prostatic discomfort).

Pumpkin

41. Name one of the most popular drinks of the
cowboys in the old west. The belief was false, but it was
thought to help in syphilis.

Sarsaparilla

42. Name an herb that has been used for kidney stones.

Stone root

43. Name a common food of Native Americans that
may have a blood pressure-lowering effect in some people.

Yucca

44. Fill in the blank:
Some individuals have a placebo response to drugs and herbs.
Other individuals have a _____ response with side effects
for no biochemical cause of the drug.

Nocebo

45. Name an herb that has been used to flavor
some alcoholic beverages, but use beyond minor amounts
and chronic use could result in multiple side effects including
seizures and death.

Wormwood

46. Name an herb used for fungal infections of
the foot and toenails that is usually safe and effective to some
degree.

Tea tree

47. Ice tea (black tea) has long been a favorite
drink in America. However, a new cousin has arrived and is
touted to have effects against cavities, cancer, cognitive slow-
ness, and cholesterol elevation. What is it?

Green tea

48. What is a danger of green tea?

It interacts with many, many drugs and
even a few common foods (grapefruit
juice and milk).

49. Name an herb that is used for malaria
and whose derivatives are used as prescription antimalarial
drugs in Africa, Asia, and Europe.

Sweet Annie

50. Name an herb that has been used as a
*cough suppressant.* It appears effective and safe for most
people.

Sundew

51. This herb was used by Native Americans
for cold and fever, but fresh herbs can be toxic, even causing death.

Boneset

52. Fill in the blank:
_____ is seaweed, is in several food
preparations, and acts as a laxative.

Agar

53. Name an herb that among its multiple uses
has been put on the tips of arrows to make them poison. It is
acrimonious, to say the least.

Aconite

54. Name a Polynesian herb that historically
was used to treat smallpox when applied topically.

Morinda

55. Name an herb that can damage the liver but has been touted
to possibly have interferon-like activity.

Bistort

56. Name an herb touted for several disorders
that has also been used as a cockroach repellent. It might
hold both cockroaches and the individual users more than at
bay.

Bay

57.  True or False:
     In 1994 the Dietary Supplement Health and Education Act
     was passed into law. A disclaimer must be included on herbal
     products that says, "This product is not intended to diagnose,
     treat, cure, or prevent any disease." However, herbal products
     are permitted to make general health claims as long as they
     are not therapeutic claims. The products are not required to
     list warnings, side effects, contradictions, safety data, and
     properties of the product as long as it is listed as a dietary
     supplement. The line between prescription drugs and herbs
     seems thin.

     True

58.  True or False:
     In general few herbs or supplements
     should be used by *pregnant women* or
     children.

     True—Knowledge is forever
     evolving. What may seem safe
     for some today may be found
     not to be true in the future.

59.  This vitamin has been used recently in an
     attempt to prevent *diabetes mellitus* type I.

     Vitamin D

60.  Name a drug that has been used as a *smoking
     deterrent* but its use is like burning down the barn to get rid
     of the rats. Deaths have been reported.

     Indian tobacco or lobelia

61.  Name just one herb used for *bad breath*.

     1. Cardamom
     2. Eucalyptus
     3. Parsley
     4. Peppermint
     5. Anise
     6. Sage
     7. Coriander
     8. Wild Bergamot
     9. Clove

62.  A. Name an herb that is rather new to
     America that some claim *lowers blood sugar* in both type I and
     type II diabetes.
     B. Name a second herb that is touted to
     lower blood sugar in both type I and type II diabetes but can
     thin the blood.

     A. Gymena

     B. Fenugreek

63.  Which popular herb contained in many
     current *weight-loss formulas* has proven to be dangerous for
     some, even causing death?

     Ephedra

64.  Which hormone is popular today and has
     been used for possible *antiaging effects* but
     could result in dangerous acromegaly in rare cases?

     Human Growth Hormone
     (HGH)

65.  Name the herb that has been used as an
     aphrodisiac in women and touted to have a *calming effect.*

     Passionflower

66. Name an herb that has been used for *wound healing*, though repeated topical use could possibly be related to skin cancer.

Gotu kola

67. What common mineral has been used in an attempt to *lower blood sugar and weight* but could possibly be a factor in cancer causation, especially with high dosages and long-term use.

Chromium

68. What supplement that carries the name of a gum has been used in an attempt to *decrease cholesterol?*

Guggul gum

69. Can foods improve the brain's functioning and performance, and can "*food* improve your mood and change your life"?

No, at least usually not. However, some qualifying statements need to be added. It is true that we all need a healthy diet. It is true that tryptophane (in some food) is converted to serotonin in the brain, and serotonin is the major factor in mood. It is true that tyrosine is a precursor of dopamine and that dopamine is a precursor of norepinephrine. Both dopamine and norepinephrine are involved in mood. It is true that choline plays a role in acetylcholine that is important in memory. All of these (tryptophane, tyramine, and choline) are amino acids that are in food or supplements. Then why couldn't just plain food or supplements help? Well, they might at times, but there are several potential roadblocks.

First, the gastric juices in the stomach are strong and certainly alter and break down food.

Second, the brain contains a blood-brain barrier that keeps many substances out. The blood-brain barrier (BBB) is a structural arrangement of capillaries that is very tight. While fat-soluble compounds pass the BBB as do water, oxygen, glucose, and carbon dioxide, many other substances do not or pass much more slowly.

Third, most research does not back up the theory that certain foods usually, customarily, and in double-blind studies alter mood for most people. This is not to say that they in every instance make no difference.

The above three lines of reasoning may also apply to GABA (which can now be purchased at health food stores), an inhibiting or calming neurotransmitter. The antianxiety benzodiazepines that augment the effects of GABA do much more than just the GABA effect. In reality, the benzodiazepines increase chloride ion conductance through the cell membrane and thus inhibit the firing of the nerve cell and results in a calming effect. It does this not by binding to the GABA receptor but to another related site that modulates the GABA sites. Certainly giving GABA alone is simplest and not comparable to antianxiety medications in effect.

70.  True or False:
     *Herbs* are safe *during pregnancy* and
     for children.

False. In general, few herbs or supplements should be used in pregnancy or in children. Herbs can be extremely dangerous. Some herbs (pennyroyal, goldenseal, lovage, mugwart, wormwood, yarrow, shepherd's purse, black cohosh, blue cohosh, angelica, mistletoe, tansy, wild ginger, rue, and excess coffee) are known for uterine contractions.

71.  What legume has been used in *menopause*?

Alfalfa

72.  What angel-like sounding herb has been used
     for *PMS and menopause*?

Angelica species

73.  What vegetable has been touted to help in
     a broad array of problems including indigestion,
     atherosclerosis, and liver problems?

Artichoke

74.  What spice has been touted to help in
     *wart* removal when applied topically?

Basil

75.  What "berry" was used by Native Americans
     for *urinary tract infections?*

Bearberry

76.  What "berry" has been used for *bruising?*

Bilberry

77.  What "melon" has been touted to *lower
     blood sugar?*

Bitter melon

78. Name the "walnut" that has been used in an attempt to counter *Montezuma's Revenge*.

Black walnut

79. What herb that carries the name of a "broom" has been used to treat varicose veins and has even been tried as preventive protection against poisonous *snakebites?*

Butcher's broom

80. What supplement lotion has a long history of helping skin and *bug bites?*

Calamine

81. Name another herb that has also been used in *skin problems* and has been touted to be antiviral, anti-inflammatory, antibacterial, and antifungal.

Calendula

82. Name one of two minerals that have been used in *baldness.*

1. Selenium
2. Silicon

83. *Fiber* is found in high concentration in apples, almonds, avocados, dates, grapes, mangos, pineapple, rhubarb, soybeans, turnips, walnuts, and prunes. All of these have been used for what?

Constipation

84. Name one of several common foods that have been used for *diarrhea.*

1. Tea
2. Apple
3. Berries—bilberry, blueberry, blackberry, raspberry
4. Carrot

85. Name only one of several herbs that have been used topically for *itching.*

1. Ginger
2. Jewelweed
3. Amaranth

86. What herb has an aromatic smell and has been used for *bad breath?*

Cardaman

87. What pepper in topical form has been used in various *pain problems?*

Cayenne pepper

88. Which supplement was recently revealed in medical literature (*American Family Physician,* 1 September 2000) to seemingly help with *diabetic neuropathy?*

Alpha lipoic acid

89. Name one of several common herbs often used for *nausea.*

1. Peppermint
2. Ginger
3. Cinnamon

90. Name an herb that has been used for the *pain of diabetic neuropathy.*

Evening primrose oil

91. Name an herb that has been used topically for *arthritis pain.*

Red pepper or capsicum

92. What adrenal-like substance has been used
for *mood-lifting effects* that can result in insulin resistance,
hypertension, deep voice, hair loss, and hirsutism?

DHEA

93. What herb has been touted to clear *red eyes*
and hay fever?

Eye bright

94. What zinc oxide powder used in a lotion
became the number one treatment of all time for poison ivy?

Calamine lotion

95. What herb is popular with chefs for seasoning
but has also been used for bad breath, *gas*, and indigestion?

Fennel

96. Name one of several herbs used topically for *pain*.

1. Lavender
2. Ginger
3. Turmeric
4. Eucalyptus

97. Name one of several herbs that have been
applied topically for *sunburn*.

1. Aloe vera
2. Calendula
3. Cucumber
4. Tea
5. Plantain
6. Eggplant

98. Name only one of several herbs that have
been used for *varicose veins*.

1. Bilberry
2. Horse chestnut
3. Butcher's broom
4. Onion
5. Lemon
6. Gingko
7. Gotu kola

99. True or False:
Herbs have no *side effects*.

False—Side effects range from
minor ones to death.

100. Complete the following:
Argin Max is a mixture of herbs touted for *sexual dysfunction*.
It contains ginseng; gingko; damiana; calcium; iron; vitamins A,
B, C; minerals zinc, niacin, selenium; and _____, which
stimulates nitric oxide synthesis as Viagra does.

L-arginine

101. Bonus Question
I was recently answering questions on
Christian radio when a caller asked how I
could talk about the possible benefits of prescription
medications. She felt I should recommend only herbs.
She felt that would be more godly.

Neither herbs nor prescription medication is godly or
ungodly in and of themselves. Either might be effective. Either

N. Unfortunately, all of the
above have been reported.

might have side effects. But neither usually has a pro or con Christian stance. It depends on how they are used.

Now, having stated the above, my caller would have been surprised that herbs sometimes do have a sordid past with demonic suggestions at times in history that Christians should strictly avoid. Which of the following is not correct?

A. Mistletoe—Standing under it considered casting a spell of love from antiquity.
B. Basil—Considered warding off evil in ancient Greece.
C. Parsley—Considered emblematic of death in ancient Greece.
D. Fo-ti—Considered "a mountain spirit" in ancient China.
E. Garlic—Considered "the devil did it" by ancient Muslims.
F. Horehound—Dedicated to "the god of light" in ancient Egypt.
G. Peppermint—Pertained to "feuding gods" of Greek mythology.
H. Saint-John's-wort—Medieval herbalists used it as "an herbal exorcist."
I. Sweet violet—Tales told pertaining to the Greek god Zeus.
J. Rose—Pertained to "the Greek goddess of flowers."
K. Witch hazel—Possible early association with witchcraft.
L. Linden—Tales told pertaining to the Greek god Zeus.
M. Vanadium—Named for the Norse goddess, Vanadis.
N. All of the above.

## Grade—Chapter 14

Number correct _____ + bonus points _____ = _____ Score

## Chapter 15

# More Questions and Answers about Herbs

Following are more questions about herbs. You may want to cover the right side of the page as you answer each of the questions to see how much you really know. Give yourself one point for each correct answer. There are two bonus questions.

| QUESTION | ANSWER |
|---|---|
| 1. What *"antiaging" supplement* may cause women to sound more like men in their voice tone and men to look more feminine in their appearance? | DHEA |
| 2. In benign prostatic hypertrophy (*BPH*), a combination of three herbs is often used: saw palmetto, pygeum, and nettle. What common medical test for men can this combination make inaccurate or difficult to read? | PSA for prostate cancer |
| 3. What is probably the most common undesirable side effect for *omega-3 fatty acids,* which is often touted to help in mood disorders and the heart? | A fishy smell |

Herbs and supplements and the condition they are often said to treat are listed below. Pick out the ones that do not match with what they are touted to treat.

| QUESTION | ANSWER |
|---|---|
| 4. Pick the wrong match:<br>A. *Anxiety*—magnesium<br>B. *Depression*—B$_6$ + Folic Acid for women<br>C. *Bipolar Disorder*—omega-3 fatty acids<br>D. *Insomnia*—guarana<br>E. *Fibromyalgia*—magnesium + Malic acid | D is incorrect. Guarana has high caffeine and tends to keep people awake. Melatonin is one of the most common supplements for insomnia. |

5.  Pick the wrong match:
    A. *High cholesterol—guggal gum*
    B. *Hepatitis—milk thistle*
    C. *Menopause—soy*
    D. *Migraines—ginseng*
    E. *Obesity—psyllium*

D is the wrong match. Feverfew is the herb that has been used most for migraines. Ginseng can result in severe headaches, especially in high doses.

6.  Pick the wrong match:
    A. *Diabetes mellitus—bee pollen*
    B. *Osteoarthritis—glucosamine-chondroitin*
    C. *PMS—evening primrose and red clover*
    D. *Indigestion—artichoke*
    E. *Car sickness—barley*

A is the wrong match. Bee pollen would make diabetes worse. *Gymnema* is an herb that has been touted to decrease blood sugar in diabetes.

7.  Pick the wrong match:
    A. *Varicose veins—bilberry and butcher's broom*
    B. *Itching and infected skin—topical use of calamine, calendula, hermanelis virginiana, menthol cream, and jewelweed*
    C. *Bad Breath—fennel*
    D. *Fatigue—valerian*
    E. *Irritable bowel syndrome—peppermint, ginger, and colostrum*

D is the wrong match. Valerian would most likely have a calming effect. It would not energize. Coffee with its drawbacks usually energizes.

8.  Pick the wrong match:
    A. *Urinary tract infections—cranberry juice*
    B. *The common cold—echinacea and zinc*
    C. *Body odor—garlic*
    D. *Athlete's foot—lavender (topical)*
    E. *Herpes—lupine*

C is the wrong match. Body odor is not helped by garlic. It is often made worse.

9.  Pick the wrong match:
    A. *Sore throat—slippery elm*
    B. *Nail infections—tea tree oil (topical)*
    C. *Bug Bites—vinegar (topical)*
    D. *Diarrhea—prunes*
    E. *Constipation—fiber, flaxseed*

D is the wrong match. Herbalists often recommend tea, apples, and various berries (blueberry, bilberry, raspberry, blackberry) for diarrhea.

10. Pick the wrong match:
    A. *OCD (obsessive compulsive disorder)—inositol*
    B. *Schizophrenia and psychosis—ephedra*
    C. *ADHD—Feingold diet*
    D. *Panic disorder—hops*
    E. All of the above are common matches.

B is the wrong match. As with the previous question, we do not always agree with some of these matches, but B is a gross mismatch. Ephedra has caused psychosis in some cases.

11. This natural hormone has been touted to lift mood and *decrease anxiety*. However, it may also possibly cause depression and weight gain. Name it.

Natural progesterone

12. Name a mouth-watering juice and an old

Cranberry

folk remedy that has often been used in *urinary tract infections* more than any other herb.

13. Name the most commonly used herb for *PMS*.    Evening primrose oil

14. This is a great herb—tasty for breakfast, *lowers cholesterol,* and nutritious. Name it.    Oats

15. This herb tastes good in custard pies, and it has been used for *bad breath* and for various gastrointestinal problems, but it can be dangerous, even causing death in certain instances.    Nutmeg

16. Of the various herbs and supplements used for depression, which one may have the *least interactions* with other drugs, but may cause mania in a few?    SAMe

17. Of all the herbs that have been used as *aphrodisiacs,* which one has been tried the most?    Ginseng

18. Of the different supplements used for the *common cold,* which one might prove dangerous in a young female during reproductive years?    Echinacea

19. Name three herbs that are often used together in benign prostatic hypertrophy (*BPH*) in males.    Saw palmetto, string nettle, pygeum

20. Which rapidly growing herb for *anxiety* used throughout the years may turn the skin yellow and may also result in a coma for those on Xanax?    Kava

21. Which two herbs commonly used for *anxiety* could be potentially addicting?    Kava, valerian

22. Of all herbs, which one has been used the most for nutritional support in *liver diseases?*    Milk thistle

23. Which supplement has probably been used the most for *insomnia* and is a hormone excreted by the pineal gland?    Melatonin

24. This amino acid has been used by some in an attempt to help with *herpes.* It certainly is no Zovirax.    Lysine

25. Of all herbs tried for *Alzheimer's,* which has been tried the most?    Gingko biloba

26. This herb is touted to help in *beauty* in spite of its name. However, it can cause nicotine-like poisoning. It has also been used for osteoporosis. Name it.    Horsetail

27. What common candy uses the name of    Peppermint

one of the most popular herbs in the treatment of *various gastrointestinal issues* such as gastritis, irritable bowel syndrome, and stomach aches?

28. Cleopatra floated down the Nile trying to *slow aging* with this herb. What was it?

Grapes

29. Of all herbs tried for *high blood pressure,* which one has been tried the most?

Garlic

30. Name a famous wine that bears this name. It has been touted to help in *the common cold.* The bark and leaves have a cyanide toxicity.

Elderberry

31. Name the herb that comes from the tallest tree in the world and is found in Vicks VapoRub used as *a decongestant.* The oil is toxic and could be lethal.

Eucalyptus

32. Which herb in a seed form has been used for *weight loss?*

Psyllium seed

33. Parkinsonism is a condition resulting in loss of the pigmented nuclei in the substantia niagra of the midbrain that produces dopamine. The treatments for *parkinsonism* are becoming more and more advanced. They include Sinemet (a dopamine containing drug) and Requip (a dopamine agonist). Name a common food that contains L-dopa (a precursor of dopamine) and has been used by some in early parkinsonism. It is no match for the more advanced medicines.

Fava bean (bean sprouts)

34. Name an herb that has been used to flavor everything from alcoholic beverages to ice cream and candy and has been touted to help in *women's issues*—PMS, menopause, uterine cramps, low sex drive. It comes from China and has a beautiful name.

Angelica (dang-quai)

35. Name an herb which carries the name of betel that might act like an antidepressant (MAO inhibiting effects) but possibly at great cost (psychosis).

Betel palm

36. Name an herb that was used by Native Americans for *urinary tract infections.* It was in the U.S. Pharmacopoeia until 1936 for urinary tract infections. It is no match for antibiotics of today that are gram negative antibacterial specific such as third-generation cephalosporins.

Bearberry (uva ursi)

37. A. Which supplement in the vitamin category has been recommended for use in ADHD, but in some of the medical literature note is made of possible increase in *lung cancer* and cardiovascular mortality?

A. Beta carotene

   B. What vitamin has been used in an

B. Vitamin D

attempt to prevent diabetes in children?

38. *The use of herbs* or supplements has *increased* during the past decade by over:
A. 20%
B. 30%
C. 40%

C

39. The *percent of Americans using herbs* or supplements is over:
A. 10%
B. 20%
C. 30%

C

40. The *number of deaths* from herbs or supplements in America is over:
A. 70
B. 80
C. 100

C

41. The number of *adverse effects* reported to the FDA from herbs or supplements over a six-year period (1993–1998) was over:
A. 500
B. 1,500
C. 2,500

C. However, overall the number of adverse effects with prescription medication is far higher.

42. What common mineral has been touted to decrease pain in *fibromyalgia* and decrease anxiety?

Magnesium

43. Name a supplement that has been used for *anxiety* but would create extreme anxiety in your cat.

Catnip

44. The following statement (actual words are altered) recently appeared on an advertisement promoting an herb. How many *jumps in logic* can you find?
"Depression can, as documented by popular magazines and television specials, be treated with a medically proven herb which is effective, safe, and inexpensive."

Six at least.

First, popular magazines are not exactly equivalent to professional medical journals.

Second, everyone has depression to some degree (upset, frustrated). Do they mean major medical depression?

Third, does *treated* mean a remission of most of the medical symptoms of depression for a substantial period of time?

Fourth, does *medically proven* mean with repeated double-blind scientific studies?

Fifth, does *safe* mean no side effects? This is almost impossible. Better questions would be: What side effects have been reported? How many dangerous drug interactions have been listed?

Sixth, how inexpensive is inexpensive? Some herbs cost several hundred dollars per month, and most of the expense is not covered by insurance.

45. Name one of seven herbs used to treat *menopause*.

Red clover, black cohosh, licorice, vilex, hops, blue cohosh, chasteberry

46. What naturally occurring brain substance, which is a B vitamin, has been used to help in *obsessive compulsive disorder?*

Inositol

47. Pregnant women are often given a substance to prevent neural tube defects. In some research when this substance plus B$_6$ was added to Prozac, it showed a *mood-lifting* effect for some study participants. Name this substance.

Folic acid

48. Name a plant with a hot-tasting root used to make sauce that is often eaten with prime rib but has also been used to open up sinuses in *allergies*.

Horseradish

49. Name an herb that is hot, red, and tasty and has been used for *arthritis*.

Red pepper

50. Name one of several herbs that have been used for *breast enhancements*.

1. Fenugreek
2. Fennel
3. Saw palmetto
4. Cumin
5. Wild yams

51. Almost any herb could be potentially dangerous, but in general the danger of herbs increases with:
    A. Large or excessive dose.
    B. Pregnant women and children.
    C. Long, known track record of dangers.
    D. Dangerous interactions with concurrent medications.
    E. All of the above.
    F. None of the above.

E. All of the above are true.

52. What ingredient from hot peppers has been used topically for *arthritic pain?*

Capsaicin

53. Name one of several herbs or supplements that have been used for *irritable bowel syndrome*.

1. Ginger
2. Peppermint
3. Tea
4. Onion
5. Psyllium
6. Cinnamon
7. Garlic
8. Valarian
9. Colostrum

54. What delicious fruit has been used for *gout*?

Cherry

55. Name a supplement that has gained recent popularity for everything from *irritable bowel syndrome* to anti-aging. (Hint—After a baby's birth it is the first food from the mother's breast.)

Colostrum

56. What amino acid can be bought over-the-counter and is the amino acid in the central nervous system that has been touted to have *a calming effect*? Can you give reasons it might not work?

GABA. It might not work because of gastric acids, the blood-brain barrier, and because it is probably not the GABA itself that calms.

57. Good genes, not smoking, avoiding the sun, and worrying less are the best wrinkle prevention. However, herbs applied topically have abounded in an attempt to *prevent wrinkles* for years. Name one of them.

1. Cocoa butter
2. Horse chestnut
3. Carrot oil
4. Cucumber
5. Purslane
6. Almond oil
7. Aloe
8. Castor oil
9. Olive oil

58. Name only one of several herbs often used in shampoo and said to offer *dandruff prevention*.

1. Comfrey
2. Rosemary

59. True or False:
*The use of herbs* and supplements is increasing at almost an unbelievable rate.

True

60. While the use of herbs dates back to antiquity, *the establishment of the Office of Dietary Supplements* dates only to what recent year?

1995

61. Name one of several *reasons people use herbs* and supplements.

1. They believe they are safe.
2. They believe natural is better.
3. They believe they cost less.
4. They believe they are stigma free.
5. They believe they are easier to obtain.
6. They believe their mechanism of action is different from present-day

medicine.

7. They are influenced by advertisements.

8. They believe they are not drugs.

9. They believe they work.

10. They do work at times.

62. Which herbs and supplements should be
used by *pregnant women and children?*

Very, very, very few

63. Name one of several topical herbs that have
been used for *poison ivy* and poison oak.

1. Aloe vera
2. Calamine lotion
3. Jewelweed
4. Plantain

64. Name a natural organic acid that has been
used with magnesium in *fibromyalgia.*

Malic acid

65. *Stress* can alter the hypothalamic-pituitary-
adrenal system that results in sustained increase in cortisol
that suppresses brain-derived neurotrophic factor that may
result in atrophy of nerve cells in the hippocampus and
thereby inhibit at times the ability to recognize that a stress is
gone—instead the body remains on high alert as in PTSD
(post-traumatic stress disorder). Name the herb that has been
shown to effectively treat this complex cascade of events.

None

66. Through *PET scans* the uptake of glucose and thus brain
functioning can be visualized in the brain. Patterns consistent
with major depression, ADHD, schizophrenia, OCD,
Alzheimer's, dementia, bipolar highs and lows can be seen
today. Name a major scientific study that shows great promise of altering these patterns with herbs and supplements.

None

67. What famous herb when ingested can
cause *fatal poisoning?*

Mistletoe

68. Name a food that is used for its seasoning
ability and has been touted to help in *high cholesterol,* colds,
and coughing but not for bad breath.

Onion

69. True or False:
Herbs work by different *mechanisms of action* in the body
from regular medications.

False

70. Name the herb that has been used for anxiety
that recently caused some cases of *liver failure.*

Kava

71. Beans and cabbage are said by some to help
in *osteoporosis.* Name an extremely common spice that is on
almost every table that has been touted by some to be of

Black pepper

some help in osteoporosis. Of course, research is lacking, but it is enjoyed by many.

72.   Name one of the most famous and effective                    Digitalis from foxglove plant
      of current *heart medicines* that is derived from a plant.

73.   Although unproved, what potato that grows                    African wild potato
      wild in Africa has been used for treatment of HIV?

74.   Nootropic compounds such as piracetam,                       Smart
      aniracetam, and pramiracetam have been touted as "_____
      drugs" even though numerous human studies have not shown
      memory improvement.

75.   What soybean derivative has been touted                      Phosphatidye serine
      to improve concentration, memory, and mood.

76.   Psychiatric medications today are highly                     None
      specific and often highly selective in how they work. They
      may affect only one neurotransmitter (as the selective sero-
      tonin reuptake neurotransmitters). They may affect subneuro-
      transmitter sites as Remeron does with its $5HT_2$ and $5HT_3$
      post-receptor site antagonism effect. They may affect sub-sub-
      neurotransmitter sites as Imitrex does for migraines. They
      may selectively affect the basal ganglia so there are fewer
      parkinsonian side effects as the new atypical neuroleptics do.
      Name an herb used for emotional purposes that is highly
      specific and highly selective.

77.   Popeye touted that it was good for *nutrition,*               Spinach
      energy, and stimulating growth in children. In reality it does
      contain several vitamins. What is it?

78.   Name a pie that carries this herb's name.                    Rhubarb
      The herb has been touted to help in *gastrointestinal problems.*
      Chronic use could accelerate bone destruction.

79.   Many people like these. A few die annually                   Peanuts
      from them. One president was known for raising them.
      Studies are conflicted in whether they *lower* or raise *choles-
      terol.* Name them.

80.   Although it is important in several body                     Iron
      functions (kreb cycle, hemoglobin function, dopamine activ-
      ity), it will not do all it is touted to do (ADHD, depression,
      *athletic enhancement,* infertility). Name it.

81.   It is used to make bread rise in cooking. A standardized      Brewer's yeast
      product of it has been used in *traveler's diarrhea.* Name it.

82.   It has been used topically to relieve pain and                Camphor
      *itching* by a local vasoconstrictive effect. Through absorption

through the skin, too much of it could be toxic. Name it.

83. It is not effective for autism. It is probably        Vitamin B$_6$—pyridoxine
not effective for *PMS* in most. However, it might help at times
with the nausea of pregnancy. Name this common vitamin.

84. This mineral might help to *lower blood pressure*        Potassium
a little in some people but certainly should not be used as a
major treatment of high blood pressure. Name it.

85. This contains statins and could react with drugs        Red yeast
such as Zocor that contain statins and are often used to
*lower cholesterol* today. Name it.

86. This comes from soy. It has been used for *osteoporosis.*        Ipriflavone
It is touted to have no estrogenic activity, but it has been
shown to increase the effects of estrogen in some studies.

87. It is an FDA-approved drug. It is used in *emergency rooms*        Ipecac
around America. Many mothers whose children have inadver-
tently swallowed the wrong drug are thankful for it. It comes
from South America. Name the herb.

88. It has been touted to decrease *high blood*        Indian snakeroot
*pressure* and was even tried in snakebites by Native
Americans from which it derives its name. However, side
effects are many, even hypertension and depression. Name it.

89. It has been touted to help *insomnia* but may        Nerve root
cause insomnia and hallucinations in some. Name it.

90. This vitamin has been used in helping prevent        Riboflavin—Vitamin B$_2$
*migraines* in some. Name it.

91. It is touted to increase *mental sharpness,* but        RNA/DNA
significant research is lacking. It is touted to help in recovery
time after surgery and serious illness. It carries the ultimate
in strong implications biochemically with its name but fails to
live up to the name implied.

92. It is used for flavoring and as a perfume.        Vanilla
However, the claim that it is an *aphrodisiac* is not substanti-
ated by research.

93. It tastes good. It is bright red. It might even        Strawberry
*slow the aging of the nervous system* a little according to some.
A famous cake carries its name. Name it.

94. One component of this herb has been tried        Potato
for weight loss although it is generally known for weight gain.
One vice president became famous for misspelling this herb.

95. This herb is interesting. Although more research        Astragalus

is needed, some research indicates it might help in the common cold and hepatitis. It has even been given to individuals receiving radiation therapy and chemotherapy for breast cancer.

96. Name an herb that has been touted to help with anxiety. Typically it has been used for *hemorrhoids*. It can be dangerous when combined with alcohol or sedatives.

Catnip

97. What herb is used as a flavoring substance and touted to reduce *gastrointestinal distress* but thins the blood?

Ginger

98. Name a common food crop grown in the south and used orally by some for *dandruff*.

Soybean

99. What tea is extremely popular in China and the USA and has been touted to have *cancer preventing effects*?

Green tea

100. What herb has been used to treat *yeast infections*?

La pacho

101. Bonus Question
True or False:
Concerns about potential long-term carcinogenicity to the bladder have been raised in regard to saccharin.

True

102. Bonus Question
Match the following:
1. Tap Water
2. Hard Water
3. Fluorinated Tap Water
4. Spring Water
5. Purified Drinking Water
6. Distilled Water
7. Carbonated Water
A. Concern of possible osteoporosis.
B. From underground source naturally coming to the surface, not necessarily filtered.
C. Concerns over chlorine, possible pesticides, possible parasites.
D. Contains high concentrations of calcium and magnesium.
E. Various processes are involved to produce this such as reverse osmosis, carbon filtration, ozonation, etc.
F. Can irritate the gastrointestinal tract in those with ulcers.
G. Boiled water that is then condensed (reverse osmosis). This is similar to purified drinking water.

1. C
2. D
3. A
4. B
5. E
6. G
7. F

# Grade—Chapter 15

Number correct _____ + bonus points _____ = _____ Score

*Chapter 16*

# Still More Questions and Answers about Herbs

Following are more questions about herbs. You may want to cover the right side of the page as you answer each of the questions to see how much you really know. Give yourself two points for each correct answer. There are three bonus questions.

| QUESTION | ANSWER |
|---|---|
| 1. What amino acid used in *depression* and insomnia is a precursor of the neurotransmitter serotonin but due to contamination resulted in eosinophilia and death in some? | L-tryptophane |
| 2. What herb has been used topically to treat *athlete's foot?* | Lavender |
| 3. What candy has been used to treat *peptic ulcers* but can carry dangers of high blood pressure? | Licorice |
| 4. Are many of the beliefs about herbs flawed with *a lack of complete understanding* and a lack of sound research? | Yes |
| 5. What common amino acid has been used to treat *cold sores?* | Lysine |
| 6. Name a supplement for hair loss that might help you to *lose your hair* in mega doses. | Selenium |
| 7. Name the *center of the brain for logic,* reason, volition, impulse control, personality, motivation, and action. Any herb or supplement (Saint-John's-wort, SAMe, etc.) or supplement that might increase mood and motiva- | Cerebral cortex |

tion would have to have some effect at this level.

| | | |
|---|---|---|
| 8. | Name *the emotional brain* involved in pain, pleasure, anger, depression, affection, sexuality, and the signal for danger. If inositol ever helps OCD, it would seem to work at this level or at the basal ganglia level. | Limbic system |
| 9. | Name an herb that has been used topically for *blisters* on the feet. | Moleskin |
| 10. | Name the part of the brain that controls *the fight-or-flight experience,* hormonal response, eating habits, and sleep patterns. Any herb that had a calming effect (Valerian, etc.) would have some effect here. | Hypothalamus |
| 11. | This part of the brain produces some important *neurotransmitter* chemicals of the brain such as nor-epinephrine, dopamine, and serotonin. These neurotransmitters are felt to be low in depression, but the lifting of mood is probably much more complex than just increasing these chemicals in the brain, and thus one probably often cannot just give a neurotransmitter or a precursor of a neurotransmitter as often sold at health food stores. The actual antidepressant effects probably have to do with complex secondary messengers with the nerve cell. Name the part of the brain that produces the neurotransmitters. | Midbrain |
| 12. | What herb was used by Native Americans to help as *a smoking deterrent?* It may well illustrate the principle of "burning down the barn to get rid of the rats" since deaths have been reported with its use. | Lobelia or "Indian tobacco" |
| 13. | Name a berry that has incorrectly been thought to be a vegetable. It has high *antioxidant effects.* | Tomato |
| 14. | True or False: The nervous system functions closely with the endocrine system in producing hormones with their effects. *Hormone*-like chemicals are in a delicate balance. Therefore, just taking hormone-like herbal preparations over-the-counter such as DHEA could be dangerous. | True |
| 15. | Many herbs have been tried over the years in an attempt to enhance erections by men. Name one of many herbs tried for *impotence.* | 1. Fava bean<br>2. Yohimbin<br>3. Ginseng<br>4. Gingko<br>5. Velvet bean<br>6. Oat<br>7. Cinnamon<br>8. Anise<br>9. Ginger<br>10. Cardamom |

11. Country mallow
12. Muira puama
13. Quebracho
14. Wolfberry
15. Ashwaganda
16. Guarana

16. Name one of six popular treatments for
    Premenstrual Syndrome (*PMS*).

    Evening primrose oil, dong quai,
    magnesium + B$_6$, calcium, L-tryptophane,
    vilex

17. What percentage of modern-day *medications*
    are *derived from herbs?*

    25 percent

18. True or False:
    Herbs are not *drugs.*

    False—*Herb* means a plant used
    for medicinal purposes.

19. Researchers at UCLA recently documented
    on PET scans that ____ percent of people given placebo
    actually showed increased activity in the frontal lobes of the
    brain, reflecting a true physiologic response to placebo alone.

    25 percent

20. For a psychiatric prescription drug to
    be permitted by the FDA for a disease process, it might need
    to show as much as a _____ percent response rate, a rate
    significantly higher than a placebo response.

    70 percent

21. Fill in the blank:
    When a drug and a placebo are compared in such
    a way that neither the patient nor the doctor knows which
    preparation is being given, the test is called _____.

    Double-blind

22. True or False:
    Most herbs have been studied with
    double-blind tests.

    False

23. Prescription medications must have been
    subjected to animal studies and then four
    phases of human studies with many individuals,
    including placebo-controlled comparisons.
    By contrast, how many phases of human studies
    are mandatory for herbs?

    None. This does not necessarily
    mean they are not effective.
    However, the scientific studies
    are often lacking. Herbs will be
    evaluated more in the future
    with double-blind studies. Some will
    prove effective while others will not.

24. True or False:
    Scientific, double-blind studies back up the
    use of supplements of amino acids for significant *bodybuilding*
    and muscle development.

    False

25. True or False:
    Herbs never work by a *placebo effect.*

    False

26. True or False:
In general, herbs are as *effective* as modern
medicines.

False—At times they do work
but not with the same efficiency overall.

27. True or False:
Overall, herbs have more *side effects* than
modern medicine.

False—Overall they have fewer
side effects and are less effective.

28. Why are herbs and supplements so
*enormously popular?*

The popular belief that natural is better,
safer, and easier.

29. Name a vitamin touted *to help the heart and
skin*. It is touted to scavenger free radicals
and thus might have a protective effect in the brain. It is
touted to help at times in movement disorders (tardive diski-
nesia).

Vitamin E

30. Name the herbal tea that has been used typically
for *yeast infections*.

Chamomile

31. Many herbs have been used for *gas*.
Name just one.

1. Savory
2. Ginger
3. Peppermint
4. Fennel
5. Nutmeg
6. Clove
7. Basil
8. Cinnamon
9. Lemon
10. Sage
11. Thyme
12. Allspice
13. Tarragon
14. Caraway
15. Dill
16. Lavender
17. Onion
18. Rosemary
19. Marjoram

32. Herbs have been used in an attempt to
decrease *gas*. In fact, soaking beans in wormwood as the
Chinese do has been said to work, or soaking beans in
wormseed as the Mexicans do has been said to work, or
soaking beans in a common American vegetable has been
touted to help. Name the vegetable.

Carrot

33. The American Indians knew that corn
might be good for more than food. What part of corn has
been used for its reported *diuretic effect?*

Corn silk

34. Name an herb that is often found in

Comfrey

over-the-counter topical preparations for bruises. According to folklore this may be the best known.

35. Name an herb eaten worldwide that is touted by some to have *antihypertensive and anticonvulsant effects*.

Celery
Celery would pale into insignificance compared to the new antiseizure medications such as Depakote, Dilartin, Tegretol, Trileptal, Lamictol, Topama, and many more. They are specific in how they work. They are usually highly effective along with the skill of a neurologist.

36. True or False:
Herbs that are touted to do simply everything would be akin to *the old medicine man* who roamed from town to town.

True

37. What herb along with its close cousin, blueberry, has been touted to help in *cataract prevention*? It certainly should not be used with aspirin or nonsteroidial anti-inflammatory drugs. It also could be dangerous with insulin since it might lower blood sugar.

Bilberry

38. Pick the one of the following that does not match up as usual touted helps with herbs:
A. *Athlete's foot*—topical garlic and ginger
B. *MS*—nettle, blueberry, black current, magnesium, evening primrose, and pineapple.
C. *Insomnia*—coffee

C. Coffee is a stimulant. It tends to cause insomnia.

39. Name an herb often found in beauty lotions that is touted to reduce *wrinkles*.

Sea buckthorn

40. Milk thistle has been used in *hepatitis*. Name another herb that has been used in hepatitis.

Schisandra

41. True or False:
Many herbs (garlic, ginger, licorice, teatree, echinacea, goldenseal, lemongrass, arrowroot, cinnamon, turmeric, etc.) are touted to help various infections with either antiseptic, antifungal, or antiviral qualities. However in some cases side effects are severe, and they rarely hold the degree of effectiveness or specificity of modern-day antibiotics.

True

42. What herb is touted to be over 100 times *sweeter than sugar*? It has been used in baking and is calorie free. This is number one in sweetness.

Stevia

43. What Mediterranean herb has been used in *sinusitis*?

Thyme

44. Every child used to live in dreaded fear of

Caster oil

this terrible herbal laxative on the old grocery store shelf. What was it?

45.  *Heartburn* has been touted to be helped by angelica, chamomile, and licorice. Why not just go to these when the pain is severe?

Gastroesophageal reflux disease can usually be treated successfully today by an internist with several different new medications such as $H_2$ receptor antagonists and proton pump inhibitors.

Licorice can have dangerous side effects as can angelica.

Why not be under the care of a medical doctor anytime a significant medical disease exists?

46.  Psychiatric medications work by various mechanisms other than just altering neurotransmitter levels. Name one.

1. Regulating receptor site.
2. Altering ion transport at the cell membrane.
3. Altering secondary messenger system.
4. Altering BDNF (brain-derived neurotrophic factor).
5. Altering DNA with the nucleus of the brain cell.

47.  There are many different classes of antidepressants today. Also, while not classified as antidepressants, several drugs have been used for their reported antidepressant effects. Several drugs are currently being tested for their antidepressant effects. Name one drug that has been used for its antidepressant effects.

1. TCAs (tricyclic antidepressants)
     Amitriptyline (Elavil, Endep)
     Clomipramine (Anafranil)
     Doxepin (Adapin, Sinequan)
     Imipramine (Tofranil)
     Trimipramine (Surmontil)
     Desipramine (Norpramin)
     Nortriptyline (Pamelor, Aventyl)
     Protriptyline (Vivactil)
2. Tetracyclic antidepressants
     Amoxapine (Asendin)
     Maprotiline (Ludiomil)
     Mirtazapine (Remeron)
3. SSRIs (selective serotonin reuptake inhibitors)
     Citalopram (Celexa)
     Fluoxetine (Prozac, Sarafem)
     Fluvoxamine (LuVox)
     Paroxetine (Paxil)
     Sertraline (Zoloft)
4. MAOIs (monoamine oxidase inhibitors)
     Phenelzine (Nardil)

Tranylcypromine (Parnate)

5. Atypical antidepressants
   Bupropion (Wellbutrin and Wellbutrin SR)
   Nefazodone (Serzone)
   Trazodone (Desyrel)
   Venlafaxine (Effexor and Effexor XR)
6. Benzodiazepine
   Xanax (Alprasolam)
7. Mood Stabilizers
   Eskalith, lithobid (Lithium Carbonate)
   Topamax (Topiramate)
8. Psychostimulants
   Adderall
   Ritalin
   Dexedrine
9. Major tranquilizers (Neuroleptics)
   Geodon
10. Minor tranquilizers
    BuSpar (Buspirone)
11. Duel dopamine/serotonin reuptake Antagonist
    Minaprine
    Bazinaprine
12. Serotonin 1D antagonist
    CP–448, 187
13. 5HT1A Agonist
    Gepirone ER
14. Substance P
15. Reversible MAOIs
    Broforamine
    Befloxatone
    RS–8359
16. Hormones
    Thyroid hormones
    Estrogen
17. Provigil (Modafinil)
18. Ultram (Tramadol)
19. Lexapro (Escitalopram)
20. Sigma/5HT1A Agonist/5HT Reuptake Inhibitors

48. Name the enzyme system of the liver that metabolizes many of the top-selling drugs and herbs and therefore could be important in potential drug-herb interactions.

P450 (CYP)

49. Twelve gene families have been identified

Saint-John's-wort

in the P450 (CYP) enzyme system. Three especially are often of significance in drug-herb interactions (CYP2C, CYP2D6, and CYP3A4). Which herb touted for depression could be dangerous when used with other drugs that inhibit CYP3A4?

50.  Psychotherapy alone may work in some
      cases through
      a.
      b.
      to improve brain chemistry as revealed
      in PET scans of the brain in depression
      and OCD.

      a. Hope (placebo study)
      b. Behavioral-cognitive choices

51.  Bonus Question
      Life is filled with paradoxes. Here is one. A common food
      often served with Mexican meals is high in cholesterol but
      can lower bad blood cholesterol. What is it?

      Avocado

52.  Bonus Question
      The rain forests of South America are
      quickly being destroyed. This is unfortunate
      since perhaps 25 percent or more of our current medicines
      were originally derived from herbs. All of the following are
      current herbs from the rain forest except which one?
      Incidentally, for herbs to become accepted medicines, they
      usually must show effectiveness in double-blind studies, have
      official recognition by medical associations, have wide use by
      physicians, and have publications in medical journals. These
      herbs do not have that yet.
      A.  Annato in skin care products for wrinkles
      B.  Jatoba touted for infections
      C.  Shiitake
      D.  Sangre de grado touted for infections

      C. Shiitake from Japan.
      The rest are from the rain
      forests of South America.

53.  Bonus Question
      True or False:
      There are several types of ginseng (Korean, American,
      Siberian, etc.), and they can vary widely in their effects.

      True

# Grade—Chapter 16

Number correct _____ + bonus points _____ multiplied by 2 = _____ Score

## Chapter 17

# Questions and Answers about Vitamins

The following questions review your knowledge of vitamins. You may want to cover the right side of the page as you answer each of the questions to see how much you really know. Give yourself four points for each correct answer. There is one bonus question.

| QUESTION | ANSWER |
|---|---|
| 1. Name substances that are essential to life, regulate metabolism, assist in biological processes, are considered micronutrients, are required in minimal amounts to ward off some diseases, and have been touted in recent years in larger amounts for many ailments. | Vitamins |
| 2. Name a vitamin that has been used topically for acne. | Vitamin A |
| 3. Name a compound related to vitamin A that has been touted for cancer prevention, but some studies point to it possibly causing some forms of cancer. | Beta carotene |
| 4. Name a vitamin often given to alcoholics. | Vitamin B (thiamine) |
| 5. Name a vitamin that has been touted for migraine headaches and cataract prevention. | Vitamin $B_2$ (riboflavin) |
| 6. Name a vitamin that has been touted for lowering cholesterol, schizophrenia, and memory enhancement. It might elevate blood sugar in diabetics and in large amounts could damage the liver in some. | Vitamin $B_3$ (niacin) |
| 7. What vitamin is known as "the antistress vitamin" and is involved in the production of some neuro-transmitters? | Vitamin $B_5$ (pantothenic acid) |

8.  Name a vitamin that has been touted to help in PMS, depression, and kidney stones.

Vitamin $B_6$ (pyridoxine)

9.  A deficiency of this vitamin can cause a severe (pernicious) anemia. Name it.

Vitamin $B_{12}$ (cyanocobalamin)

10. A deficiency of this vitamin could cause seborrheic dermatitis (cradle cap) in infants. Name it.

Biotin

11. This vitamin is important in pregnancy in preventing neural tube defects and has been used with $B_6$ to help in some depression. Name it.

Folic acid

12. Name the vitamin that has been tried for OCD but in rare cases has induced mania. It has also been touted to lower cholesterol.

Inositol

13. Name the vitamin that has been used topically to protect against sunburn. It has even been touted in certain cases to turn gray hair to its original color.

PABA (para-aminobenzoic acid)

14. What vitamin is required for many, many metabolic functions; is needed for the metabolism of folic acid, tyosine, and phenylalanine; is touted to lower cholesterol and high blood pressure; protects against bruising; and is found in citrus fruit?

Vitamin C (ascorbic acid)

15. This vitamin has been touted to help in preventing diabetes mellitus type I in children. Name it.

Vitamin D

16. This vitamin has become popular in recent years because of several touted benefits in various diseases: dementia, cardiovascular disease, cancer, PMS, fibrocystic disease, high blood pressure, and cataracts. Often significant research is lacking, but it may have benefit. It is a good antioxidant. Name it.

Vitamin E

17. This vitamin is necessary for blood clotting. It can be toxic in large doses for the fetus during the last few weeks of pregnancy. It can interfere with blood thinning medications. Name it.

Vitamin K

18. Name a vitamin-like substance that has been used much in athletic injuries.

Bioflavonoids (citrin, eriodictyol, flavones, hesperetin, hesperidin, quercetin, quercetrin, and rutin)

19. Name a popular vitamin-like substance that has been touted for heart disease, high blood pressure, diabetes mellitus, aging, obesity, MS, and ulcers. It is a strong antioxidant and thus has been touted to boost the immune system.

Coenzyme Q10

20. Which vitamin does not match up with
the stated deficiency disease:
A. Rickets—Vitamin D
B. Pernicious Anemia—Vitamin $B_6$
C. Scurvy—Vitamin C
D. Tooth decay—Vitamin C
E. Pellagra—Niacin

D is the wrong match. Too
much chewable vitamin C might
damage tooth enamel.

21. Name a vitamin that has been tried in
Alzheimer's dementia because of deficiencies of the neurotransmitter acetylcholine in this dementia. It has also been
tried in TD (tardive depkinesia) and parkinsonism.

Choline

22. This vitamin would not be
recommended in ovarian cancer. Name it.

Folic acid

23. Name the vitamin that should be taken
with calcium.

Vitamin D

24. Name a popular vitamin-like substance that
might preserve health when a small amount of vitamin E is
present with it.

Coenzyme Q10

25. True or False:
Usually oil-soluble vitamins (A, D, E, K) should be taken
before meals, and water-soluble vitamins (C, Bs) should be
taken after meals.

True

26. What B vitamin has been used for mixed
hyperlipidemia?

Niacin (vitamin $B_3$)

27. What vitamin can inhibit the hypopro-
thrombinemic effect of the anitcoagulant drug warfarin?

Vitamin K

28. What vitamin can induce hypercalcemia and
increase the effects of the heart medicine digoxin and,
thereby, lead to cardiac arrhythmias?

Vitamin D

29. Tobacco decreases the body's ability to absorb
which vitamins?

Vitamins $B_6$ and C

30. If one is on Sinemet for parkinsonism, what
vitamin should be avoided for the most part?

Vitamin $B_6$

31. Oral contraceptives decrease the body's
ability to absorb which vitamins and minerals?

Vitamins $B_1$, $B_2$, $B_3$, $B_6$,
$B_{12}$, folic acid ($B_9$)
Minerals calcium, magnesium, zinc

32. Antacids decrease the body's ability to
absorb which vitamins and minerals?

Vitamins A, $B_1$, folic acid ($B_9$)
Minerals calcium, copper, iron, phospho-
rus

33. Diuretics such as thiazides, furosemide, and

Vitamins $B_2$ and folic acid ($B_9$)

triamterone decrease the body's ability to absorb which vitamins and minerals?

Minerals calcium, magnesium, potassium, zinc

## Grade—Chapter 17

Number correct _____ + bonus points _____ multiplied by 3 = _____ Score

# Chapter 18

# Questions and Answers about Minerals

The following questions review your knowledge of minerals. You may want to cover the right side of the page as you answer each of the questions to see how much you really know. Give yourself four points for each correct answer.

| QUESTION | ANSWER |
|---|---|
| 1. What are naturally occurring elements found in the earth and rock formations, are involved in chemical processes in the body, and touted for various health issues. | Minerals |
| 2. Name one of several bulk minerals. | 1. Calcium<br>2. Magnesium<br>3. Sodium<br>4. Potassium<br>5. Phosphorus |
| 3. Name one of several trace minerals. | 1. Boron<br>2. Chromium<br>3. Copper<br>4. Germanium<br>5. Iodine<br>6. Iron<br>7. Manganese<br>8. Molybdenum<br>9. Selenium<br>10. Silicon<br>11. Silver<br>12. Vanadium<br>13. Zinc |
| 4. Why are trace minerals called "trace," | Only minute amounts are |

and what implications does that have
for consumption?

needed, and they could be
toxic in large amounts.

5.  What trace element mineral has been
    touted as "the missing" one and has been touted as "a foun-
    tain of youth" although significant research is lacking in
    regard to effectiveness and side effects?

    Indium

6.  What trace mineral has been touted to
    lower blood sugar but carries some question of cancer, espe-
    cially in high dosages?

    Chromium

7.  What mineral has been touted for
    strong bones, teeth, and counteracting osteoporosis?

    Calcium

8.  What trace mineral in excess might be
    associated with depression?

    Copper

9.  What trace mineral has been touted
    for a healthy thyroid gland?

    Iodine

10. What trace mineral is sometimes given to
    those with one form of anemia?

    Iron for iron
    deficiency anemia

11. What mineral has been touted for
    anxiety and fibromyalgia?

    Magnesium

12. What mineral is important in a regular
    heartbeat?

    Potassium

13. What trace mineral has been used for hair
    loss but in excess might contribute to it further?

    Selenium

14. What trace mineral is often restricted in
    high blood pressure?

    Sodium

15. What trace mineral has been touted to
    help in colds?

    Zinc

16. What trace mineral has been touted for
    types I and II diabetes mellitus but has serious problems in a
    few?

    Vanadium

17. What line of antibiotics involved this
    trace mineral?

    Sulfur (the sulfur drugs)

18. What trace mineral is found in avocados,
    whole grains, blueberries, egg yolks, green vegetables, pineap-
    ples, and alfalfa? It is touted to be important in a healthy
    immune system.

    Manganese

19. This trace mineral is important in healthy
    nails, and some have touted that since it might have an antag-

    Silicon

onist effect on aluminum it might help prevent Alzheimer's disease (this is without research backing).

20. What trace mineral might help calcium                    Boron
    absorption in the elderly and is touted to help prevent post-
    menopausal osteoporosis?

21. Name a mineral that has been the backbone                Lithium carbonate
    of the treatment of manic depressive disorder for over 50
    years.

22. Name a disease due to a mineral deficiency               Pica
    characterized by children eating dirt.

23. True or False:                                           True
    Fiber might decrease the absorption of minerals.

24. Which of the following possibilities does not            G. They all possibly could
    match the diseases with excess amounts?                  match at times.
    A. Germanium—kidney disease
    B. Chromium—cancer
    C. Zinc—suppressed immune system
    D. Vanadyl—liver disease
    E. Sodium—high blood pressure
    F. Molybdenum—gout
    G. They all could match.

25. An excess of this mineral could result in                Iron
    constipation for some.

# Grade—Chapter 18

Number correct _____ + bonus points _____ multiplied by 4 = _____ Score

*Chapter 19*

# Questions and Answers about Amino Acids

How much do you know about amino acids? You may want to cover the right side of the page as you answer each of the questions to see how much you really know. Give yourself four points for each correct answer. There is one bonus question.

| QUESTION | ANSWER |
|---|---|
| 1. What are the building blocks of proteins that provide the structure of every living organism and support for metabolic pathways to keep us healthy? Supplements of these have become very popular in recent years. | Amino acids |
| 2. Some have claimed that taking this amino acid at bedtime can help prevent nighttime hypoglycemia (although significant research is lacking). | Alanine |
| 3. Some claim that this amino acid in large doses might produce side effects such as an increase of any already present herpes infection, worsening of schizophrenia, and thickening of the skin. Name it. | Arginine |
| 4. The artificial sweetener aspartame is made from this amino acid plus phenylalanine. This amino acid is touted to be good in depression and fatigue and to help the immune system. | Aspartic acid |
| 5. This is one of the more popular amino acids because it has been touted to help in weight loss, fatigue, high triglycerides, Alzheimer's dementia, aging, peripheral neuropathy of diabetes, and depression. However, there are different forms and the DL form can be toxic. Name it. | Carnitine |

6.  Name an amino acid that has been touted to promote energy, protect the liver, and enhance energy.                                    Citrulline

7.  Name an amino acid that is touted to help protect the liver when it has been damaged by alcohol, to help the skin look younger, to promote wound healing, and to help in RA (rheumatoid arthritis). However, it could be dangerous for those with diabetes since it can inactivate insulin.                                    Cysteine

8.  What amino acid is a neurotransmitter that is involved in a relaxing effect? It has been used for anxiety, high blood pressure, enlarged prostate, ADHD, and alcohol cravings. It does not appear addicting, but it could possibly paradoxically increase anxiety at times and even cause seizures.                                    GABA (gamma-aminobutyric acid)

9.  What amino acid is an excitatory neurotransmitter? It has been touted for personality disorders and hypoglycemia. It has trouble crossing the blood-brain barrier.                                    Glutamic acid

10. What amino acid is the most abundant in muscles of the body, passes the blood-brain barrier, and has been touted for a variety of mental disorders?                                    Glutamine

11. What amino acid has been touted for seizures, bipolar disorders, and a healthy prostate? However, research is lacking.                                    Glycine

12. This amino acid is touted to aid in sexual arousal. Name it.                                    Histidine

13. High levels of this amino acid might be associated with increased risk of heart disease. Name it.                                    Homocysteine

14. What amino acid is a branched-chain amino acid (along with isoleucine and valine) and is touted to lower high blood sugar?                                    Leucine

15. What amino acid has been touted to help fight cold sores and herpes viruses?                                    Lysine

16. What amino acid has been touted to help protect the liver and to help in schizophrenia by lowering histamine? Research is lacking.                                    Methionine

17. Sometimes amino acids might make certain conditions worse. Pick the correct answer of the condition possibly made worse by the amino acid.
    A. Herpes—arginine
    B. Diabetes—cysteine
    C. Migraines precipitated by MSG—glutamic acid
    D. Bipolar disorder—histadine                                    G. All of the above.

E. Schizophrenia—ornithine
F. Major depressions treated with
MAO inhibitors—tyrosine
G. All of the above

18. What amino acid has been touted to          Phenylalanine
elevate mood, decrease pain, enhance memory, and suppress
appetite? It has been touted for schizophrenia, PMS, and
parkinsonism. Significant research is lacking.

19. This amino acid is touted to produce          Proline
healthy-looking skin. Name it.

20. This amino acid is a component of          Serine
many skin care preparations. Name it.

21. This amino acid is touted for high          Taurine
blood pressure, anxiety, prevention of cardiac arrhythmias,
hypoglycemia, and seizures. Research is lacking. Name it.

22. This amino acid is touted to enhance          Threonine
the production of antibodies, help in depression, and help to
prevent fatty buildup in the liver.

23. Name the amino acid that, probably          Tryptophane
because of contaminants, resulted in more than 30 deaths in
the United States.

24. This amino acid is a precursor of the          Tyrosine
neurotransmitters adrenaline, norepinephrine, and dopamine.
It has been touted for fatigue, narcolepsy, depression, drug
withdrawal, parkinsonism, and low sex drive. It is dangerous
with MAO inhibitors.

25. High levels of this amino acid might          Valine
produce hallucinations. Name it.

26. Bonus Question          Methyl alcohol
Fill in the blank:
Aspartame consists of two amino acids (phenylalanine and
aspartic acid) and methanol, which is also called _____
_____. The question of toxicity has arisen with methanol,
especially in larger than modest amounts. The question of
increased aggression has arisen with aspartic acid in bipolar
disorders.

# Grade—Chapter 19

Number correct _____ + bonus points _____ multiplied by 4 = _____ Score

## Chapter 20

# Questions and Answers about Antioxidants, Enzymes, and Hormones

The following review questions cover antioxidants, enzymes, and hormones. You may want to cover the right side of the page as you answer each of the questions to see how much you really know. Give yourself four points for each correct answer.

| **QUESTION** | | **ANSWER** |
|---|---|---|
| 1. | Fill in the blank: | Antioxidants |
| | _____ are naturally occurring substances that help to neutralize free radicals that are touted to cause cancer, aging, and other diseases. | |

In questions 2–13 indicate whether the following substances are high in antioxidants or high in free radical production.

| 2. | Alpha-lipoic acid | | Antioxidants |
|---|---|---|---|
| 3. | Tobacco | | Free radicals |
| 4. | Bilberry | | Antioxidants |
| 5. | The sun | | Free radicals |
| 6. | Coenzyme Q10 | | Antioxidants |
| 7. | Hydrogen peroxide | | Free radicals |
| 8. | Grape seed, gingko, glutathione | | Antioxidants |
| 9. | Radiation | | Free radicals |
| 10. | Polluted air | | Free radicals |

| | | |
|---|---|---|
| 11. | Melatonin and methionine | Antioxidants |
| 12. | Flavonoids | Antioxidants |
| 13. | Vitamins A, C, E, and Zinc | Antioxidants |
| 14. | Fill in the blank: | Hormones |

14. Fill in the blank:

_____ are substances that have become popular in recent years. They are secreted by the endocrine glands, but plant forms of similar substances are often sold as supplements. Sometimes the substances decrease with age, and various replacements are in vogue. They can have powerful effects as well as side effects at times.

In questions 15–20 indicate true or false for the following touted combinations:

| QUESTION | ANSWER |
|---|---|
| 15. Natural progesterone—menopause and depression | True |
| 16. Estrogen-like substances (evening primrose oil, dong quai, chasteberry)—PMS | True |
| 17. DHEA—Diabetes Mellitus | False—DHEA can cause an insulin resistance and thus make diabetes worse. |
| 18. Wild yams—menopause | True |
| 19. Human growth hormone—aging | True |
| 20. Estrogen-like hormones (soy, red clover, black cohosh)—menopause | True |
| 21. Fill in the blank: | Enzymes |

21. Fill in the blank:

_____ are necessary in all biochemical activities and functions in the body. Some may decrease with age, so replacement has become popular.

| | |
|---|---|
| 22. True or false: Digestive enzymes—pancreatin and pepsin | True |
| 23. True or false: Enzymes that dissolve protein—pepsin, trypsin, rennin, pancreatin, chymotrypsin | True |
| 24. True or false: Pancreatin has been touted to help in digestion, injuries, and viral infections. | True |
| 25. All of the following are enzymes except one. Which one is not an enzyme? | K. Plasma is not an enzyme. Rather, it is a blood product. |

A. Amylace
B. Lipace
C. Lactase
D. Bromelain
E. Cellulose
F. Maltase
G. Papain
H. Pepsin
I. Pectinase
J. Plasmin
K. Plasma

## Grade—Chapter 20

Number correct _____ + bonus points _____ multiplied by 4 = _____ Score

# Chapter 21

# Questions and Answers about the Dangers of Herbs

The following questions review the dangers of herbs. You may want to cover the right side of the page as you answer each of the questions to see how much you really know. Give yourself two points for each correct answer. There are six bonus questions.

Following each herb and its possible matches in questions 1–37, indicate whether the whole match is true or false. Use T for true and F for false.

| Herb | Possible Country of Original Use | Time of Original Use | One Disease Touted to Help | One Possible Side Effect | True or False |
|---|---|---|---|---|---|
| 1. Kelp | North America | 1800s | Hypothyroid | Hyperthyroid | T |
| 2. Horsetail | Europe | 1700s | Sprained muscle | Kidney damage | T |
| 3. Passion-flower | South America | 1600s | Anxiety | Sedation | T |
| 4. Schizandra | China | 1400s | Low sex drive | Gastrointestinal upset | T |
| 5. Shiitake mushroom | Japan | 1300s | Poor health | Not known | T |
| 6. Anise | Greece | 1400s | Cough | Toxic | T |
| 7. Dong quai | China | 2000 BC | Menopause | Estrogen-like side effects | T |
| 8. Evening primrose | North America | 1700s | Female problems | Seizures | T |
| 9. Fenugreek | Egypt | 1500 BC | Diabetes mellitus | Uterine stimulant | T |
| 10. Milk thistle | Rome | First century AD | Liver problems | Allergic reactions | T |

| | | | | | |
|---|---|---|---|---|---|
| 11. Mustard | Rome | First century AD | Common cold | Accentuate asthma | T |
| 12. Parsley | Greece | | Bad breath | Heart disease in high doses | T |
| 13. Pumpkin | North America | For centuries | BPH | | T |
| 14. Aloe | Greece | 30s | Topically for skin irritations | Death with IV use | T |
| 15. Boneset | North America | 1800s | Common cold | Coma and death | T |
| 16. Cardamom | India | 100s | Gas | Gallstone colic | T |
| 17. Cayenne | North America | 1400s | Topically for arthritis | Possible skin cancer with repeated use | T |
| 18. Cleavers | Britain | 1600s | Constipation | Complications in diabetes | T |
| 19. Dandelion | Arabia | 900s | Swelling of PMS | Poisoning from herbicides | T |
| 20. Echinacea | North America | 1300s | Common cold | Damage to reproductive cells in females | T |
| 21. Feverfew | Greece | 1000 BC | Migraine headaches | Mouth sores | T |
| 22. Garlic | Both West and East | Antiquity | High blood pressure | Odor pressure | T |
| 23. Gentian | Bosnia | 200 BC | Gas | Gastrointestinal irritation. This herb often grows next to hellebore, which is highly toxic. | T |
| 24. Ginger | Greece | 2000 BC | Gastrointestinal distress | Gastrointestinal distress | T |
| 25. Ginseng | China | 2000 BC | Low sex drive | Insomnia | T |
| 26. Horse-radish | Controversial | First century AD | Sinus congestion | Especially dangerous with ulcers | T |
| 27. Kava | Polynesia | First century AD | Anxiety | Liver failure | T |
| 28. Lemon balm | Rome | First century AD | Depression | Interfere with thyroid medication | T |
| 29. Licorice | China ("The grandfather of Chinese herbs") | 1000 BC | Peptic ulcers | High blood pressure | T |
| 30. Marsh-mallow | Syria | 1000 BC | Mouth irritations | None for most | T |
| 31. Mother-wort | Rome | First century AD | Rapid heart rate | Uterine contractions | T |
| 32. Mugwort | Germany | Middle Ages | Insomnia | Possible poisoning in high doses | T |
| 33. Turmeric | India | First century AD | Inflammation | Stomach irritation | T |
| 34. Valerian | Greece | Fourth century AD | Anxiety | Addiction | T |
| 35. Bilberry | North America | 1300s | Bruising | Hypoglycemia | T |

| | | | | | |
|---|---|---|---|---|---|
| | | | | in diabetics | |
| 36. Winter-green | North America | 1200s | Sore throat | Possible Reye's Syndrome in children since it contains salicylates | T |
| 37. Gingko | Asia | One of the oldest many believe | Dementia | Spontaneous brain hemorrhage and death | T |

Yes, unfortunately, they all can be true at times. Any herb can have almost any side effect known to man. This chapter does not begin to detail all the possible side effects of the many herbs, vitamins, minerals, amino acids, hormones, and supplements. Some herbs and supplements are just plain dangerous. Others become more dangerous as the dose is increased. Some are all right topically but not internally. Most are not safe for pregnant women and children. Some are dangerous to a select populous with a specific disease or physiology. Overall herbs usually have fewer side effects than prescription medications, but either can potentially be dangerous. Even peanuts result in a few deaths every year. For more information on possible dangers please see the Natural Medicines Comprehensive Database 2002 (phone: 209–472–2244; fax: 209–472–2249). At times all of the dangers are just not known. So while herbs have helped many through the years and can be safe at times, the above are just a few of the reasons never to pick up any herb book, including this one, for specific health needs.

And yes, herbs come from almost every part of the plant and almost every country.

The following questions address more of the dangers of herbs.

**QUESTION**

38.  Which of the following is not an especially dangerous herb?
A. Cannabis sativa (marijuana)
B. Tobacco
C. Opium poppy
D. Hallucinogenic mushrooms
E. Spinach
F. Moldy rye (ergot)

39.  Which combination is not considered potentially dangerous?
A. Saint-John's-wort and antidepressants
B. Gingko and aspirin
C. Licorice and digoxin
D. Ephedra and MAOs
E. Belladonna and anticholinergics
F. Inositol and lithium
G. Omega-3 fatty acids and Coumadin
H. Echinacea and reproductive females
I. Saint-John's-wort and Indinavir (for AIDS)
J. Maca and prostate cancer history
K. Eucalyptus and seizure history
L. Wild marshmallow and diabetes mellitus
M. Herbal laxatives and beta blockers
N. Echinacea and immunosuppressants

**ANSWER**

E. Spinach, although not always loved, is not usually dangerous. In fact, it is very healthy.

L. Wild (not commercial) marshmallow might even lower blood sugar a little in some.

O. Gingko and Trazadone
P. Kava and Alprazolam
Q. Passa Flora Incanta and SSRIs
R. Reserpine and antihypertensives
S. Inositol and Lithium
T. Gingko and Coumadin or nonsteroidal
   Anti-inflammatory drugs
U. Omega-3 fatty acids and Coumadin

40. All of the following herbs are inclined
    to raise blood sugar except which one?
    A. Bee pollen
    B. Glucosamine
    C. Sugar
    D. Fenugreek

D. Fenugreek

41. All of the following herbs and minerals
    are inclined to raise blood pressure
    except which one?
    A. Ephedra
    B. Caffeine
    C. Guarana
    D. Potassium
    E. Yohimbe
    F. Ginseng
    G. Goldenseal

D. Potassium has been touted
to lower blood pressure. This
seems minimal at best.
It should be noted that ginseng
might have paradoxical effects
in blood pressure. In low doses
it might increase blood
pressure, but in higher doses it
might lower blood pressure.

42. All of the following have had cases of liver
    damage reported with use except which one?
    A. Kava
    B. Valerian
    C. Topical comfrey

C. I was recently in an old
country store and noted that
they had an ointment for sale
for chapped lips. It contained
vitamin E plus comfrey. It should be
noted that oral comfrey is highly toxic
and can cause liver damage. It has been
touted for short-term topical use.

43. All of the following are well known for
    their interactions with other drugs except which one?
    A. Saint-John's-Wort
    B. Grapefruit juice
    C. Coffee
    D. Folic acid + $B_6$

D. Folic acid + $B_6$

44. Questions of causing cancer at excessive
    levels have been raised with all of the
    following except which one?
    A. Beta carotene
    B. Chromium
    C. SAMe
    D. Vitamin C
    E. Strawberry

E. Strawberry. This herb has
not had any questions raised in
regard to cancer.

45.  All of the following have estrogen-like
     components except which one?
     A.  Soy
     B.  Black cohosh
     C.  Vitex
     D.  Chasteberry
     E.  Red clover
     F.  Stevia
     G.  Licorice
     H.  Evening primrose oil
     I.  Dong quai

F. Stevia

46.  All of the following can cause increased bleeding
     except which one?
     A.  Potassium
     B.  Ginseng
     C.  Ginger
     D.  Garlic
     E.  Gingko
     F.  Fenugreek
     G.  Willow
     H.  Omega-3 fatty acids

A. Potassium

47.  Herbs and supplements may become more
     dangerous with all of the following except:
     A.  Large doses
     B.  Use in pregnant females and children
     C.  Contamination
     D.  Long use
     E.  Under the care of a physician
     F.  Known as dangerous
     G.  Idiosyncratic reactions
     H.  Certain combinations

E. Under the care of a physician.
Medical doctors understand the
complexities of the human
body. They understand disease.
They understand potential drug
interactions. They usually know
the scientific research behind
the validity of various herbs
and supplements.

48.  Herbs that are especially contraindicated
     during pregnancy because they stimulate
     uterine contractions include all of the following
     except which one?
     A.  Pennyroyal
     B.  Goldenseal
     C.  Lovage
     D.  Mugwood
     E.  Yarrow
     F.  Shepherd's purse
     G.  Black cohosh
     H.  Blue cohosh
     I.  Angelica
     J.  Mistletoe
     K.  Tansy
     L.  Folic acid

L. Folic acid. All of the rest can
stimulate uterine contractions.

M. Wild ginger
N. Rue
O. Coffee in excess

49. Fill in the blank:
While natural products are safe for
many people, side effects are possible. Over _____ deaths
have been reported to the FDA and over _____ serious
side effects.

Over 100 deaths.
Over 1,000 serious side effects.

50. All of the following natural products are
currently (2002) being reviewed by the
FDA because of health concerns except
which one?

| Natural Product | Possible Concern |
| --- | --- |
| A. Chaparral | Liver toxicity |
| B. Chromium | Kidney toxicity |
| C. Glucosamine | Increased blood glucose in diabetics |
| D. Melatonin | Impurities |
| E. Saw palmetto | Heart problems |
| F. Shark cartilage | Hepatitis |
| G. Potato | Weight gain |

G. While too many potatoes
can certainly cause weight gain,
they are not under review by
the FDA.

51. Bonus Question
Fill in the blank:
_____, an herbal supplement with estrogen-like effects, is
sold for "prostate health," but in some cases it has been
found to be contaminated with warfarin, a strong prescription blood-thinning medication. It has also been found contaminated with Xanax, a minor tranquilizer, and indocin, an
antiinflammatory drug.

PC Spes

52. Bonus Question
True or False:
In 1991 and 1992, approximately 100 women in Brussels who
had taken a preparation of Chinese herbs for weight loss
developed impairment in renal function with 70 requiring
dialysis or transplantation. Aristolochic acid, a known nephrotoxin, had apparently contaminated the preparations.

True

53. Bonus Question
Which of the following herbal preparations
have recently been found to have contaminations?
A. Echinacea touted for the common cold—
possible organochlorine pesticide
contamination
B. Melatonin touted for insomnia—
possible L-tryptophane, associated with
eosinophilia and death contamination

C. Both echinacea and
melatonin have recently been
found to contain contaminants.

C. Both of the above
D. Neither of the above

54.    Bonus Question
Name dangers of herbs from exogenous sources.

Pesticides

55.    Bonus Question
A. Some store-bought fresh fish may
not be safe if consumed too frequently
because they contain mercury.
Name some of these.

1. Swordfish
2. Shark
3. Tilefish
4. King
5. Mackerel
6. Marlin

B. Name some fish that are probably safe in
regard to the lack of excessive
mercury content.

1. Salmon
2. Sardines
3. Sole
4. Freshwater catfish
5. Tilapia
6. Farm-raised trout
7. Shrimp
8. Scallops
9. Canned tuna

56.    Bonus Question
Recently (May 2004) a dirty dozen of
dietary supplements were listed on Web
MD with AOL Health. These supplements
were listed because they may cause
cancer, severe liver or kidney damage,
heart problems, or death. How many of
the twelve can you name? Number 1 is
listed as definitely hazardous, 2 through 6
are listed as very likely hazardous, and 7
through 12 are listed as likely hazardous.

1.  Aristolochic acid (snakeroot
and other names)—cancer,
kidney failure
2.  Comfrey (black root and
other names)—liver
damage, death
3.  Androstenedione—cancer
risk, lower HDL (the good
cholesterol)
4.  Chaparral—abnormal liver
function
5.  Germander—abnormal liver function
6.  Kava—abnormal liver function
7.  Bitter orange—high blood pressure, heart arrhythmias, myocardial
infarction, stroke
8.  Organ/glandular extracts—theoretical risk of mad cow disease
9.  Lobelia (wild tobacco and other
names)—rapid heartbeat, difficulty
breathing
10.  Pennyroyal oil (mosquito plant,
squaw balm, stinking balm, tickweed,
and other names)—liver failure,
kidney failure, nerve damage, convulsions, abdominal tenderness,

death
11. Scullcap (mad dog herb, skullcap, and other names)—liver damage
12. Yohimbe—heart arrhythmias, increased blood pressure, myocardial infarction

## Grade—Chapter 21

Number correct _____ + bonus points _____ multiplied by 2 = _____ Score

## Chapter 22

# Natural Products from A to Z—
# a Fair Approach

In the following chapter natural products are covered from A to Z. Each product is given one salient claim and one possible concern. The claims are not intended to be exhaustive, and neither are the dangers. I trust it is fair and balanced. For those who desire a more detailed account of possible benefits and dangers with interesting and historical data, see Appendix A.

More than eleven hundred natural products are covered in this chapter. Many natural products have been covered in other chapters of this book. Some are repeated here although many have not previously been discussed.

This chapter can serve as a quick reference regarding many natural products. A question format and alphabetical sequence make it easy to reference and learn the most popular and many less common natural products.

| QUESTION | ANSWER |
|---|---|
| 1. Name a natural product that has been touted for depression, although at least 10 cases of eosinophilia-myalgia have occurred worldwide. | 5-HTP |
| 2. Name a natural product that is possibly effective to increase metabolism and to boost memory, although more research is needed. | 7-Keto-DHEA |
| 3. Name a natural product that is touted for fever but can cause GI upset. | Abscess root |
| 4. Name a natural product touted for acne that lacks significant research. | Abuta |
| 5. Name a natural product that is touted to lower cholesterol but can precipitate severe asthmatic attacks. | Acacia |

6.  Name a natural product that is touted for
    infections and is rich in vitamin C but can cause GI upset.

    Acerola

7.  Name a natural product that is possibly
    effective for slowing the rate of Alzheimer's but can cause
    nausea, vomiting, and agitation.

    Acetyl-L-carnitine

8.  Name a natural product that has been used
    in drug-associated diarrhea.

    Acidophilus

9.  Name a natural product that has been used
    orally for colds, fever, and epilepsy but can cause hypo-
    glycemia, convulsions, and even death when the unripe fruit
    and seeds are ingested.

    Ackee

10. Name a natural product that has been used in
    China for cancer but is extremely toxic.

    Aconite

11. Name a natural product that has long been
    used in emergency in the management of poisoning.

    Activated charcoal

12. Name a natural product that has been touted
    to treat liver and gallbladder disorders but might cause dys-
    pepsia.

    Adam's needle

13. Name a natural product that has been touted
    for fatigue, but since it is derived from slaughtered animals,
    contamination is a concern.

    Adrenal extract

14. Name a natural product that has been used
    orally for digestive disorders and as a sedative; however,
    there is insufficient reliable information available about its
    effectiveness.

    Adrue

15. Name a natural product that has been touted
    for HIV, but reliable data in regard to its effectiveness and
    safety is not available.

    African wild potato

16. Name a natural product that has been used
    as a hallucinogen and for nerve pain and anxiety but can
    cause dizziness, spasms, delirium, and even coma.

    Aga

17. Name a natural product that has another name
    for seaweed that has been used as a laxative and has been
    touted to decrease cholesterol. It is high in thyroid content
    and should not be used by those on thyroid medication.

    Agar

18. Name a natural product that is possibly effective
    for sore throat and upset stomach but can affect blood pres-
    sure.

    Agrimony

19. Name a natural product that is possibly

    Agropyron

effective for inflammatory diseases of the urinary tract but can cause hypokalemia when used excessively.

20. Name an amino acid that some claim can help prevent nighttime hypoglycemia although significant research is lacking.

Alanine

21. Name a natural product that has been used for diarrhea and heavy menstrual flow although effectiveness is not proven. It can cause liver damage in rare cases.

Alchemilla

22. Name a substance found in beer, wine, and liquor that with chronic use can cause cirrhosis of the liver, peripheral neuropathy, dementia, cardiomyopathy, and hypertension. Blood levels of 8–150 mg/dl can cause intoxication, levels of 300 mg/dl can cause blackouts, and levels above 400 mg/dl can cause death.

Alcohol

23. Name a natural product that has been touted as a laxative, but it can cause cramp-like discomfort.

Alder buckthorn

24. Name a natural product that is possibly effective for menstrual disorders but can cause colic and vertigo.

Aletris

25. Name a natural product that has been touted to help in PMS and menopause but can trigger a recurrence of systemic lupus erythematosis.

Alfalfa

26. Name a natural product that is possibly effective to reduce cholesterol and blood pressure. It is also used in foods such as candy, gelatins, and puddings.

Algin

27. Name a natural product that was used by the ancient Greeks to heal skin wounds. It may be effective when used topically to enhance healing of leg ulcers, but there is insufficient information regarding its effectiveness for other uses.

Alkanna

28. Name a natural product that has been used to treat indigestion, but high doses of it can induce seizures.

Allspice (clove pepper)

29. Name a natural product that is purported to be a potential cholesterol reducer. It is also used in moisturizers to soften skin.

Almond

30. Name a natural product that has been used topically for skin irritations.

Aloe vera

31. Name a natural product that is used for fibromyalgia. Topically this product is used as a moisturizer and for rejuvenating skin. Side effects include gastrointestinal symptoms such as nausea and diarrhea. Topically, with

Alpha hydroxy acid

long-term use, this product can increase the risk of skin cancer.

32.  Name a natural product that is used for                          Alpha-ketoglutamate
     chronic kidney disease, bacterial overgrowth, and liver dys-
     function. Intravenously this product is used for preventing
     ischemic heart injury, but significant scientific research is lack-
     ing.

33.  Name a natural product that has been                             Alpha-lipoic acid
     touted to help in diabetic neuropathy.

34.  Name a natural product that is used for                          Alpine cranberry
     urinary disorders, gout, and arthritis. It is also an antiviral and
     diuretic. It releases hydroquinones, thus when ingested may
     cause liver damage.

35.  Name a natural product that is used as a                         Alpine lady's mantle
     diuretic, cardiovascular agent, and an antispasmodic. No sig-
     nificant side effects are known to occur though insufficient
     data is available.

36.  Name a natural product that has been touted                      Alpinia
     as an antiflatulent, antibacterial, and antispasmodic.

37.  Name a Chinese herb rich in vitamin C,                           Amalaki
     touted to boost immune function and has the Western name
     of phyllanthus emblica.

38.  Name a natural product that has been                             Amaranth
     touted for ulcers and diarrhea, but research is lacking as to
     its effectiveness. It may be effective in lowering cholesterol.

39.  Name a natural product that has been                             Ambrette
     used in snake bites, but reliable research is lacking.

40.  Name a natural product that is used                              American adder's tongue
     topically for ulcers. No significant side effects are known to
     occur.

41.  Name a natural product that was historically                     American bittersweet
     used as a diuretic, for arthritis, and menstrual and liver disor-
     ders, but is rarely used today due to tannin content, and
     insufficient scientific data is lacking.

42.  Name a natural product that is used                              American chestnut
     for respiratory illnesses, a sedative, and antirheumatic. As
     such regular ingestion of these herbs with tannins can
     increase the chances of esophageal and nasal cancer.

43.  Name a natural product that has been touted                      American dogwood
     to help in headaches and fatigue, but sufficient scientific
     research is lacking.

44. Name a natural product that has been touted
to help in hypertension but is extremely toxic.

American hellebore

45. Name a natural product that is touted to
help in digestive disorders but is considered poisonous.

American ivy

46. Name a natural product that is used as a
smooth muscle stimulant for increasing blood pressure and
uterine and intestinal contractions. It may cause bradycardia,
hypertension, hallucinations, delirium, vasoconstriction, and
cardiac arrest.

American mistletoe

47. Name a root that is an expectorant and
is used for respiratory disorders, arthritis, stimulates tissue
renewal, and is used for dermatological treatments. It is
unsafe in pregnancy.

American spikenard

48. Name the natural products that are the raw
material for the building of human protein, but excessive
amounts can be toxic.

Amino acids

49. Name a natural product that has been
touted to help in herpes and various skin problems, but significant research is lacking.

Andiroba

50. Name a natural product that is touted
to help in the common cold but might inhibit male and
female fertility.

Andrographis

51. Name a natural product that has been
used to increase testosterone and has been touted to
increase athletic performance. It could possibly be a factor in
cancer.

Androstenedione

52. Name a natural product that has been
used in PMS and menopause because of its estrogen-like
activities but would raise considerable concerns regarding
cancer.

Angelica (dong quai)

53. Name a natural product that is used for
asthma and can induce feelings of elation and hallucinations.
Orally it is severely toxic. It can cause acute anticholinergic
poisoning such as tachycardia, audiovisual disassociation, urinary retention, convulsions, coma, and respiratory arrest. It
can also exacerbate congestive heart failure due to its
atropine and scopolamine content.

Angel's trumpet

54. Name a natural product that has been
used as an antidiarrheal and antispasmodic but can cause
nausea and vomiting in large doses.

Angostura

55. Name a natural product that has been

Aniracetam

touted to improve brain functioning although significant
research is lacking.

56. Name a natural product that has been
used in America for the flu, but in oil form could cause pulmonary edema and seizures.                                          Anise

57. Name a natural product that has been
used topically in South America in hopes of preventing wrinkles.                                                               Annatto

58. Name a natural product that is a fruit and
is possibly effective to help with diarrhea and constipation.
Ingestion of large amounts of the seeds can cause cyanide
poisoning and even death.                                          Apple

59. Name a natural product that is often
consumed in the winter, tastes good, and is touted to help in
weight loss although significant research is lacking.              Apple cider vinegar

60. Name a natural product that is used
for infertility, bleeding disorders, and vaginal infections. The
kernels are unsafe to use due to a content of cyanide. Acute
poisoning may lead to respiratory failure, coma, and death
within 15 minutes.                                                 Apricot

61. Name a natural product that is used
in the Far East for schizophrenia but has been associated
with oral cancer and heart disease.                                Areca

62. Name an amino acid that in high
doses might increase already present herpes infection and
schizophrenia.                                                     Arginine

63. Name a natural product that is a
mixture of herbs that is touted to help in sexual dysfunction,
but research is lacking.                                            ArginMax

64. Name a natural product that has been
used as an immune-system stimulant and to promote menstruation but is probably ineffective for any use. It can cause
vomiting, kidney damage, and even death.                           Aristolochia

65. Name a natural product that is used for pain
but can irritate mucous membranes.                                 Arnica

66. Name a group of products that are found
in glue, paint thinner, gasoline, kerosene, and fingernail polish
that can cause intoxication and possibly even dementia with
enough repeated use.                                               Aromatic hydrocarbons

67. Name a natural product that has been
touted orally to relieve cramps and induce menstruation, but   Arrach

significant research is lacking.

| | | |
|---|---|---|
| 68. | Name a natural product that is used as a nutritional food for infants, but significant research is lacking. | Arrowroot |
| 69. | Name a natural product that has been touted to help in indigestion, but significant research is lacking. | Artichoke |
| 70. | Name a natural product that has been touted to help in weight loss but can result in renal failure. | Artistolochic acid |
| 71. | Name a natural product that is touted to help inflammations of the throat but can cause severe mucous membrane irritation. | Arum |
| 72. | Name a natural product that is touted for asthma and dyspepsia but can cause diarrhea, headache, and convulsions in large amounts. | Asafoetida |
| 73. | Name a natural product that has been used for bronchitis and bronchial spasms but can cause nausea and vomiting. | Asarabacca |
| 74. | Name a natural product that is used to treat gout, bladder complaints, constipation, and is a diuretic. No significant side effects are known to occur, but some cases have reported confusion. | Ash |
| 75. | Name a natural product that is known as an all-purpose tonic without any significant research. | Ashwaganda |
| 76. | Name a natural product that is touted to help in kidney stone prevention. | Asparagus |
| 77. | Name a natural product that increases absorption of minerals and enhances athletic performance. No significant side effects are known to occur. | Aspartates |
| 78. | Name an amino acid that is used to make the artificial sweetener aspartame. Some claim that it helps in depression and fatigue. | Aspartic acid |
| 79. | Name an herb that is used to treat prostate disorders, sciatica, and rheumatic disorders. It is a precursor to salicylate. Avoid the usage of any herbs with anticoagulant potential. It can induce an increase in bleeding. | Aspen |
| 80. | Name a natural product that comes from China and is touted to help in fatigue, hepatitis, and AIDS. | Astragalus |

81. Name an herb that is used for arthritis,      Autumn crocus
gout, and Mediterranean fever. Orally it causes nausea, vomiting, diarrhea, liver necrosis, multiorgan failure, hypovolemic
shock, and death.

82. Name a root that is used for ulcerative      Avens
colitis, uterine bleeding, diarrhea, and fever, with no significant
adverse effects reported.

83. Name a natural product that is touted to      Avocado
decrease cholesterol but can decrease the effects of the drug
warfarin.

84. Name a natural product that has been      $B_{12}$
touted to lift mood but has no research to back this up.

85. Name a natural product that is touted      Bael
for constipation and diarrhea but can cause GI upset and
constipation when taken in large amounts.

86. Name a root that appears to bind with Gaba      Baikal skullcap
receptors with possible benzodiazepine-like effects. It also
appears to have antibacterial and antiviral properties. It is
generally known to be nontoxic, though several case reports
have found it hepatotoxic.

87. Name a natural product that has been      Bamboo
used in China for asthma, coughs, and gallbladder disorders,
but information regarding its effectiveness is insufficient.

88. Name a natural product that has been      Barberry
used topically for skin infections.

89. Name a natural product that has been      Barley
used in car sickness although significant research is lacking.

90. Name a natural product that is a folk      Basil
remedy used for warts when applied topically.

91. Name a root that is thought to work      Ba ti tian
in depression by increasing serotonergic effects. It also has
diuretic properties and is an antihypertensive. This root may
exacerbate urinary difficulties.

92. Name a natural product that has been      Bay
touted for ulcers but can cause perforation of the gastrointestinal tract.

93. Name a natural product that was used by      Bayberry
early settlers for sore throat, but it can cause high blood
pressure.

94. Name a natural product that is possibly      Bean pod

effective in the promotion of urine flow but can cause vomiting and diarrhea when eaten raw in large amounts.

| | | |
|---|---|---|
| 95. | Name a natural product that some feel might help in early parkinsonism. | Bean sprouts |
| 96. | Name a natural product that was listed in the *U.S. Pharmacopoeia* until 1936 for urinary tract infections but can cause gastrointestinal upset. | Bearberry |
| 97. | Name a natural product that has been touted to help in impotence but can raise blood sugar. | Bee pollen |
| 98. | Name an extremely popular natural product that has been used for preventing cardiovascular disease. Unfortunately, it may have sundry side effects such as incoordination, drowsiness, respiratory depression, central nervous system depression, hypoglycemia, hypokalemia, arrhythmias, and seizures. Chronic heavy use may result in encephalopathy and cancer of the mouth. | Beer |
| 99. | Name a natural product that has been touted for various inflammations, but significant research is lacking. | Beeswax |
| 100. | Name a natural product that has been touted to help in liver disease but in large amounts could cause kidney damage. | Beet |
| 101. | Name a natural product that is used for bee sting allergy and for rheumatoid arthritis, multiple sclerosis, and neuralgia. It is a potent hemolytic and can cause swelling at the site of injections. It can also cause anaphylaxis. | Bee venom |
| 102. | Name a natural product that has been used as a sedative but can interfere with the metabolism of several prescription medications and can cause dry mouth, dilation of the pupils, and even hallucinations at times. | Belladonna |
| 103. | Name a natural product that has been used topically for wounds but can cause allergic reactions. | Benzoin |
| 104. | Name a natural product that is possibly effective for treating mycosis fungoides when used in combination with long-wave ultraviolet light but can cause blisters, skin rash, and pigment spots. | Bergamot oil |
| 105. | Name a natural product that has been touted to help in cancer, but scientific research is lacking. | Beta-1, 3-glucan |
| 106. | Name a natural product that is possibly effective in preventing breast cancer in premenopausal women but can cause yellow or orange skin pigmentation | Beta-carotene |

when taken in large amounts.

107. Name a natural product that is touted to
help in prostatitis and gallstones but can cause gastrointestinal upset.

Beta-sitosterol

108. Name a natural product that has been
used in homocynstinuria.

Betaine anhydrous

109. Name a natural product that has been
touted to help in depression but acts similar to an MAO
inhibitor antidepressant and can thus have significant side
effects.

Betal palm

110. Name a natural product that has long
been used for the pain of menstruation but in pregnant
women could cause uterine contractions.

Beth root

111. Name a natural product that has been
touted for diarrhea, headaches, bronchitls, and asthma. It may
be effective when taken in small doses for headaches.

Betony

112. Name a natural product that has been
used for traveler's diarrhea.

Bifidobacterium bifidum

113. Name a natural product that has been
touted to help in various eye disorders.

Bilberry

114. Name a natural product that has been
touted to help in athletic injuries.

Bioflavonoids

115. Name a natural product that has been
touted to help in weight gain. It has also been used in brittle
nails.

Biotin

116. Name a natural product that comes
from a common tree and is touted to help in urinary tract
infections.

Birch

117. Name a natural product that is touted
to help in asthma but might increase liver enzymes.

Bishop's weed

118. Name a natural product that has been
touted to help in hepatitis C but can also damage the liver.

Bistort

119. Name an oil that is used as an antispasmodic,
a local anesthetic, and has narcotic properties. It is highly
toxic and fatal, causing central nervous system depression
and respiratory failure.

Bitter almond

120. Name a natural product that is touted
to lower blood sugar in diabetes.

Bitter melon

121. Name a root that has expectorant properties and is used for respiratory disorders. No significant side effects are reported.

Bitter milkwort

122. Name a natural product that has been touted to help in dyspepsia but might increase blood pressure.

Bitter orange peel

123. Name a natural product that has been touted for eczema but is toxic when consumed orally.

Bittersweet nightshade

124. Name a natural product that is touted to help in sore throat.

Black alder

125. Name a root that is used as an emetic and can stimulate external nerve endings. As such it can induce diarrhea, decrease kidney function, and cause respiratory depression.

Black bryony

126. Name a natural product that is touted to help in PMS and menopause but can increase the actions of blood pressure medications and could therefore lead to dangerously low blood pressure.

Black cohosh

127. Name a natural product that has been touted to help in colds and flu and is high in omega-6 fatty acids.

Black currant

128. Name a natural product that was used for menstrual cramps by Native American females.

Black haw

129. Name an herb that is used for nausea, parasite infestation, and constipation. It has a digitalis-like effect, and it is a gastrointestinal irritant. Symptoms of poisoning include vomiting, diarrhea, shortness of breath, and even asphyxiation.

Black hellebore

130. Name a natural product that is touted to help in nausea and nervous disorders.

Black horehound

131. Name an herb that has been used as a laxative.

Black mulberry

132. Name a natural product that has been used for upper respiratory infections. It has been included in liniment preparations to treat lung congestion. It seems to have antimicrobial properties. Large amounts can be toxic and even cause death.

Black mustard seed

133. Name a natural product that has been used for gastric irritation and cramps but causes nausea, vomiting, paralysis, and even death when taken in large doses.

Black nightshade

134. Name a natural product that has been
used for upset stomach and bronchitis. Topically, it has been
used for pain. It is a flavoring agent.

Black pepper

135. Name a natural product that is possibly
effective as a laxative and for lowering cholesterol but can
cause flatulence.

Black psyllium

136. Name a natural product that has been used
as a diuretic but can be toxic to the central nervous system.

Black root

137. Name a natural product that has been
used for treating gastrointestinal upset but can be associated
with liver toxicity.

Black seed

138. Name a natural product that has been used
for improving cognitive performance. It is a common caffeinated beverage. Possible side effects include GI upset, anxiety, insomnia, heart palpitations, elevated cholesterol, ringing
in the ears, hepatoxicity, and convulsions.

Black tea

139. Name a natural product that has been
used for Montezuma's revenge but could possibly be carcinogenic.

Black walnut

140. Name a natural product that is a fruit and
has been touted to help with cataracts and macular degeneration. The leaves have been touted to help in diarrhea.
Significant research is lacking in its effectiveness.

Blackberry

141. Name a natural product that is possibly
effective for mild inflammation of the oral mucosa when used
as a mouth rinse but can be unsafe when used orally for long
periods of time.

Blackthorn berry

142. Name a natural product that has been touted
for urinary tract infections and kidney stones, although
research is lacking.

Bladderwort

143. Name a natural product that has been touted
to help in thyroid disorders but could induce hyperthyroidism.

Bladderwrack

144. Name a natural product that has been used
by breast-feeding mothers to stimulate milk production but
could produce allergic reactions and aggravate ulcers.

Blessed thistle

145. Name a natural product that is possibly
effective for diarrhea but can cause abdominal pain, constipation, and nausea.

Blond psyllium

146. Name a natural product that is a product
in many toothpastes to reduce plaque.

Bloodroot

147. Name a natural product that has been used for ulcers, urinary tract infections, hemorrhoids, and as a laxative, but sufficient reliable information is lacking.    Blueberry

148. Name a natural product that has been touted for various gynecological problems but is potentially a dangerous herb.    Blue cohosh

149. Name a natural product that is used as a laxative but is likely unsafe when used orally.    Blue flag

150. Name a natural product that is a good source of dietary proteins, B-vitamins, and iron. Hepatotoxicity is possible.    Blue-green algae

151. Name a natural product that is possibly effective for stimulating appetite but can cause diarrhea, nausea, and vomiting in large doses.    Bogbean

152. Name an herb that has been used for diarrhea. Large amounts can cause poisoning.    Bog bilberry

153. Name a natural product used as a flavoring agent in foods.    Bois de rose oil

154. Name a natural product that has been used in South America but can be toxic to the kidneys and liver.    Boldo

155. Name a natural product used by the Native Americans for the common cold, but it can be toxic even causing death.    Boneset

156. Name a natural product that is often found in potpourri in bathrooms.    Borage

157. Name a natural product that is a trace mineral and is touted for osteoporosis.    Boron

158. Name a natural product that has been touted for ringworm, but the claims are unproved.    Boswellia

159. Name a natural product that has been used topically for poison ivy but can cause allergic reactions when used topically.    Bovine cartilage

160. Name a natural product that has been used for treating diarrhea in people with AIDS. Allergic reactions are possible. Mad cow disease is always a concern here.    Bovine colostrum

161. Name a natural product that has been    Boxwood

touted for HIV/AIDS and for boosting immunity. It is possibly safe when the leaf extract is used but can cause vomiting, paralysis, and even death when the whole leaf is used orally.

| | | |
|---|---|---|
| 162. | Name a natural product that has been touted to help in asthma. | Brahmi |
| 163. | Name a natural product that is the coat of the seed of cereal grains and might help in lowering cholesterol when combined with a low-fat diet. | Bran |
| 164. | Name a natural product that has been reputed to enhance performance, decrease fatigue, increase muscle mass, and improve concentration. | Branched-chain amino acids |
| 165. | Name a natural product that has been used for diarrhea. | Brewer's yeast |
| 166. | Name a natural product that comes from pineapples and has been touted to help in arthritis. | Bromelain |
| 167. | Name a natural product that has been used as a sedative but can have significant psychiatric side effects. | Bromide |
| 168. | Name a natural product that has been touted for liver complaints, dysentery, and bleeding gums, but scientific information is lacking. | Brooklime |
| 169. | Name a natural product touted to help in arrhythmias but could be dangerous because of possible serious side effects on the heart. | Broom |
| 170. | Name a natural product that has been used as a laxative but in large doses can cause paralysis and even death. | Bryonia |
| 171. | Name a natural product that comes from Africa that has long been used in bladder and prostate infections. | Buchu |
| 172. | Name a natural product that is possibly effective for skin inflammation but is an allergen. | Buckhorn plantain |
| 173. | Name a natural product from which a type of pancakes is made and is touted to help varicose veins. | Buckwheat |
| 174. | Name a natural product that has been touted for both hypothyroidism and hyperthyroidism and thus the claims seem contradictory. | Bugle |
| 175. | Name a natural product that has | Bugleweed |

been touted for mild hyperthyroidism and bleeding, but significant research is lacking.

176. Name an herb that has been used for arthritis and gout, but it can cause GI upset. Topically it can cause blisters.                                   Bulbous buttercup

177. Name a natural product from China that has been used for the flu although significant studies are lacking at best.                                   Bupleurum

178. Name a natural product that has been used in anorexia nervosa, but significant research is lacking.                                   Burdock

179. Name a natural product that is touted for varicose veins.                                   Burnet

180. Name a natural product that is used in China for skin inflammations but can cause a phototoxicity.                                   Burning bush root

181. Name a natural product that has been touted for hair loss and to promote sweating but can cause allergic reaction in those sensitive to the ragweed family.                                   Burr marigold

182. Name an herb that has been used in body building. It is converted to GHD (gamma hydroxybutyrate) in the body and as such can cause coma, agitation, seizures, and even death.                                   Butanediol (BD)

183. Name a natural product from Europe that has been touted for varicose veins.                                   Butcher's broom

184. Name a natural product that has been touted for migraine headaches but raises possible concerns about liver damage.                                   Butterbur

185. Name a natural product that is touted for arthritis but can cause severe irritation to the gastrointestinal tract.                                   Buttercup

186. Name a natural product that is touted for use in gallbladder disorders, hemorrholds, and skin diseases, but there is insufficient information regarding its effectiveness.                                   Butternut

187. Name a natural product that is a common food and has been touted for gastritis.                                   Cabbage

188. Name a natural product that has been used for many years for flavoring food and drinks and is touted for its stimulating effects.                                   Cacao (chocolate)

189. Name a natural product the oil of which                                   Cade oil

is used topically for itching and psoriasis.

190.  Name a natural product that is
      contained in many drinks that are common in America and is
      touted for increasing mental alertness. In spite of possible
      side effects and the fact that interactions with other drugs
      are legion, it remains one of the top herbs.                    Caffeine

191.  Name a natural product that is
      possibly effective as an expectorant and also when used topi-
      cally to relieve discomfort from arthritis and rheumatism but
      can lead to dyspepsia when used orally and hypersensitivity
      when used topically.                                            Cajeput oil

192.  Name an herb that acts as an
      acetylcholine agonist. Thus, it increases parasympathetic activ-
      ity which can increase GI peristalsis, slow heart rate, and
      cause pupil constriction. Overdose can cause a cholinergic
      crisis and death.                                               Calabar bean

193.  Name a natural product that has
      been used for many years in lotion form for calming itching
      skin and bug bites.                                             Calamine

194.  Name a natural product that is touted
      for respiratory illnesses and colds with fever, but insufficient
      information is available.                                       Calamint

195.  Name a natural product that is touted for
      digestive disorders, and some even chew it to remove the
      odor of tobacco, but it contains a known carcinogen.            Calamus

196.  Name a natural product that has been
      used in antacids and in helping in osteoporosis. Serious side
      effects are possible, especially in high dosages with long-term
      use.                                                            Calcium

197.  Name a natural product that has been
      touted without significant research to help in cancer preven-
      tion.                                                           Calcium D-glucarate

198.  Name a natural product that has been
      used topically for fungal skin infections.                      Calendula

199.  Name a natural product that has been
      used for insomnia and, in combination with other herbs, has
      been used for depression and various psychiatric conditions,
      although research is lacking in regards to its effectiveness.   California poppy

200.  Name an herb that has been used for
      cancer, but it contains cardiac glycosides, and high doses
      could cause death.                                              Calotropis

201.  Name a natural product that has been                    Calumba
      touted for diarrhea, although research is lacking.

202.  Name a natural product that has been                    Camphor
      used topically to help with hemorrhoids, cold sores, and bug
      bites.

203.  Name a natural product that has been                    Canada balsam
      touted to help topically with hemorrhoids.

204.  Name an herb that has been used for                     Canadian fleabane
      bronchitis and diarrhea although research is lacking.

205.  Name an herb that has been used to                      Canadian hemp
      strengthen an aging heart, but it can cause bradycardia and
      reflex hypertension.

206.  Name a natural product, which is an                     Canaigre
      inexpensive alternative to ginseng, that has been used to
      increase physical stamina, cognitive function, and as an antide-
      pressant, although research is lacking regarding its effective-
      ness.

207.  Name a natural product that is used as                  Cananga oil
      a flavoring agent in beverages and puddings.

208.  Name an herb that is used as a cooking                  Canella
      spice and is purported to have stimulant and antimicrobial
      activities.

209.  Name a natural product that has been used to            Canthaxanthin
      reduce the photosensitivity of erythropoietic protoporphyria.

210.  Name a natural product that is a food and               Capers
      has been used topically for skin disorders and dry skin but
      may cause contact dermatitis.

211.  Name a natural product that is the active               Capsaicin
      ingredient in hot peppers and has been touted for arthritic
      pain.

212.  Name a natural product that is part of the              Capsicum
      pepper family and is used to make cayenne. Topically it has
      antipain effects but can also cause burning.

213.  Name a natural product that has been used               Caramel color
      as a coloring agent in medications, foods, and cosmetics.
      Large doses might suppress the immune system.

214.  Name a natural product that has been used               Caraway
      to reduce gas and is often found on rye bread.

215.  Name a natural product that has been                    Cardamom

used for bad breath and mouth inflammations.

216. Name a natural product that has been used for gallbladder disease and poor digestion but can cause allergic reactions in those sensitive to the ragweed family.

Carlina

217. Name a popular amino acid that some claim helps in weight loss, fatigue, high triglycerides, dementia, peripheral neuropathy of diabetes, and depression. There are different forms of this amino acid, and the DL form can be toxic.

Carnitine

218. Name a natural product that has been reputed to have antiaging effects and to be of help in diabetes mellitus.

Carnosine

219. Name a natural product that has been used for indigestion and has been touted as a chocolate substitute.

Carob

220. Name a natural product that is possibly effective for peptic ulcers but can cause bleeding, cramping, diarrhea, and can lead to infection.

Carrageenan

221. Name a natural product that is a vegetable touted to prevent cancer, lower cholesterol, and promote eye health.

Carrot

222. Name a natural product that is found in many laxatives.

Cascara sagrada

223. Name a natural product that has been used in GI complaints although effectiveness is not known.

Cascarilla

224. Name a natural product that has been used for GI complaints. Topically it can cause blisters.

Cashew

225. Name a natural product that has been touted for gastrointestinal problems.

Cassia

226. Name a natural product that has been used as an antispasmodic, antidiarrheal, and topically for dry skin, but research is lacking in regards to its safety and effectiveness.

Cassie absolute

227. Name a natural product that has been used for anxiety, insomnia, and painful menses.

Castoreum

228. Name a natural product that has long been used as a strong laxative.

Castor oil

229. Name a natural product that has been used for contraception although it can be extremely toxic

Castor seed

and even can cause death.

230. Name an herb that has antibacterial and astringent effects and has been used for dysentery.    Catechu

231. Name a natural product that has been touted to help in anxiety but can have dangerous interactions with alcohol and sedatives.    Catnip

232. Name a natural product from South America that is touted to enhance the immune system, but some species of this plant are toxic.    Cat's claw

233. Name an herb that has been used to treat internal disease although significant research is lacking. Allergic reactions are possible.    Cat's foot

234. Name a natural product that is touted as an aphrodisiac, but scientific research is lacking.    Catuaba

235. Name a pepper that is touted to reduce the likelihood of arteriosclerosis, but research is lacking for this claim.    Cayenne pepper

236. Name a natural product that comes from a common tree and is used topically for warts but used orally could result in seizures or even death.    Cedar

237. Name a natural product that is possibly effective for alopecia areata when combined with other essential oils but can be a local irritant.    Cedarwood oil

238. Name a natural product that has been purported to help in cancer and liver disease, although it can cause fatigue, nausea, low blood pressure, and liver damage.    Celandine

239. Name a natural product that is a food eaten worldwide that is touted to lower blood pressure, but research is lacking.    Celery

240. Name a natural product that has been touted for ADHD, but scientific research is lacking.    Centaury

241. Name a natural product that has been touted to help in angina, but research is lacking.    Cereus

242. Name a natural product that is touted for different kinds of arthritis, but research is lacking.    Cetyl myristoleate

243. Name a natural product that is touted to have calming effects, but since it is related to the ragweed family, allergic reactions are possible.    Chamomile

244. Name a natural product found in the rain forest that is touted to help with kidney stones.

Chanca piedra

245. Name a natural product that is touted to promote hair growth but is likely unsafe with the possibility of liver or kidney damage.

Chaparral

246. Name a natural product that has long been used for PMS. Side effects (GI upset, headaches, alopecia, tiredness, tachycardia, dry mouth) are possible but relatively rare.

Chasteberry

247. Name a natural product that has been used topically for centuries for leprosy.

Chaulmoogra oil

248. Name an herb that has been used as a general tonic and as a diuretic although effectiveness is not known.

Cheken

249. Name a natural product that has been used as a dietary mineral supplement.

Chelated minerals

250. Name a natural product that is possibly effective for diarrhea, but the vitamin C found in this product can cause nausea, abdominal cramps, and insomnia.

Cherokee rosehip

251. Name a natural product that is a fruit that has been used in colds, cough, and gout.

Cherry

252. Name a natural product that has been used as a sedative and pain reliever although significant research is lacking. An overdose could cause death.

Cherry laurel water

253. Name a natural product that is a flavoring agent in foods and beverages and in folk medicine is touted as a diuretic, expectorant, and digestive aid.

Chervil

254. Name a natural product that has been used to treat various arthritic conditions although research is lacking, and its effectiveness seems unlikely. Allergic reactions are possible.

Chicken collagen

255. Name a natural product that has been used as a diuretic and for weight loss, but the use is purely based on folklore.

Chickweed

256. Name a natural product that is an ingredient in hair preparations and a gum base in chewing gum.

Chicle

257. Name a natural product that has been touted to slow rapid heart rate.

Chicory

258. Name an herb that has been used
in memory disorders. It does have acetylcholinerase inhibitor
activity, which most of the drugs for Alzheimer's dementia do.

Chinese club moss

259. Name a natural product that has been
touted for use in diabetes but without significant research.

Chinese cucumber

260. Name an herb that has antibacterial
activity, anti-inflammatory activity, and might be hepatoprotective activity and possibly antituberculous activity.

Chirata

261. Name a natural product that is likely
effective for weight loss but should be used cautiously by
those with shellfish allergies.

Chitosan

262. Name a natural product that has been used
for intestinal worms without significant research.

Chive

263. Name an herbal preparation, which is a
combination of echinacea extract, propolis, and vitamin C,
that is an over-the-counter product used in Israel reputedly
to reduce colds in children.

Chizukit

264. Name a natural product that has been
touted for fibromyalgia but can cause gastrointestinal upset,
and research is lacking.

Chlorella

265. Name a natural product that is touted for
wound healing, but significant research is lacking.

Chlorophyll

266. Name a natural product that is possibly
effective for controlling body and fecal odors.

Chlorophyllin

267. Name a natural product that is high in
antioxidants and is best used as a stimulant.

Chocolate

268. Name a natural product that has been
touted to help mood stabilizing properties but at best is a
weak mood stabilizer.

Choline

269. Name a natural product that has been
touted for osteoarthritis, but research is lacking.

Chondroitin sulfate

270. Name a natural product that is a mineral
and has been touted to lower blood sugar, but there has
been a question of cancer in high doses, as well as a plethora
of other possible side effects.

Chromium

271. Name a natural product that has been
touted for prostate cancer, but more research is needed and
allergic reactions are possible.

Chrysanthemum

272.  Name a natural product found in the rain                    Chuchuhuasi
      forest of South America and is touted to stimulate sex drive,
      but research is lacking.
      _____

273.  Name a natural product that is effective                    Chymotrypsin
      for reducing trauma to the eye during cataract surgery and
      possibly is effective for treating burns, but in rare cases ana-
      phylactic reaction is possible when taken orally, even leading
      to death.
      _____

274.  Name a natural product that is                              Ciguatera
      inadvertently consumed through eating tainted fish and is
      poisonous.
      _____

275.  Name a natural product that has                             Cinchona
      been touted for appetite stimulation, bloating, fullness, and
      hemorrhoids but can cause bleeding, hives, and fever.
      _____

276.  Name a natural product that is a                            Cinnamon
      popular spice that is touted for bronchitis and may lower
      blood sugar.
      _____

277.  Name a natural product that has been                        Citronella oil
      touted as an insect repellent, although research is lacking.
      _____

278.  Name an amino acid that some claim                          Citrulline
      promotes energy and protects the liver.
      _____

279.  Name a natural product that has been                        Civet
      used as a flavoring agent in foods and also used in China for
      pain relief and as a sedative.
      _____

280.  Name a natural product that has been                        Clary sage
      added to beverages and foods because of its fragrance but in
      high doses could cause dizziness and headaches.
      _____

281.  Name a natural product that is a relative                   Cleavers (lady's bedstraw)
      of coffee and has been touted to help in high blood pressure.
      _____

282.  Name a natural product that has been                        Clematis
      touted for migraine headaches but can irritate the gastroin-
      testinal tract and has been known to cause seizures and even
      death.
      _____

283.  Name a natural product that has been used                   Clivers
      for enlarged lymph nodes although research is lacking. The
      more important question would be, what is causing the
      enlarged lymph nodes?
      _____

284.  Name a natural product used to dull                         Clove
      pain as in toothaches.
      _____

285.  Name a natural product that is touted for                   Clown's mustard plant

irritable bowel syndrome but can itself cause nausea.

286. Name a natural product that has been used in folk medicine as a diuretic and for bladder and kidney disorders, but significant research is lacking.

Club moss

287. Name a natural product that is a fatty acid that is touted to help in arthritis.

CMO (cerasomal-cis-9-cetylmyristolcate)

288. Name a natural product that has been used in cough syrups, but significant research is lacking.

Cocillana

289. Name the plant that is the source of cocaine that has been so much abused because of its mind-altering effects.

Coca

290. Name a natural product that is a CNS stimulant and a heart stimulant. It can cause tremors and rapid heartbeat.

Cocoa

291. Name a natural product that has been touted to help in high blood lipids and hypertension.

Cod liver oil

292. Name a natural product that is touted to increase energy and to increase the immune system although significant research is lacking.

Coenzyme A

293. Name a natural product that has been touted to help in congestive heart failure. It is an important enzyme in many reactions in the body.

Coenzyme Q10

294. Name a natural product that is the number one drink in America that is touted to help with fatigue.

Coffee

295. Name a natural product that is the number one cold drink and is also touted for its stimulating effects.

Cola

296. Name a natural product that comes from India that is touted to lower high blood pressure, but great caution is warranted in regard to this herb.

Coleus forskohlii

297. Name a natural product that is described as a wellness product that helps in weight loss, but significant research is lacking.

CollagenPlus

298. Name a natural product from shale deposits that has been used as a supplement source of trace minerals.

Colloidal minerals

299. Name a natural product that has been touted for use topically for fungal infections, but significant research is lacking.

Colloidal silver

300.  Name a natural product that has been
      touted for constipation and liver and gallbladder ailments but
      causes bloody diarrhea, kidney damage, convulsions, paralysis,
      and even death.                                         Colocynth

301.  Name a natural product that has been
      touted for gastritis, dyspepsia, and diarrhea but in large doses
      could cause vomiting, paralysis, and unconsciousness.   Colombo

302.  Name a natural product that is the first
      food that comes from a mother's breast and is touted to
      have many health benefits, but when it comes from the cow,
      caution is warranted in regard to such diseases as mad cow
      disease.                                                Colostrum

303.  Name a natural product that has been
      used as a cough suppressant, but it can damage the liver.   Coltsfoot

304.  Name a natural product that has
      been touted for gastrointestinal disorders and for jaundice,
      although significant research is lacking.                Columbine

305.  Name a natural product that was
      used by Native Americans for respiratory infections but can
      be highly toxic.                                        Comfrey

306.  Name a natural product that has been
      touted for high blood pressure, but research is lacking.   Common stonecrop

307.  Name a natural product that is possibly
      effective as an appetite stimulant, although anaphylaxis is pos-
      sible when the bark of this product is used.             Condurango

308.  Name a natural product that may lower
      cholesterol, lower triglycerides, lower weight, and help in
      arthritis.                                              Conjugated linoleic acid (CLA)

309.  Name an herb that has been used as a
      snakebite antidote although significant scientific research is
      lacking.                                                Contragerva

310.  Name a natural product that has been
      used for urinary tract disorders and indigestion, but signifi-
      cant research is lacking.                               Coolwort

311.  Name an herb that has been used for
      upper respiratory infections, urinary tract infections, and con-
      stipation. Preliminary research reveals that indeed it might
      have some antibacterial, anti-inflammatory, and stimulating
      properties. It can cause stomach pains and tremors. Large
      doses can cause diarrhea.                               Copaiba balsam

312.  Name a natural product that has been                    Copper

touted for copper deficiencies.

313.  Name a natural product that has been                    Coral
      used as a base in orthopedic surgery for new bone growth.

314.  Name a natural product that has been                    Cordonopsis
      touted to help in fatigue, but significant research is lacking.

315.  Name a natural product that is touted                   Cordyceps
      to increase energy.

316.  Name a natural product that has been                    Coriander
      touted to help stimulate appetite.

317.  Name a natural product that has been                    Coriolus mushroom
      reputed to improve the quality of cancer chemotherapy and
      to help in hepatitis.

318.  Name a natural product that has been                    Corkwood
      used in motion sickness but in large doses could result in
      confusion.

319.  Name a natural product that has been                    Corn cockle
      used topically for warts but could result in poisoning.

320.  Name a natural product that has long                    Corn silk
      been used for its diuretic effects.

321.  Name a natural product that has been                    Cornflower
      touted for fever and as an expectorant, although it may cause
      an allergic reaction in those sensitive to the ragweed family.

322.  Name an herb that has been used for                     Corn poppy
      insomnia and pain. Sufficient scientific data is lacking.

323.  Name an herb that has been used for                     Corydalis
      depression and tremors. Its effectiveness is not known.
      Ironically, in high doses it might induce tremors.

324.  Name a natural product that has been                    Cosamin
      touted for osteoarthrits, but the risk of transmission of
      bovine spongiform encephalopathy is a concern.

325.  Name an herb that has been touted for                   Costus root
      antinematode therapy. Sufficient scientific data is lacking. It
      might be carcinogenic.

326.  Name an herb that has been used for                     Cotton
      menstrual problems (amenorrhea, dysmenorrhea, pain, and
      bleeding). It seems to stimulate menstrual flow. It is also
      reputed to have some male contraceptive effects.
      Effectiveness is not known. Poisoning and death are conceiv-
      able, especially in long-term use.

327. Name a natural product that has been
touted for urinary tract infections, but significant research is
lacking.

Couch grass

328. Name a natural product that has been
touted for weight loss but has an ephedrine constituent that
would be of significant concern.

Country mallow

329. Name a natural product that is
possibly effective to help in Parkinson's disease when combined with other medications, although more research is
needed.

Cowhage

330. Name a natural product that has
been touted for anxiety but could possibly cause either
hypotension or hypertension.

Cowslip

331. Name a natural product that has been
touted for muscle spasms, but significant research is lacking.

Cramp bark

332. Name a natural product that has been
used in urinary tract infections.

Cranberry

333. Name a natural product that has been
tried in Alzheimer's dementia, but serious side effects are certainly possible in high doses.

Creatine

334. Name a natural product that is possibly
effective when used as a purgative, although it can cause
vomiting, dizziness, and painful bowel movements.

Croton seeds

335. Name an herb that has been used as a
diuretic, for urinary tract infections, and for amoebic dysentery. Effectiveness is not known.

Cubebs

336. Name a natural product that has been
touted for high blood pressure, but significant research is
lacking.

Cucumber

337. Name a natural product that has
been used as a gargle in sore throats, but since it is related to
the ragweed family, allergic reactions are possible.

Cudweed

338. Name an herb that has been used for
upper respiratory infections, but its effectiveness is not
known.

Cupmoss

339. Name an herb that has been used for
digestive disorders, but its effectiveness is not known.

Cup plant

340. Name a natural product that is a common
spice that has been touted as an antiflatulent, although it has

Cumin

phototoxic effects.

341. Name a natural product that has been touted
for treating pernicious anemia.

Cyanocobalamin (Vitamin B$_{12}$)

342. Name an herb that has been used for
menstrual problems and anxiety. It can cause GI upset and
even asphyxiation at high doses.

Cyclamen

343. Name a natural product that has been
used topically as an ointment when one has a cold.

Cypress

344. Name an herb that has been used for
diarrhea, but ironically it is a GI irritant. It contains carcinogenic agents.

Cypress spurge

345. Name an amino acid that some claim helps
in alcoholic liver damage, in wound healing, rheumatoid
arthritis, and in aging skin. However, it could be dangerous for
those with diabetes since it can inactivate insulin.

Cysteine

346. Name a natural product that has been
touted to aid in wound healing but can cause shivering, vomiting, and paralysis.

Daffodil

347. Name a natural product that has been
touted to be antimicrobial and antifungal, but significant
research is lacking.

Daisy

348. Name a natural product that is a Mexican
herb touted to increase sex drive, although significant
research is lacking. One of its constituents is similar to
cyanide.

Damiana

349. Name a natural product that has been
touted to help in hepatitis, but dangerous interactions with
various medications are possible.

Dandelion

350. Name a natural product that has been
touted for circulatory problems but can cause itching and
stomach upset.

Danshen

351. Name a Chinese herb that has been
touted to help in hepatitis and prostate cancer, although significant research is lacking.

Da qing ye

352. Name a natural product that has been
used for upper respiratory infections, but its effectiveness
and dangers are not known.

Date palm

353. Name a natural product that has been
touted to help in attention deficit disorder, but significant
research is lacking. It can have many side effects including

Deanol

drowsiness, depression, increased blood pressure, hypomania, an increase in schizophrenic symptoms, and tardive dyskinesia.

354.  Give another name for lu rong that contains hormones and is thus reputed as an aphrodisiac.     Deer antler

355.  Name an herb that has been used for malaria, but its effectiveness is not proven, and it can cause liver hemorrhage.     Deer tongue

356.  Name a natural product that is touted to help antiaging effects but contains sex hormones.     Deer velvet

357.  Name a natural product that has been used as a diuretic, sedative, and appetite stimulant but can cause cardiac arrest and respiratory failure.     Delphinium

358.  Name a natural product that has been touted for arthritis.     Devil's claw

359.  Name an herb that has been used for a variety of ailments such as arthritis, fever, and upper respiratory infections, but so far scientific studies have found no significant results.     Devil's club

360.  Name a natural product that is derived from licorice and is touted to help in the treatment of ulcers but can elevate blood pressure.     DGL

361.  Name a natural product that has been touted to help in cancer although significant research is lacking.     D-glucarate

362.  Name an herb that has been used as a supplement in preterm infants, for reducing anger, for improving night vision in dyslexic children, and to improve movement disorders in children with dyspraxia.     DHA (docosahexaenoic acid) (omega-3 fatty acids)

363.  Name a natural product that has been touted to have antidepressant effects but can cause hair loss, voice deepening, and even liver damage.     DHEA

364.  Name an herb that is another name for coenzyme $B_{12}$.     Dibencozide

365.  Name a natural product that has been touted for congestive heart failure but could cause heart arrhythmias and even death.     Digitalis

366.  Name a natural product that has been used for gas, but significant research is lacking.     Dill

367. Name a natural product that is possibly
effective for improving athletic performance although it may
react with nitrates in the gastrointestinal tract forming carcinogenic substance.                                          Dimethylglycine

368. Name a natural product that is possibly
effective for treating internal hemorrhoids but can cause
abdominal pain and diarrhea.                                  Diosmin

369. Name a natural product that has been
touted for fever and diabetes, but significant research is lacking.                                                          Divi-divi

370. Name a natural product that is derived
from broccoli and is touted to help in cancer.               DIM

371. Name a natural product that is
made from wood and is touted to help in various kinds of
pain, but significant research is lacking.                   DMAE

372. Name a natural product that is touted
to lower cholesterol, but significant research is lacking.   DMG

373. Name a natural product that is
possibly effective when used topically for symptoms associated with osteoarthritis and rheumatoid arthritis, although it
can cause sedation, nausea, and constipation.               DMSO

374. Name an herb that has been used in
diseases of the liver, but its effectiveness is not known.  Dodder

375. Name a natural product that is possibly
effective when used as a supplement of calcium and magnesium, although some product may be contaminated with
heavy metals.                                                Dolomite

376. Name a natural product that comes
from China and has been used in PMS but contains estrogen-
like compounds. There are concerns with any such compounds.                                                      Dong quai

377. Name a natural product that is a
neurotransmitter and is touted to increase energy.          Dopamine

378. Name a natural product that has been
tried in diarrhea, although insufficient reliable information is
available.                                                   Dragon's blood

379. Name an herb that has been used in upper
respiratory infections, but its effectiveness is not known. Duckweed

380. Name an herb that has been used in                      Dusty miller

migraines, but it can be toxic to the liver.

381. Name a natural product that has been
touted for arthritis and weight reduction, although excessive
amounts could cause vomiting, bloody diarrhea, cyanosis, and
even death.

Dwarf elder

382. Name an herb that is used as a
flavoring agent.

Dwarf pine needle

383. Name a natural product that has been
touted for digestive disorders and to remove bladder stones,
although it can cause nausea and vomiting.

Dyer's broom

384. Name a natural product that has been
touted to help in the common cold, although it might damage
reproductive cells.

Echinacea

385. Name a natural product that is
effective in treating lead poisoning when used intravenously
but can cause abdominal cramps, nausea, and anorexia.

EDTA

386. Name a natural product that is used
to make a famous wine, although the bark and leaves are
toxic.

Elderberry or elder

387. Name an herb that has been used to
treat sinusitis. It does seem to have some antiviral and anti-
inflammatory effects.

Elderflower

388. Name a natural product that has been
touted for use in hookworms, although large doses can cause
gastrointestinal upset and even paralysis.

Elecampane

389. Name an herb that has been used
as a flavoring agent in beverages.

Elemi

390. Name a natural product that has been
used for digestive disorders and diarrhea, although significant
research is lacking.

Elm bark

391. Name a natural product that has been
used topically for stretch marks after pregnancy, although significant research is lacking.

Emu oil

392. Name an herb that has been used to
treat ulcers although effectiveness is not known.

English adder's tongue

393. Name an herb that has been used for
flatulence. Effectiveness is not known.

English horsemint

394. Name a natural product that has been
touted for bronchitis, although effectiveness is not known.

English ivy

395.  Name a natural product that is possibly
      effective to lower cholesterol as part of a special diet but
      may cause soft stools and mild bloating.

English walnut

396.  Name a natural product that is another
      name for omega-3 fatty acids and has been touted for schizo-
      phrenia.

EPA (elcosapentaenoic acid)

397.  Name a natural product that has been
      used in many weight loss preparations but can have many
      serious side effects including anxiety, headache, heart palpita-
      tions, and even death.

Ephedra

398.  Name a natural product that has been
      used for impotence and memory loss although some species
      can cause respiratory arrest, and research is lacking regarding
      its effectiveness.

Epimedium

399.  Name a natural product that has been
      used in ob-gyn conditions, although it can be poisonous in
      chronic use.

Ergot

400.  Name a natural product that has been
      touted for urinary tract and kidney inflammation, although
      significant research is lacking.

Eryngo

401.  Name a natural product that has been
      touted for use in the common cold, although there is insuffi-
      cient reliable information available.

Esberitox

402.  Name a natural product that has been
      touted for use in cancer, although reliable information is lack-
      ing.

Essiac

403.  Name a natural product that comes from
      the tallest tree in the world and has been touted for use in
      congestion, although the oil can be lethal.

Eucalyptus

404.  Name a natural product that has been
      touted for asthma, bronchitis, hay fever, and tumors but may
      cause nausea and vomiting.

Euphorbia

405.  Name a natural product nicknamed
      "eyebright" that has been used for bloodshot eyes.

Euphrasia

406.  Name an herb that has been used in a
      wide array of disorders: urinary tract infections, gastrointesti-
      nal upset, respiratory infections, and narcotic withdrawal.
      Large doses can cause lethargy, hypotension, kidney damage,
      cardiac arrest, and death.

European barberry

407.  Name a natural product that is possibly

European buckthorn

effective for constipation but can cause abdominal pain and
watery diarrhea.

408.  Name an herb that has been used topically                          European fiber-fingergrass
to treat open wounds. Its astringent effects are probably sec-
ondary to tannin contents.

409.  Name an herb that has been used as a                               European mandrake
painkiller and also as an aphrodisiac. It contains several anticholinergic alkaloids and can be dangerous.

410.  Name a natural product that has been                               European mistletoe
tried for cancer, although these claims are unlikely. High
doses can cause severe toxicity.

411.  Name a natural product that is extremely                           Evening primrose oil
popular and has been touted for PMS. Compelling evidence
that it is better than placebo seems to be lacking.

412.  Name a natural product that has been used                          Eyebright
in hay fever and to make the eyes look less red, although significant research is lacking.

413.  Name a natural product that has been                               False unicorn root
used in menstrual problems, although its effectiveness has not
been proven.

414.  Name a natural product that has been                               Fennel
used for bad breath.

415.  Name a natural product that has been                               Fenugreek
touted for diabetes, but it can also thin the blood.

416.  Name an herb that has been used to treat                           Fever bark
high blood pressure and fever. It contains reserpine and
yohimbine that can cause psychosis and renal failure.

417.  Name a natural product that has been                               Feverfew
touted for migraine headaches. It might work similarly to the
nonsteroidal anti-inflammatory drugs.

418.  Name a natural product that comes from                             Fiber
oat bran, whole grain cereals, rice, and vegetables that might
help lower cholesterol in some people.

419.  Name a natural product that has been                               Ficin
used as a digestive aid, although significant reliable information is unavailable.

420.  Name an herb that has been purported to                            Field scabions
help when taken orally for cough and when used topically for
skin conditions such as anal fissions and eczema. It contains
triterpene saponins that might have astringent, antiseptic, and

expectorant properties.

421. Name a natural product that has been
used as a laxative, although research is lacking.

Fig

422. Name a natural product that has
been used for various skin disorders because it may have
some anti-inflammatory activity when used topically.

Figwort

423. Name a natural product that has been
used for upper respiratory infections, but significant research
is lacking.

Fir

424. Name a natural product that has been
touted for inflammations, although there is insufficient reliable
information available.

Fireweed

425. Name a natural product that has been
touted to lift mood and also stabilize mood, lower cholesterol, and lower triglycerides, although it can thin the blood.

Fish oils

426. Name a natural product that has been
touted to be antiaging because of its antioxidant effects.

Flavonoids

427. Name a natural product that is high
in omega-3 fatty acids and therefore has been touted in
depression and for lowering blood lipids. The question of
possible prostate cancer has been raised.

Flaxseed

428. Name a natural product that has been
touted for rheumatoid arthritis but is possibly ineffective for
this use.

Flaxseed oil

429. Name a natural product that has been
used in pernicious anemia and in pregnant women to prevent
neural tube defects. High doses can have numerous adverse
side effects.

Folic acid

430. Name a natural product that has been
touted for gastrointestinal complaints although there have
been reported cases of death with this plant.

Fool's parsley

431. Name a natural product that is touted
for respiratory disorders and nosebleeds, although it can be
toxic.

Forget-me-not

432. Name a natural product that has been
used for asthma, allergies, congestive heart failure, and glaucoma but can cause throat irritation, cough, tremors, and
stinging of the eyes.

Forskolin

433. Name a natural product that is possibly
effective as a laxative, although it may cause diarrhea, nausea,

Fo-ti

and vomiting.

434. Name a natural product that was the forerunner of one of the most famous heart medicines of all time.

Foxglove

435. Name a natural product that is used for colic and flatulence and topically in hand cream.

Frankincense

436. Name a natural product that has been touted for gallstones, although significant research is lacking.

Fringetree

437. Name a natural product that has been used for digestive disorders, but research is lacking.

Frostwort

438. Name a natural product that has been touted to reduce serum cholesterol but can cause abdominal cramps.

Fructo-oligosaccharides

439. Name a natural product that has been used in biliary colic but is dangerous in large doses, even causing convulsions and death.

Fumitory

440. Name a natural product that is the primary inhibitory or calming neurotransmitter in the brain, and it has been used for anxiety.

GABA (Gamma-aminobutyric acid)

441. Name a natural product that is reputed for fungal infections and rheumatism, but research is lacking.

Galangal

442. Name a natural product that was used to develop the drug Reminyl, which is used for Alzheimer's disease.

Galanthamine

443. Name a natural product that has been used for digestive disorders and flatulence, although significant research is lacking.

Galbanum

444. Name an herb that has been touted for constipation and intestinal worms, but it can cause nausea and vomiting. Sufficient scientific data is lacking.

Gamboge

445. Name an herb that has been purported to calm anxiety but has been associated with life-threatening adverse effects.

Gamma butyrolactone (GBL)

446. Name a natural product that is possibly effective for narcolepsy, although it can cause dependence and also hallucinations, confusion, agitation, and diarrhea.

Gamma hydroxybutyrate (GHB)

447. Name a natural product that has been touted for rheumatoid arthritis and diabetic neuropathy,

Gamma linolenic acid (GLA)

although significant research is lacking.

| | | |
|---|---|---|
| 448. | Name a natural product that has been used in menopause, although reliable information is lacking. | Gamma oryzanol |
| 449. | Name a natural product that has been touted for multiple uses including anxiety, insomnia, URIs, AIDS, and even cancer but can also have multiple side effects. | Ganoderma |
| 450. | Name a natural product that has been touted for weight loss, although significant research is lacking. | Garcinia |
| 451. | Name a natural product that has been used for coughs and vitamin C deficiency but may cause gastrointestinal irritation in large amounts. | Garden cress |
| 452. | Name an herb that has been touted for bronchitis, though significant scientific research is lacking. | Garden violet |
| 453. | Name a natural product that is often used for seasoning and has been touted for use in high blood pressure. | Garlic |
| 454. | Name a natural product that has been touted for migraine headaches but can cause double vision, dizziness, muscle weakness, seizures, and even death. | Gelsemium |
| 455. | Name a natural product that has been touted to help in digestive disorders, although it can also cause gastrointestinal irritation. | Gentian |
| 456. | Name a natural product that has been used in China for hepatitis, although research seems non-existent. | Gentiana |
| 457. | Name a natural product that may be effective topically for mucositis induced by radiation therapy but can cause an allergic reaction in those sensitive to the ragweed family. | German chamomile |
| 458. | Name a natural product that has been used as a mouthwash and for gallbladder disorders but may cause hepatitis and even death. | Germander |
| 459. | Name an herb that has been used in kidney disorders, dysmenorrhea, bruising, and edema but may cause paralysis and cardiac arrest. | German ipecac |
| 460. | Name a natural product that is a mineral touted to help reduce pain, though significant research is lacking, and side effects such as weakness, neuropathy, and even death can occur. | Germanium |

461. Name an herb that has been used for preventing gout but can cause irritation. Sufficient scientific data is lacking.

German sarsaparilla

462. Name a natural product that has been used for motion sickness but may cause abdominal discomfort in some.

Ginger root

463. Name a natural product that has been widely used and touted to help in dementia, although it can increase the risk of bleeding. The actual benefits in dementia are minimal at best.

Gingko biloba

464. Name a natural product that has been used as an aphrodisiac but can have multiple side effects including hypoglycemia, skin rashes, increased heart rate, nervousness, mania, and even infant death.

Ginseng
There are different types of ginseng: Panax, Siberian, and American. Panax ginseng has been purported to enhance cognitive functioning. Siberian ginseng has been purported to increase the capacity for physical work. American ginseng has been purported to be a general tonic. There are multiple potential adverse side effects to all types.

465. Name a natural product that has been used in scurvy, although it can cause severe irritation in the gastrointestinal tract.

Globe flower

466. Name an herb that has been reputed to promote hair growth and darkening of hair although significant research is lacking. Respiratory allergies from this herb are conceivable.

Glossy privet

467. Name a natural product that comes from Asia and is touted for weight loss, although significant research is lacking.

Glucomannan

468. Name two natural products that have been touted for use in osteoarthritis but definitely should not be used in those with diabetes.

Glucosamine-chondroitin

469. Name an amino acid that is an excitatory neurotransmitter. Some claim it helps in hypoglycemia and in personality disorders. It has trouble crossing the blood-brain barrier.

Glutamic acid

470. Name a natural product that is possibly effective for chemotherapy-induced mucositis and is generally well tolerated.

Glutamine

471. Name a natural product that is high in antioxidants and is touted for antiaging effects, but significant research is lacking.

Glutathione

472. Name an amino acid that has been used as an adjunct to conventional antipsychotics in schizophrenia. It is a coagonist with glutamate at the NMDA receptor.

Glycine

473. Name a natural product that has been touted for weight loss and as a laxative, although it may cause headache, dizziness, nausea, thirst, and diarrhea.

Glycerol

474. Name a natural product that has been touted to help psoriasis, although it can cause redness and swelling of the skin. Research is lacking in regard to its effectiveness.

Goa powder

475. Name a natural product that has been touted to lower blood sugar in diabetics, although it can be toxic.

Goat rue

476. Name an herb that has been purported to help in diabetes mellitus, but it can cause hepatic necrosis.

Golden ragwort

477. Name a natural product that has been touted for urinary tract infections.

Goldenrod

478. Name a natural product that was used by the Native Americans to fight various infections but can have many serious side effects including death.

Goldenseal

479. Name a natural product that has been touted for digestive disorders but can cause nausea and vomiting.

Goldthread

480. Name a natural product that has been touted as a male contraceptive but can produce heart failure and paralysis in some.

Gossypol

481. Name a natural product that has been used for years for wound healing, but the question of skin cancer from repeated topical exposure has been raised.

Gotu kola

482. Name a natural product that has been touted for gout, although insufficient reliable information is available.

Goutweed

483. Name a natural product that has been touted as a stimulant.

Grains of paradise

484. Name a natural product that is a

Grape juice (red)

juice and has been touted to have protective effects on the heart.

485. Name a natural product that has been used for vascular and circulatory disorders but can cause diarrhea and dyspepsia.

Grape leaf

486. Name a natural product that is possibly effective for chronic venous insufficiency.

Grape seed

487. Name a natural product that is a fruit that tends to interfere with many prescription medications.

Grapefruit

488. Name a natural product that has been touted for kidney stones.

Gravel root

489. Name a natural product that is possibly effective for treating symptoms of the common cold but can have a laxative effect in large amounts.

Great plantain

490. Name an herb that is touted for fever, increasing bile production, and urinary tract disorders. In large amounts it may cause stomach pain. It is contraindicated in gastrointestinal conditions.

Greater bindweed

491. Name an herb touted for menstrual irregularities, heavy menstrual flow in menopause, hot flashes, phlebitis, and varicosities. It appears to be low on side effects.

Greater burnet

492. Name an herb that is used to reduce inflammation of the mouth and throat. It can prolong the effects of hexobarbital.

Greek sage

493. Name a natural product that is a popular tea in China and becoming more so in America, and although research is seriously lacking, it has been touted for cancer prevention. It does have a stimulating effect from the caffeine content.

Green tea

494. Name a natural product that has been touted for sinusitis, although it can have significant side effects including congestion, edema, and turning blue.

Ground ivy

495. Name a natural product that has been used for gout, rheumatism, malaria, and inducing menstrual flow. It is also a stimulant and a diuretic. Topically it is used for wounds. Sufficient scientific data is lacking.

Ground pine

496. Name an herb that is touted for parasite infestation and colic. The pressed juice is used for epilepsy and dysmenorrhea. Symptoms of acute veno-occlusive disease with chronic exposure are seen with nausea, vomiting, dull abdominal pain, and marked abdominal distension.

Groundsel

497.  Name a natural product that is used as a preventive treatment for gout and rheumatism. It is also used for skin disorders and syphilis. Topically it is used as a bacteriostatic mouthwash. It is a diagnostic tool for occult blood.

Guaiac wood resin

498.  Name a natural product from South America that is considered the greatest source of caffeine in the world and as such can potentially cause many side effects.

Guarana

499.  Name a natural product that has been touted to help to lower blood sugar in diabetics, although significant research is lacking.

Guar gum

500.  Name a natural product that is a natural rubber and is not used medically. It can induce erythema on contact.

Guayule

501.  Name an herb that has diuretic effects, can lower blood pressure, could be dangeous, and has the Western name of tinospora cordifolia.

Guduchi

502.  Name a natural product that comes from a tree native to Arabia and is touted to lower blood sugar.

Guggal gum

503.  Cammiphora muskul is also known as what? It is touted to lower cholesterol and triglycerides. It is touted to stimulate thyroid function.

Guggulipid

504.  Name a natural product that has been touted for dental care.

Gum arabic

505.  Name a natural product that has been touted for cough and bronchitis but can cause diarrhea, kidney irritation, and allergic reaction in those sensitive to the ragweed family.

Gumweed

506.  Name a natural product that has been touted to lower blood sugar in diabetics.

Gymnema

507.  Name a natural product that can cause hallucinations although related, safe products are epicurean delights.

Hallucinogenic mushrooms

508.  Name a group of related substances that can cause altered consciousness, visual hallucinations, flashbacks, depression, psychosis, seizures, and renal failure.

Hallucinogens including:
LSD (lysergic acid diethylamide)
DMT (dimethyltryptamine)
STP (2, 5–dimethoxy–4–methylamphetamine)
DMA (dimethoxyamphetamine)

MDMA or "Ecstasy" (3–4–methyl-
enedioxymeth-amphetamine)
Psilocybin
Mescaline

509. Name a natural product that is
native to North America and is
touted for various skin problems, although research is lacking
in regard to its effectiveness.

Hamamelis virginiana
(devil's claw)

510. Name a natural product that
may be effective for mild exocrine pancreatic insufficiency,
although photosensitivity is possible.

Haronga

511. Name a natural product that
comes from Africa and has been touted to help with arthritis
but can have undesirable side effects such as ulcers, high
blood pressure, and heart disease.

Harpagophytum procumbers

512. Name a natural product that has been
touted to help in urinary tract infections, although there is
insufficient reliable information available.

Hartstongue

513. Name a natural product that promotes
sweating and is used for pain and as a hallucinogen. It may
cause vomiting, auditory hallucinations, dizziness, tachycardia,
and high blood pressure.

Hawaiian baby woodrose

514. Name a natural product that has been
touted for congestive heart failure but definitely should not
be used with digitalis because of possible dangerous interactions.

Hawthorne

515. Name a natural product that has been
touted to help in arthritis, although significant research is
lacking.

Hay flower

516. Name a natural product that is a
common nut used to reduce cholesterol and as an antioxidant, although it can cause allergic reactions in some individuals.

Hazelnut

517. Name a natural product that is used
for respiratory disorders and as a laxative. Topically it is used
for seborrheic skin disorders. Sufficient scientific data is lacking.

Heart's ease

518. Name a natural product that has been
used for diarrhea, gastrointestinal spasm, liver and gallbladder
disease, gout, and arthritis, although significant research is
lacking.

Heather

519.  Name an herb that is used as an emetic, stimulates bowel movements, and eliminates intestinal parasites. In large amounts it can cause spasms, paralysis, and circulatory collapse.

Hedge hyssop

520.  Name an herb that is used for the treatment of bronchitis, urinary tract disorders, and to decrease inflammation of the gallbladder. Digitalis-like effects are possible such as vomiting, headache, and arrhythmias.

Hedge mustard

521.  Name a natural product that has been used as a sedative but is unsafe and can cause cardiovascular collapse and death.

Hemlock

522.  Name a natural product that has been touted for coughs and the common cold, although there is insufficient reliable information available.

Hemlock spruce

523.  Name an herb that is used for cold, fever, and liver and gallbladder disorders. Chronic toxicity may cause veno-occlusive liver disease.

Hemp agrimony

524.  Name a natural product that has been touted for bronchitis, although significant research is lacking.

Hempnettle

525.  Name a natural product that has been touted for spasms of the gastrointestinal tract but contains a poisonous alkaloid and can cause death.

Henbane

526.  Name a natural product that is used topically for dandruff but can cause contact dermatitis, swelling, scaling, blisters, and scarring.

Henna

527.  Name a natural product that has been used for headaches, but the plant and berries are poisonous and can cause nausea, vomiting, and respiratory paralysis.

Herb Paris

528.  Name an herb that decreases inflammation of the gallbladder, bladder, and kidneys. It prevents formation of calcium. It has hypotensive effects.

Herb Robert

529.  Name a natural product that is used for hemorrhoids but can cause abdominal pain, diarrhea, and gastritis.

Hesperidin

530.  Name a natural product that is a hormone of pituitary origin that has been touted as having antiaging effects, although the effectiveness and safety are not known.

HGH (human growth hormone)

531.  Name a natural product that has been used as an antispasmodic, although significant research is lacking.

Hibiscus

532. Name a natural product that is possibly effective for rheumatoid arthritis and anemia associated with dialysis.

Histidine

533. Name a natural product that has been touted to lower both blood pressure and cholesterol, although the effectiveness and safety are not known.

HMB

534. Name a natural product that has been used for coughs, digestive disorders, jaundice, and as a diuretic, although there is insufficient reliable information available.

Holly

535. Name an amino acid that at high levels might be associated with increased risk of heart disease.

Homocysteine

536. Name a natural product that is a sweetener and has been used for coughs, asthma, and as an expectorant, but it can cause allergic reactions in some and even botulism poisoning in infants.

Honey

537. Name a natural product that has been used for digestive disorders and as a laxative but may irritate the gastrointestinal tract, kidneys, and urinary tract.

Honeysuckle

538. Name a natural product that has been touted for years to decrease anxiety and improve sleep.

Hops

539. Name a natural product that has been touted to lower blood sugar, but it can interact with migraine medications, diabetic medications, and antiarrhythmias.

Horehound

540. Name a natural product that has been used for varicose veins, although the pure forms may be toxic and may even cause death.

Horse chestnut

541. Name a natural product that has been used for digestive disorders and to promote menstruation, although more research is needed.

Horsemint

542. Name a natural product that has been used for sinus congestion. Some people love the taste, and others hate the taste. It should not be used by those with ulcers.

Horseradish

543. Name a natural product that has been touted as a beauty aid for the hair, skin, and nails, although it can cause nicotine-like poisoning.

Horsetail

544. Name a natural product that has been used for diarrhea, bronchitis, and as a cough sedative, although research is lacking.

Hound's tongue

545. Name a natural product that has been
used for severe diarrhea, although more research is needed.

Houseleek

546. Name a natural product that has been
touted for Alzheimer's disease, although it can cause vomiting, diarrhea, cramping, and bradycardia.

Huperzine A

547. Name a natural product that has been
touted for urinary tract infections, although it can cause dizziness and its effectiveness is not yet known.

Hydrangea

548. Name a natural product that is used
for treating metastatic colorectal cancer when used as a single agent. It can cause confusion, irregular breathing, violent
behavior, seizures, and coma. It can cause renal toxicity and
is hepatotoxic.

Hydrazine sulfate

549. Name a natural product that has been
touted for high blood pressure and is often found in small
amounts in alcoholic beverages. However, in larger amounts it
can cause seizures.

Hyssop

550. Name a natural product that is from Spain
that is touted for irritable bowel syndrome.

Iberis amara

551. Name a natural product that has been
touted to help in indigestion, although there is insufficient
reliable information available.

Iberogast

552. Name a natural product that has been
touted as an aphrodisiac and for fever and flu, although it can
cause convulsions, paralysis, and respiratory arrest.

Iboga

553. Name a natural product that has been
touted to help in HIV, although research is lacking. This product can irritate the gastrointestinal tract.

Iceland moss

554. Name a natural product that has been
touted to help those who are prone to fainting, although it
can cause anxiety and even seizures.

Ignatius bean

555. Name a natural product that has been
touted for liver and gallbladder disorders, although it may
cause colic in those with gallstones and allergic reaction in
those sensitive to ragweed.

Immortelle

556. Name a natural product that has been
touted for various cardiovascular problems, although it can
cause hepatic and renal damage.

Indian almond

557. Name a natural product that comes
from the bark of the boswellia tree that is touted for arthritis, although research regarding its effectiveness is not known.

Indian frankincense

558. Name a natural product that has been
touted to help in various kinds of pain, although effectiveness
is not known.

Indian gooseberry

559. Name a natural product that according
to folk medicine was used to treat various kinds of pain,
although sufficient scientific research is lacking.

Indian long pepper

560. Name a natural product that has been
used for digestive disorders, although sufficient information is
lacking.

Indian physic

561. Name a natural product that has been
touted for both hypertension and schizophrenia, although it
may have many side effects including drowsiness, sexual dysfunction, and hypertension, which it is touted to help.

Indian snakeroot

562. Name a natural product that has been
touted to help in liver toxicities, although it can also be toxic
to the liver.

Indigo

563. Name a natural product that has been
touted as "a fountain of youth," although significant scientific
research is lacking.

Indium

564. Name a natural product that has been
touted to help in the prevention of cancer, although there
might be a risk that it might actually cause cancer.

Indole-3-carbinol

565. Name a natural product that has been
used by weight trainers but has also been used to help in
stroke recovery. Significant research is lacking.

Inosine

566. Name a natural product that has been tried
in a number of psychiatric disorders, although most research
shows it is no better than placebo. However, it may have possibly helped at times in OCD.

Inositol

567. Name a natural product that may be
effective for hyperlipidemia.

Inositol nicotinate

568. Name a natural product that has been
touted to help in obesity, although some people have severe
allergic reactions to it.

Inulin

569. Name a natural product that is a
mineral used for treating goiter and hyperthyroidism.

Iodine

570. Name a natural product that has been
touted to help in cancer, although scientific research does not
back this up.

IP-6

571.  Name a natural product from South America that has been used as an expectorant in many emergency rooms. Chronic use can cause death.

Ipecac

572.  Name a natural product that has been touted for many ailments including coughs, diarrhea, headache, bronchitis, chills, gonorrhea, hemorrhoids, and ringworm, although reliable information is not available.

Iporuru

573.  Name a natural product that has been touted for osteoporosis, but more studies are needed.

Ipriflavone

574.  Name a natural product that has been touted for the common cold and bronchitis, although it can cause bleeding, cramping, and dizziness.

Irish moss

575.  Name a natural product that is used in iron-deficiency anemia.

Iron

576.  Name a natural product that has been touted to reduce intraoccular pressure in glaucoma, although it can have several side effects including hypertension, dizziness, and headaches and should definitely not be used by those with angle-closure glaucoma.

Jaborandi

577.  Name a natural product that has been touted for fever and inflammation, although research is lacking.

Jacob's ladder

578.  Name a natural product that has been used as a diuretic, although information regarding its effectiveness is insufficient.

Jalap

579.  Name a natural product that has been touted for insomnia, although it can cause sedation, vomiting, and tremors.

Jamaican dogwood

580.  Name a natural product that is possibly effective when used topically for mild inflammation of the skin.

Jambolan bark

581.  Name a natural product that has been touted to lower blood sugar, although effectiveness is highly in doubt and research is lacking.

Jambul

582.  Name a natural product that is possibly effective for improving gastrointestinal and gallbladder function and when used topically for myalgia, although it can cause stomach upset when taken orally and contact dermatitis when used topically.

Japanese mint

583.  Name an herb that is used for hepatitis and for hepatic and abdominal pain. Other species of this

Jasmine

plant have been used as a sedative and cancer treatment. It
may cause hypersensitivity.

584.  Name a natural product that is found in                    Jatoba
      the rain forests of South America and is touted for many
      uses including infections, although research is lacking and its
      effectiveness is not known.

585.  Name a natural product that is possibly                    Japanese turmeric
      effective for peptic disorders, although it can cause gastric
      irritation and nausea in large amounts.

586.  Name a natural product that has been                       Java tea
      used for genitourinary disorder. Scientific data regarding its
      effectiveness is lacking.

587.  Name a natural product that is used for mild               Jewelweed
      digestive disorders and poison ivy, although research is lack-
      ing.

588.  Name a natural product that has been                       Jiaogulan
      touted for hypertension and hyperlipidemia, although it can
      cause severe nausea and increase the risk of bleeding.

589.  Name a natural product that has been                       Jimsonweed
      touted for use in parkinsonism, although it is highly toxic and
      can even cause death.

590.  Name a natural product that has been                       Jojoba
      used topically for chapped lips.

591.  Name a natural product that has been                       Jujube
      touted to help in liver disease, although significant scientific
      research is lacking.

592.  Name a natural product that has been used                  Juniper
      for years for flavoring alcoholic beverages and has been
      touted for urinary tract infections.

593.  Name a natural product that has been                       Kamala
      touted for treating tape worm infestation, although research
      is lacking.

594.  Name a natural product that has been                       Kan jang
      touted to help in the common cold, although scientific infor-
      mation is lacking.

595.  Name a natural product that has been                       Kaolin
      touted for use in diarrhea, although it can cause constipation.

596.  Name a natural product that has been                       Karaya gum
      used as a laxative, although it might cause gastrointestinal dis-
      tress.

597. Name a popular product that has been touted for use in anxiety, although there have been reports of serious liver toxicity.     Kava

598. Name a natural product that is exceptionally high in nutritional value of many trace elements, several amino acids, and several vitamins.     Kelp

599. Name a natural product that is touted to help in depression, although side effects can be serious including manic behavior, psychosis, myocardial infarctions, and cerebral hemorrhage.     Khat

600. Name a natural product that has been used in angina in Egypt and Pakistan, although it can cause insomnia and liver disease.     Khella

601. Name a natural product that has been used topically to reduce the effects of aging and for skin roughness, although it may cause dry skin.     Kinetin

602. Name a natural product which is an extract of Saint-John's-wort that has been touted for use in depression, although there is insufficient reliable information in regard to its effectiveness.     Kira

603. Name a natural product that is high in serotonin and vitamin C and is often added to some drinks.     Kiwi

604. Name a natural product that has been touted for bronchitis and inflammation of the mouth and pharynx, although significant research is lacking.     Knotweed herb

605. Name a Chinese herb touted to help in sore throats, often found as a tea, and has the Western name of curburbitaceae fruit.     Lo han kuo

606. Name a natural product used to make a popular soft drink that is also touted to help with asthma, diarrhea, depression, and migraines.     Kola

607. Name a natural product that has been touted for fatigue, although it can have serious side effects including jaundice and even possibly death.     Kombucha tea

608. Name an herb that has been used for tapeworms. Sufficient scientific data is inadequate. It is a gastrointestinal irritant and can cause acidosis and shock.     Kousso

609. Name a natural product that has been touted to improve blood flow in angina, although it can be dangerous when used with other cardiac medicines.     Kudzu

610. Name a natural product that is an odor-free
garlic and has been used in high blood pressure, although it
could conceivably thin the blood.                                    Kwai

611. Name a natural product which is another
form of garlic and has been used in high blood pressure.             Kyolic

612. Name a natural product that has been used
for bronchitis and as an expectorant, although research is
lacking.                                                             Labdanum

613. Name a natural product that has been used
as an expectorant but can cause spasms, paralysis, and even
death.                                                               Labrador tea

614. Name a natural product that has been
used as a pesticide.                                                 Laburnum

615. Name a natural product that has been used to
prevent the symptoms of lactose intolerance such as cramps,
diarrhea, and gas.                                                   Lactase

616. Name a natural product that has been used
to treat and prevent diarrhea but can cause mild flatulence.         Lactobacillus

617. Name a natural product that has been
touted to stimulate the immune system, although significant
research is lacking.                                                 Lactoferrin

618. Name a natural product that has been
touted to help in wound healing, although scientific research
is not available.                                                    Lady's bedstraw

619. Name a natural product that has been used for
respiratory and GI disorders. Its effectiveness is not known.        Lady's fern

620. Name a natural product that has been used to
decrease bleeding, although it can cause liver damage.               Lady's mantle

621. Name a natural product that is possibly
effective as a bulk laxative when the derivative, sodium algi-
nate, is used.                                                       Laminaria

622. Name a natural product that has been touted to
help in yeast infections, although it can cause severe anemia
in chronic use.                                                      La pacho

623. Name a natural product that has been used
diversely from the common cold to AIDS. Its effectiveness is
not known. It can cause GI side effects.                             Larch arabinogalactan

624. Name a natural product that is used                             Larch turpentine

topically for neuralgia, fever, and upper respiratory infections. It is unsafe in large quantities and can cause kidney and central nervous system toxicity. When inhaled, it can cause acute airway inflammation.

625. Name a natural product that is possibly effective for congestive heart failure when combined with conventional treatment, although it can cause abdominal pain, diarrhea, and gout.

L-arginine

626. Name a natural product that has been used as a sedative and appetite stimulant, although research is lacking.

Larkspur

627. Name a natural product that is used in foods such as unleavened Indian bread. The flowers are used for color and fragrance. It is unsafe when used orally. It can be neurotoxic.

Lathyrus

628. Name a natural product that has been touted to help in HIV infections but can cause dizziness and headaches.

Laurelwood

629. Name a natural product that has been used topically for fungal infections of the feet, although scientific research is lacking.

Lavender

630. Name an herb that is used for premenstrual syndrome, worm infestation, and digestive disorders. Topically it is an insect repellant. Scientific data is inadequate.

Lavender cotton

631. Name a natural product that has been touted to help in weight loss, is often used by body builders, and has even been used in chronic fatigue syndrome, although the racemic mixture is toxic.

L-carnitine

632. Name a natural product that has been tried in Alzheimer's disease, although it can cause hepatitis and research is lacking in regard to its effectiveness.

Lecithin

633. Name a natural product that is an insect and has been used for stimulating blood flow at surgical reattachment sites. Its saliva does inhibit platelet aggregation and contains several substances with anticoagulant properties. They can cause infections, bleeding, and even tracheal obstruction.

Leech

634. Name a natural product that has been used as a source of vitamin C for scurvy and the common cold. Its effectiveness is not known.

Lemon

635. Name a natural product that has a folklore

Lemon balm

reputation for lifting mood, although it is contraindicated in
hypothyroidism and contraindicated in other herbs or drugs
that might have sedative properties.

636.  Name a natural product that has been                      Lemongrass
      touted to help in upper respiratory infections, although its
      effectiveness is not known.

637.  Name a natural product that has been                      Lemon verbena
      touted to help in digestive disorders, agitation, and insomnia,
      although research is lacking.

638.  Name a natural product that has been                      Lentinan
      touted to help in HIV infections by a possible augmentation
      of natural killer cells and enhanced T-helper cell functioning,
      but significant research is lacking.

639.  Name a natural product that has been used                 Lesser celandine
      orally for scurvy and topically for warts and bleeding wounds
      but can cause GI irritation and skin irritation.

640.  Name a branched-chain amino acid that                     Leucine
      some claim helps to lower blood sugar.

641.  Name a natural product that has been used                 Levent berry
      orally for dizziness and topically for scabies. With this herb
      there have been cases of uncoordination, depression, and
      muscle spasms. Cases of coma and death have occurred.

642.  Name a natural product that is touted for                 Licorice
      use for peptic ulcers, although it can have estrogen-like side
      effects and can be especially dangerous for those with any
      kidney damage.

643.  Name a natural product that has been                      Lily of the valley
      touted for use in heart failure, but its effectiveness seems
      lacking.

644.  Name a natural product that is a                          Lime fruit
      fruit and has been used as a source of vitamin C for scurvy.
      Scientific use is inadequate.

645.  Name a natural product that is used in                    Lime oil
      cosmetics and as a flavoring agent in food and beverages.
      Topically it can cause hypersensitivity.

646.  Name a natural product that has been                      Linden charcoal
      used for intestinal disorders. Scientific data is inadequate.

647.  Name a natural product that has been                      Linden dried flower
      touted for use in the common cold but could with frequent
      use damage the heart.

648.  Name a natural product that has been
      touted for indigestion, heartburn, and Crohn's disease, but in
      large amounts may cause nausea, cramping, or diarrhea.

Lipase

649.  Name a natural product that has been
      touted to help in building energy, but since extracts of this
      product come from slaughterhouses, bovine spongiform
      encephalitis is a concern.

Liver extract

650.  Name a natural product that has been used
      for liver diseases, jaundice, and hepatitis but can cause colic,
      diarrhea, and gastrointestinal irritation.

Liverwort

651.  Name a natural product that Native
      Americans used for its tobacco-like effects. Deaths have been
      reported with its use.

Lobelia

652.  Name a natural product that has been
      used for diarrhea, hemorrhage, and as an astringent, although
      research is lacking.

Logwood

653.  Name a natural product that has been
      used for scurvy and as an astringent, although its effective-
      ness is not known.

Loosestrife

654.  Name a natural product that is possibly
      effective for adrenoleukodystrophy in asymptomatic patients,
      although research is lacking.

Lorenzo's oil

655.  Name an herb that has been used as an
      astringent for bleeding. Scientific data is lacking.

Lotus flower

656.  Name an herb that has been used for
      diarrhea. Scientific effectiveness is lacking.

Lotus seed

657.  Name a natural product that has been
      used in edema, although effectiveness is not known.

Lovage

658.  Name a natural product that has been used
      in depression and touted to help insomnia, although cases of
      eosinophilia have been reported.

L-tryptophane

659.  Name a natural product that is a precursor
      to dopamine, epinephrine, and norepinephrine and has been
      touted to help in depression, although controlled studies are
      lacking.

L-tyrosine

660.  Name a natural product that has been
      touted to help with the common cold, although effectiveness
      is not known.

Luffa

661.  Name a natural product that has
      been touted to help with bronchitis, asthma, and coughs,

Lungmoss

although research is lacking.

| | | |
|---|---|---|
| 662. | Name a natural product that has been touted to help in upper respiratory infections, although effectiveness is not known. | Lungwort |
| 663. | Name a natural product that has been touted to help in cataracts, although effectiveness is not known. | Lutein |
| 664. | Name an herb that has been purported to help in diabetes, hypertension, fever, and cancer. Sufficient scientific data is lacking. It can cause nausea and vomiting. | Lycium |
| 665. | Name a natural product that has been touted to help in cancer prevention, although effectiveness is not known. | Lycopene |
| 666. | Name a natural product that is an alkaline solution of potassium carbonate originally made by leaching wood ashes and that was used in soap making. The soap, which was popular 100 years ago and still occasionally used today, is said to be helpful in decreasing the itch of chigger bites. | Lye soap |
| 667. | Name a natural product that has been used in herpes infections. | Lysine |
| 668. | Name a natural product that has been touted to enhance sexual excitement, although it might increase the risk of cancer in some individuals. | Maca |
| 669. | Name a natural product that has been used for diabetes, cancer, and coughing. Sufficient scientific data is lacking. It can cause hallucinations, seizures, liver toxicity, and hair loss. | Madagascar periwinkle |
| 670. | Name a natural product that has been touted to help in renal stones, although it could possibly cause liver cancer. | Madder |
| 671. | Name a natural product that has been used topically for necrotic skin wounds, though it can cause pain and intense itching. | Maggots |
| 672. | Name a natural product that is a mineral and has been touted to help fibromyalgia, to decrease headaches, and also to decrease anxiety, although large amounts can be dangerous. | Magnesium |
| 673. | Name a natural product that is touted as a stimulant and used for digestive disorders and to promote | Magnolia bark |

sweating. Scientific research is lacking.

674. Name a natural product that comes
from China that has been touted to help in nasal congestion.

Magnolia flower

675. Name a natural product that has
been touted to help in bronchitis, although large amounts can
result in emesis.

Maidenhair fern

676. Name a natural product that has been
touted to help in herpes, although research is lacking.

Maitake mushroom

677. Name a natural product that has been
touted to help in weight loss, although effectiveness is not
proven.

Malabar tamarind

678. Name a natural product that is touted
as an expectorant, bronchodilator, and mild spasmolytic. It has
excitatory activity when taken in large amounts.

Malabur nut

679. Name a natural product that has been
touted to help in tapeworm infections but can damage the
liver and can even result in seizures and death.

Male fern

680. Name a natural product that has
been touted to help in fibromyalgia.

Malic acid

681. Name a natural product that has been
touted to help in upper respiratory infections, although
research into effectiveness is lacking. The leaf has been touted
for types of respiratory infections. The flower has been
touted for gastroenteritis and for bladder complaints.

Mallow

682. Name a natural product that has been
touted to help in constipation, although research is lacking.

Maltsupex

683. Name a natural product that has been
used for arthritis and as a diuretic, although research is lacking.

Manaca

684. Name a natural product that has
been touted to help in PMS, although at high doses it could
be toxic. It may also be a factor in parkinsonism.

Manganese

685. Name a natural product that has been
used as a laxative and stool softener but may cause nausea or
flatulence.

Manna

686. Name a natural product that has
been touted to help in cancer, although research is lacking.

Marigold

687. Name a natural product that produces
euphoria, but over a long period of time it could produce

Marijuana

what is known as amotivational syndrome.

688. Name a natural product that has been
touted to help in insomnia, although research is lacking.

Marjoram

689. Name a natural product that has
been touted to help in kidney disease, although it can cause
liver toxicity.

Marsh blazing star

690. Name a natural product that has been
used for bronchial inflammation, menstrual irregularities, and
liver and biliary disorders. It is also used to lower cholesterol
and increase blood glucose. Topically it is used for cleaning
sores. It can cause gastrointestinal irritation.

Marsh marigold

691. Name a natural product that has been
eaten in Europe for centuries and is touted to help soothe
irritations in the mouth, throat, and stomach.

Marshmallow

692. Name a tea touted for rheumatic
discomforts, cough, whooping cough and cold, but it can
cause poisoning.

Marsh tea

693. Name a natural product that has
been used orally as a diuretic and topically for ulcers,
although research is lacking.

Martagon

694. Name a natural product that has been
touted for stomach disorders and digestive problems but may
lead to phototoxicity.

Masterwort

695. Name a natural product that has been
used topically for cuts on the skin and as insect repellent.

Mastic

696. Name a natural product that has been
used for fatigue, although long-term use can be associated
with cancer of the esophagus and other organs.

Maté

697. Name a natural product that has been
used topically to remove warts. Oral use could result in liver
toxicity.

Mayapple

698. Name a natural product that has long
been used for fever. The chemicals of this product are similar
to those found in aspirin today.

Meadowsweet

699. Name a natural product that is effective
in helping diarrhea and may be effective in
treating seizures in children but may cause diarrhea, vomiting,
irritability, and abdominal discomfort.

Medium chain triglycerides
(MCT)

700. Name a natural product that is possibly
effective when used subcutaneously for erectile dysfunction

Melanotan-II

but may cause gastrointestinal cramping, nausea, and fatigue.

701.  Name a natural product that has been
      touted to help in insomnia, although this is highly in doubt.
      Some research shows it might help in tardive dyskinesia.

Melatonin

702.  Name a natural product that has been
      used for poison ivy.

Menthol cream

703.  Name a natural product touted for
      gastric disorders, but sufficient reliable information is not
      available.

Mentzella

704.  Name a natural product that has
      been used as a laxative and a diuretic but can cause diarrhea
      and overactive bladder. Poisoning can cause nerve paralysis
      and even death.

Mercury herb

705.  Name a natural product that has been
      touted for atherosclerosis, varicose veins, and hemorrhoids
      but may cause nausea, vomiting, heartburn, or diarrhea.

Mesoglycan

706.  Name a natural product that is high
      in antioxidants and has been touted to have antiaging effects,
      although significant research is lacking.

Methionine

707.  Name a natural product that is possibly
      effective as a purgative but can cause vomiting in large
      amounts.

Mexican scammony root

708.  Name a natural product that has been
      touted for headaches and toothaches, although it may cause
      vomiting, severe diarrhea, tachycardia, and even death.

Mezereon

709.  Name a natural product that has been
      touted for boosting immune function and treating AIDS,
      although significant research is lacking.

MGN-3

710.  Name a natural product that has been
      touted for macular degeneration in the eyes, Alzheimer's,
      parkinsonism, and for some cancers, but significant research
      is lacking. Reported adverse reactions are few. Salmon con-
      tains this natural product.

Microalgae

711.  Name a natural product that has been
      used for nutritional purposes in liver disease.

Milk thistle

712.  Name a natural product that grows on
      the bark of various trees that can be fatal if taken orally.

Mistletoe

713.  Name a natural product that has been
      used for blisters on the feet.

Moleskin

714. Name a natural product that is a chelated mineral touted to improve the immune system, although significant research is lacking.

Molybdenum

715. Name a natural product that has been touted to lower cholesterol, although in rare cases it can damage the liver.

Monascus

716. Name a natural product that has been used for chronic eczema, although research is lacking.

Moneywort

717. Name a natural product that was used in the Pacific Islands for treating smallpox.

Morinda

718. Name a natural product that has been touted to help in kidney disorders, although research is lacking.

Mormon tea

719. Name a natural product that has been used to slow rapid heartbeat.

Motherwort

720. Name a natural product that has been touted to help kidney diseases, diabetes, and arthritis but can cause vomiting, diarrhea, and kidney damage in large amounts.

Mountain ash berry

721. Name a natural product used as an emetic and laxative, but it can cause gastrointestinal upset.

Mountain flax

722. Name a natural product touted for use topically for psoriasis, herpes, and fungal infections. Orally, it can cause death. Effectiveness topically is not known.

Mountain laurel

723. Name a natural product that has been touted for asthma, bronchitis, and whooping cough but can cause an allergic reaction to those sensitive to the ragweed family.

Mouse ear

724. Name a natural product that has been touted to help in arthritis, although significant research is lacking.

MSM

725. Name a natural product that is high in fiber.

Mucilage

726. Name a natural product that has been touted to help in insomnia, although research is lacking.

Mugwort

727. Name a natural product that has been touted to help in impotence, although effectiveness is not known.

Muira puama

728. Name a natural product that has been touted to help in upper respiratory infections.

Mullein

729. Name a natural product that has been used in Chinese medicine for stroke, coma, and convulsions, although research is lacking.

Musk

730. Name a natural product that has been touted to help in arthritis, although significant research is lacking.

Mussel

731. Name a natural product that has been touted to help in upper respiratory infections, although significant research is lacking.

Mustard

732. Name a natural product that has been touted to help with sore throat infections, although side effects are possible including fever, which it is touted to help.

Myrrh

733. Name a natural product that has been touted to help lower blood sugar in diabetes but could possibly damage the liver.

Myrtle

734. Name a natural product that has been touted to have antiaging effects, although significant research is lacking.

NAC

735. Name a natural product that has been touted for Crohn's disease and osteoarthritis, although research is lacking.

N-Acetyl glucosamine

736. Name a natural product that has been touted to reduce high cholesterol, although it can possibly have adverse side effects such as headaches, dizziness, liver damage, and insulin resistance.

NADH (niacin)

737. Name a natural product that has been used for urinary tract infections when combined with other herbs but may cause GI tract infections.

Nasturtium

738. Name a natural product that is in some commercial preparations of toothpaste and is touted to help in gingivitis, although the effectiveness of these claims has not been established, and it can in excessive dosages even cause death in children.

Neem

739. Name a natural product that is an oil that when breathed is touted to help with insomnia, although research is lacking.

Neroli

740. Name a natural product that has been touted for insomnia, although it can cause hallucinations.

Nerve root

741. Name a natural product that has been touted to help in hay fever.

Nettle

742. Name a natural product that has been used historically as an expectorant, clotting agent, and astringent, although reliable information is unavailable.

New Jersey tea

743. Name a natural product that has been touted for rheumatoid arthritis, although these claims are unlikely.

New Zealand green-lipped mussel

744. Name a natural product that has been touted to help lower cholesterol but may cause skin flushing and other symptoms.

Niacin

745. Name a natural product that has been touted to help in diabetes.

Niacinamide

746. Name a natural product that is possibly effective for inflammation of the upper respiratory tract mucous membrane, although it can cause nausea, vomiting, and diarrhea.

Niauli oil

747. Name a natural product that has been touted to help cramps, fever, and inflammation, although research is lacking.

Northern prickly ash

748. Name a natural product that is a neurotransmitter in the brain.

Norepinephrine

749. Name a natural product that has been used in China for nosebleeds, but its use is based on folklore.

Notoginseng root

750. Name a natural product that is found in custard pies, but in large dosages it could cause seizures and even death.

Nutmeg

751. Name two natural products used for digestive symptoms, as well as cancer and as a hallucinogen. They are used topically as an analgesic. In excessive doses they can cause neurological symptoms, impaired cognition, psychosis, seizures, shock, coma, and occassional death.

Nutmeg and mace

752. Name a natural product that has been touted for impotence but has contents of strychnine in it.

Nux vomica

753. Name a natural product that has been touted to help with kidney stones, although significant research is lacking.

Oak

754. Name a natural product that is possibly effective when used orally for acute diarrhea and when used topically for inflammatory skin diseases, although it can cause gastrointestinal disturbances and kidney damage.

Oak bark

755. Name a natural product that has been
used in folk medicine as an intestinal tonic, although it can
cause vomiting, vertigo, and convulsions.

Oak moss

756. Name a natural product that may
decrease high cholesterol.

Oat bran

757. Name a natural product that is possibly
effective when used topically for inflammatory skin conditions.

Oat straw

758. Name a natural product that is a nutritious
food and may lower cholesterol in some.

Oats

759. Name a natural product that has been
touted to help in athletic performance but can cause movement disorders.

Octacosanol

760. Name a natural product that has been
used for asthma, epilepsy, and cancer but can cause nausea,
vomiting, weakness, cardiac arrest, and even death.

Oleander

761. Name a natural product that has been
touted to help lower high blood pressure, although more
research is needed.

Olive leaf

762. Name a natural product that is likely
effective for constipation, although it may cause biliary colic
in those with gallstones.

Olive oil

763. Name a natural product that has been
touted to lift mood in some and stabilize mood in others.

Omega-3 fatty acids

764. Name a natural product that has been
used to relieve pain but can also be addicting.

Opium

765. Name a natural product that has been
touted for gallbladder and liver disease. It is no longer used
as a single entity, only in combination preparations.

Opium antidote

766. Name a natural product that has been
touted to help in the common cold, although it can cause bad
breath.

Onion

767. Name a natural product that has been
used to maintain healthy testicular function. It is derived from
raw bovine testes gathered from slaughterhouses, possibly
from diseased animals.

Orchic extract

768. Name a natural product that has been
touted to help in upper respiratory infections but can cause
gastrointestinal upset, edema, and inability to breathe.

Oregano

769. Name a natural product that has been
used traditionally for burns, sores, and cuts, although significant research is lacking.

Oregon fir balsam

770. Name a natural product that has been
touted to help in psoriasis of the skin but can be dangerous,
causing respiratory arrest and even death in high doses.

Oregon grape

771. Name a natural product that is used for
nervous disorders, ejaculatory problems, dysmenorrhea, cancer, insomnia, and rheumatism. It has also been used as a
diuretic, inducing menses, and as a pain reliever. Significant scientific data is lacking, although Thujone intoxication can cause
psychoactivity similar to marijuana.

Oriental arbortivae

772. Name a natural product that has been
touted for enhancing athletic performance.

Ornithine

773. Name a natural product that is possibly
effective for wound healing in burn patients.

Ornithine ketoglutarate

774. Name a natural product that has been used
for skin diseases, bronchitis, and as an appetite stimulant,
although significant research is lacking.

Orris root

775. Name a natural product that has been
touted for sore throat and the common cold, although
research is lacking.

Osha

776. Name an herb that is used for food. It is
considered a seasonal delicacy. The Center for Disease
Control and Prevention links outbreaks of severe food poisoning to consumption of lightly cooked fiddlehead ferns.

Ostrich fern

777. Name a natural product that has been
touted to help in digestive disorders such as flatulence.

Oswego tea

778. Name a natural product that has been
used for the common cold, cough, and as a diuretic, although
research is lacking.

Ox-eye daisy

779. Name a natural product that has been
used for dysentary, although long-term use of the seeds may
cause edema or even death.

Pagoda tree

780. Name a natural product that is possibly
effective when combined with seven other herbs (PC–SPES)
for prostate cancer, although it can cause dry mouth, nervousness, and vomiting.

Panax pseudoginseng

781. Name a natural product that has also been
touted to help in digestive disorders such as flatulence but in

Pancreatin

excessive doses could cause vomiting and diarrhea.

782.  Name a natural product that has been                           Pangamic acid
      used for detoxification, although it can potentially be carcino-
      genic.

783.  Name a natural product that is touted                          Pansy
      for bronchitis and rheumatism but can cause diarrhea and
      interacts with aspirin.

784.  Name a natural product that has been                           Pantethine
      touted to help lower cholesterol and high triglycerides,
      although significant information is lacking in regard to its
      effectiveness.

785.  Name a natural product that has been                           Pantothenic acid
      touted to help in rheumatoid arthritis, although large
      amounts could cause eosinophilic pleuropericardial effusion.

786.  Name a natural product that has been                           Papain
      touted to help in inflammations, although it can cause severe
      gastritis.

787.  Name a natural product that has been                           Papaya
      touted to help with intestinal parasites, although effectiveness
      is not proven. Large amounts could cause esophageal perfo-
      ration.

788.  Name a natural product that has been                           Para-aminobenzoic acid (PABA)
      approved by the FDA as a sunscreen.

789.  Name a natural product that has been                           Pareira
      touted as a diuretic and to promote menstruation, although
      research is lacking.

790.  Name a natural product that was                                Parsley
      used by the ancient Greeks for bad breath, although large
      dosages could be dangerous.

791.  Name a natural product that has been                           Parsley piert
      used to reduce fever and as a diuretic, although research is
      lacking.

792.  Name a natural product that has been                           Parsnip
      used for digestive and kidney disorders, although contact der-
      matitis is possible.

793.  Name a natural product that has been                           Parsnip root
      used as a diuretic. Scientific research is lacking. Topically it can
      cause dermatitis.

794.  Name a natural product that was used                           Partridge berry
      by the Native American females for menstrual cramps, although

effectiveness has not been proven.

795.  Name a natural product that has been
      touted for nervous restlessness and insomnia, although it can
      cause altered consciousness.

      Passionflower

796.  Name a natural product that has been
      used for colds, headaches, and abdominal pain, although
      research is lacking.

      Patchouli oil

797.  Name a natural product that has been
      used for yeast infections, although this herb can be lethal.

      Pau d'Arco

798.  Name a natural product that is a fruit
      touted to help with many ailments including constipation,
      bruises, headache, and menstrual pain, although the pits,
      seeds, leaves, flowers, and bark can cause poisoning, some-
      times leading to death.

      Peach

799.  Name a natural product that has been
      touted for lowering cholesterol, although animal studies sug-
      gest it might actually cause atheroscleretic heart disease.

      Peanut oil

800.  Name a natural product that is a
      common fruit that has been touted for mild digestive disor-
      ders, although significant research is lacking.

      Pear

801.  Name a natural product that has been
      touted to lower cholesterol, although it is probably not effec-
      tive in doing this.

      Pectin

802.  Name a natural product that has been
      touted for arthritis and as a digestive aid, although research is
      lacking.

      Pellitory

803.  Name a natural product that has been
      touted as a diuretic and laxative, although the pollen has
      been associated with seasonal allergies.

      Pellitory-of-the-wall

804.  Name a natural product that is a member
      of the mint family, is highly toxic, and has resulted in
      numerous deaths.

      Pennyroyal

805.  Name a natural product that has been
      used for gout, arthritis, and cough, although it can cause gas-
      troenteritis in overdose with vomiting, colic, and diarrhea.

      Peony

806.  Name a natural product that is often
      eaten as a candy and is touted to help in irritable bowel syn-
      drome.

      Peppermint

807.  Name a natural product that is possibly
      effective when used orally for irritable bowel syndrome and

      Peppermint oil

when it is used topically for tension headaches, although it
can cause heartburn.

808.  Name a natural product that comes
from Asia that is touted to help in asthma, although research
is lacking.

Perilla

809.  Name a natural product that has been
touted to help in dementia, although it contains toxic alkaloids that can damage the liver and kidneys.

Periwinkle

810.  Name a natural product from New Zealand
that has been touted to help in arthritis.

Perna

811.  Name a natural product from Peru that
has been touted to help in poor wound healing, although
orally it could damage the kidneys.

Peru balsam

812.  Name a natural product that has been
used for fevers, rheumatism, and paralysis, although it can
cause nausea, vomiting, and hallucinations.

Peyote

813.  Name a natural product that has been
touted for mild heart failure and arrhythmia, although it can
cause arrhythmias, nausea, and vomiting.

Pheasant's eye

814.  Name a substance that can cause
intoxication, euphoria, lethargy, agitation, increased heart rate,
ataxia, tremors, delirium, stupor, and coma.

Phencyclidine (PCP)

815.  Name a natural product that has been
touted to help in parkinsonism, although it could exacerbate
tremor, rigidity, and tardive dyskinesia and has resulted in
birth defects.

Phenylalanine

816.  Name a natural product that has been
touted to help kidney stones, although it could result in
extraskeletal calcification.

Phosphate salts

817.  Name a natural product that has been
touted to help in memory loss, although this has not been
proven.

Phosphatidyl choline

818.  Name a natural product that is
possibly effective for Alzheimer's disease and senile dementia
when used short-term, although more research is needed.

Phosphatidylserine

819.  Name a natural product that has been
touted to help in hepatitis and HIV, although its effectiveness
and safety are not known.

Phyllanthus

820.  Name a natural product that has been
touted to help in arthritis, although sufficient information is

Phytodolor

not available.

821. Name a natural product that has been touted to help in hepatitis, although effectiveness and safety are not proven.

Picrorrhiza

822. Name a natural product that has been touted to help inflammations.

Pimpinella root

823. Name a natural product that has been used for blood pressure problems, the common cold, cough, fevers, and topically for mild muscular pain.

Pine

824. Name a natural product that has been touted to help in arthritis.

Pineapple

825. Name a natural product that has been touted to treat worm infestations, although research is lacking.

Pink root

826. Name a natural product that has been touted to help digestive disorders and diseases of the mouth and throat, although research is lacking.

Pinus bark

827. Name a natural product that has been touted to help lower blood sugar.

Pipsissewa

828. Name a natural product that has been touted to help with cognitive enhancement, although effectiveness of this is not proven.

Piracetam

829. Name a natural product that has been touted for digestive disorders and urinary tract infections, although significant research is lacking.

Pitcher plant

830. Name a natural product that has been touted to help with constipation, although it can have gastrointestinal side effects.

Plantain

831. Name a natural product that has been touted to help with pleurisy, although it is probably unsafe for most people.

Pleurisy root

832. Name a natural product that has been used for warts but can cause severe abdominal pain, fever, hallucinations, renal failure, coma, and even death.

Podophyllum

833. Name a natural product used to stimulate lactation and as an antipyretic. Significant scientific data is lacking.

Poinsettia

834. Name a natural product that has been used topically as a stimulant for skin diseases, such as

Poisonous buttercup

scabies, but can cause blisters or burns with extended use.

835. Name a natural product that in folk
medicine was used to reduce pain, but it can cause severe
mucous membrane irritation and can even cause stupor and
unconsciousness.

Poison ivy

836. Name a natural product that has been
used as a laxative but can potentially cause confusion and
seizures.

Pokeweed

837. Name a natural product that has been
touted to help in hyperlipidemia, although it can cause
migraines, dizziness, weight loss, and gum bleeding.

Policosanol

838. Name a natural product that has been
used in China for schizophrenia, although there are questions
regarding its safety.

Polygonum

839. Name a natural product that has been
touted to help with intestinal worms, such as tapeworms, but
can cause liver damage.

Pomegranate

840. Name a natural product that has been
touted to help in arthritis. It contains a salicylate similar to
that in commercial aspirin and can cause increased bleeding
time and damage to the liver.

Poplar

841. Name a natural product that helps with
pain and has been used to make opiates, which is illegal.

Poppy

842. Name a natural product that has been
used for amnesia, fatigue, anxiety, urinary problems, and
tumors. Effectiveness is not known.

Poria mushroom

843. Name a natural product that has been
touted to decrease high blood pressure, although research is
lacking.

Potassium

844. Name a natural product that tends to
increase weight, but an extract of it has been tried in weight
loss.

Potato

845. Name a natural product that has been
used in PMS and diarrhea, although it can cause stomach irritation.

Potentilla

846. Name a natural product that has been
touted to improve brain functioning although significant
research is lacking.

Praminacetam

847. Name a natural product that in folk
medicine was used to quicken labor. It can cause cramping,

Precatory bean

nausea, weakness, cerebral edema, and even death.

848. Name a natural product that has been touted to be antiaging and is a precursor of all the steroid hormones such as DHEA, progesterone, cortisol, testosterone, estrogen, and aldosterone. It could potentially cause multiple steroid-like side effects.

Pregnenolone

849. Name a natural product that has been used for upper respiratory infections. Effectiveness is not known.

Premorse

850. Name a natural product that has been touted to help in high blood pressure, although the effectiveness is not proven, and it can be a uterine stimulant and result in hypotension.

Prickly ash

851. Name a natural product that is possibly effective when used short-term to reduce blood glucose in those with type 2 diabetes.

Prickly pear cactus

852. Name a natural product that may help in normal digestion for some people.

Probiotics

853. Name a natural product that is effective as a local anesthesia when the prescription-only product is used. It can cause heartburn and migraines.

Procaine

854. Name a natural product that has been touted to help in anxiety, although it carries the same potential dangers of its synthetic cousin.

Progesterone

855. Name an amino acid that some claim produces healthy-looking skin.

Proline

856. Name a natural product that has been used for intermittent claudication. Adverse reactions include nausea and ironically even angina.

Propionyl-L-carnitine

857. Name a natural product that has been touted to help in infections because of its antiviral and anti-inflammatory effects.

Propolis

858. Name a natural product that has been used as a laxative and has been used to help people lose weight.

Psyllium

859. Name a natural product that has been touted to help nosebleeds and skin disorders, although inhalation of the spores can cause respiratory illness.

Puff ball

860. Name a natural product that has been touted to help in otitis media but can cause the spillage of

Pulsatilla

protein and blood in the urine and in high doses can even cause seizures and kidney damage.

861. Name a natural product that is used to make a common pie that is touted to help in benign prostatic hypertrophy.

Pumpkin

862. Name a natural product that has been touted to help in low sex drive, although research is lacking.

Puncture vine

863. Name a natural product that has been used for diarrhea and menstrual complaints, although research is lacking.

Purple loosestrife

864. Name a natural product that is high in antioxidants.

Pycnogenol

865. Name a natural product that has been touted to help in benign prostatic hypertrophy.

Pygeum

866. Name a natural product that has been touted to help with head lice, although allergic reactions are possible.

Pyrethrum

867. Name a natural product that has been touted to help in PMS, although effectiveness is not proven.

Pyridoxine (vitamin $B_6$)

868. Name a natural product that has been touted for weight loss but can cause gas, bloating, and diarrhea in large doses.

Pyruvate

869. Name a natural product that has been used for anorexia, constipation, and fever but can cause mucous membrane irritation and in large doses may cause blindness.

Quassia

870. Name a natural product that has been touted to help asthma but in large doses can cause nausea and vomiting.

Quebracho

871. Name a natural product that has been touted to help in liver damage, although significant research is lacking. It can be sedating.

Queen Anne's lace

872. Name a natural product that has been touted as a blood purifier and for digestive disorders, although it can cause vomiting, diarrhea, and nausea.

Queen's delight

873. Name a natural product that has been touted to help in cancer, although it can cause headaches and tingling of the extremities.

Quercetin

874. Name a natural product that has been touted to help with coughs, bronchitis, and pulmonary ail-

Quillaia

ments, although research is lacking.

875. Name a natural product that has been
touted to help in gonorrhea, although significant research is
lacking.

Quince

876. Name a natural product that has been used
for malaria, although potential serious side effects are possible.

Quinine

877. Name a natural product that has been
used for peptic disorders, although it may cause irritation of
the gastrointestinal mucus membrane.

Radish

878. Name a natural product that is a fruit
with a great taste and has been touted to help with PMS,
although studies are conflicting and contradicting.

Raspberry

879. Name a natural product that is touted
to help with menstrual cramps and sore throats when made
into a tea.

Raspberry leaves

880. Name a natural product that lowers
blood pressure but has been replaced by newer, more effective medication.

Rauwolfia

881. Name a natural product that has been
touted to have antiaging effects, although research is lacking.

Red bush tea

882. Name a natural product that has been
touted to help in PMS, and indeed it does have estrogen-like
compounds, and thus the question of the possibility of
increasing cancer would arise as with other estrogen compounds.

Red clover

883. Name a natural product that Native
Americans used topically for infections of the eye, although
there is no significant reliable information.

Red maple

884. Name a natural product also known
as cayenne that has been touted to help in digestive problems, chronic pain, and headaches but can cause stomach
upset and diarrhea.

Red pepper

885. Name a natural product that has been
touted for gastrointestinal tract ailments and as a diuretic,
although research is lacking.

Red sandalwood

886. Name a natural product that is possibly
effective for inflammation of the mucous membranes in the
respiratory tract, although it can cause nausea and vomiting.

Red soapwort

887. Name a natural product that has been

Red yeast

touted to lower cholesterol, although it can be dangerous
when combined with other cholesterol-lowering drugs
because of possible interactions.

888.    Name an herb that is used for digestive                          Reed herb
        disorders. In Asia it is used for treatment of breast cancer,
        leukemia, and diabetes. Topically the juice is used for the relief
        of insect bites. Significant scientific data is lacking.

889.    Name a natural product that has been                             Reishi mushroom
        used for years in China and touted to have antiaging effects,
        although significant research is lacking.

890.    Name an herb that has been used for                             Resveratrol
        lowering cholesterol. It has been purported to have antioxi-
        dant and antitumor activity. Significant scientific data is lack-
        ing.

891.    Name a natural product that is                                  Rhatany
        possibly effective topically for mild inflammation of the oral
        and pharyngeal mucosa, although it may cause digestive com-
        plaints.

892.    Name a natural compound that is used to                         Rhubarb
        make a famous pie. It has been touted to help in digestive
        disorders, although it can also cause abdominal cramps.

893.    Name a vitamin that may help at times                           Riboflavin (vitamin B$_2$)
        with migraine headaches.

894.    Name a natural product that has been                            Ribose
        touted to increase muscle function and athletic performance
        but can cause diarrhea, nausea, and headache.

895.    Name a natural product that has been                            Rice bran
        touted for diabetes, hypertension, and cancer prevention but
        can cause flatulence and abdominal discomfort.

896.    Name a natural product that has been                            RNA/DNA
        touted to improve memory in those with Alzheimer's demen-
        tia, but significant research is lacking.

897.    Name an herb that has been used                                 Roman chamomile
        for indigestion. Ironically, it may cause vomiting. Topically it
        may cause dermatitis in a high percentage of individuals.

898.    Name a natural product that has been                            Rose geranium
        used for diarrhea. Scientific data is lacking.

899.    Name a natural product that has been                            Rose hips
        touted for upper respiratory infections and diarrhea but can
        cause gastrointestinal upset. It is a natural source of
        vitamin C.

900. Name a natural product that has been touted to help in Alzheimer's disease, but it contains camphor, which could precipitate convulsions in those with epilepsy.

Rosemary

901. Name a natural product that has been touted to increase energy, although there is no sufficient reliable information regarding it.

Roseroot

902. Name a natural product that has been touted for digestive disorders, although research is lacking.

Rosinweed

903. Name a natural product that has been touted to lower high cholesterol, although allergic reactions are possible especially for those with asthma.

Royal jelly

904. Name a natural product that has been touted to help in snakebites, although significant research is lacking, and it can cause spontaneous abortions and lower blood pressure.

Rue

905. Name a natural product that has been used for gout, arthritis, and rheumatism, although significant research is lacking.

Rupturewort

906. Name a natural product that is used in combination with other herbs for extreme muscle tension, joint rheumatism, hardening of the muscles, neuralgia, migraines, gout, biliary or urinary stones, and geriatric and aging disorders. Excessive amounts of this herb induces weakness, dizziness, hypotension, bradycardia, and transient A-V disassociation. Symptoms of toxicity include sweating, impaired consciousness, fainting, shock, seizures, and cardiac and respiratory arrest. Prolonged use may lead to hydroquinone toxicity, which is characterized by a gastroenteritis-like syndrome.

Rusty-leaved rhododendron

907. Name a natural product that has been touted to help in osteoarthritis, although it can cause headaches, flushing, rashes, and mild gastrointestinal disturbances.

Rutin

908. Name a natural product that is possibly effective for managing symptoms related to benign prostatic hyperplasia including frequency, urgency, and painful urination but can cause heartburn and nausea.

Rye grass

909. Name a natural product that is possibly effective for diarrhea.

Saccharomyces boulardii

910. Name a natural product that has been

Safflower

touted to help in arthritis.

911. Name a natural product that has been touted to help in menopausal night sweats, although significant research is lacking.

Sage

912. Name a natural product that may help in minor depression but probably does not help in major depressive disorders. It could be dangerous because of possible dangerous interactions with other medications.

Saint-John's-wort

913. Name a natural product that has been used for diarrhea, especially in children, and indigestion, although research is lacking.

Salep

914. Name a natural product that has been touted to help in depression, but an increased level of formaldehyde is found in the blood of some who take it.

SAMe

915. Name a natural product that has been touted for scurvy, although significant research is lacking.

Samphire

916. Name a natural product that is possibly effective for peptic discomforts such as dyspepsia, although it can cause an allergic reaction in those sensitive to the ragweed family.

Sandy everlasting

917. Name a natural product that is found in the rain forest of South America and is touted for various kinds of infections, although research is lacking.

Sangre de Grado

918. Name a natural product that has been touted to help with bronchitis, although large amounts can upset the stomach.

Sanicle

919. Name a natural product that has been touted to help with syphilis, but it is definitely not effective for this.

Sarsaparilla

920. Name a natural product that has been touted to be a blood purifier, but large dose could cause hallucinations, liver cancer, and even death.

Sassafras

921. Name a natural product that has been touted to help with benign prostatic hypertrophy.

Saw palmetto

922. Name three natural products that are often used together for benign prostatic hypertrophy.

Saw palmetto, pygeum, and stinging nettle

923. Name a natural product that has been touted to help with depression, although gastroenteritis may occur with large doses.

Scarlet pimpernel

924. Name a natural product that has been
used in China for hepatitis, although it can cause severe
depression at high dosages.

Schisandra

925. Name a natural product that is possibly
effective for spasms of the gastrointestinal tract, bile ducts,
and urinary tract, although the root can cause dry mouth, dry
and reddened skin, hyperthermia, and constipation.

Scopolia

926. Name a natural product that has been
touted to help in various heart disorders, but certain toxicities can occur in doses greater than 300 mg per day.

Scotch broom

927. Name a natural product that has been
used orally and by inhalation for the common cold and bronchitis, although research is lacking.

Scotch pine needle

928. Name a natural product that has been
touted as a cardiac stimulant, although significant research is
lacking.

Scotch thistle

929. Name a natural product that has been
touted for vitamin C deficiency, skin irritations, and gum disease, although it may cause skin irritation and gastrointestinal
irritation.

Scurvy grass

930. Name a natural product that is often
used in beauty lotions and is touted to decrease wrinkles,
although significant research is lacking.

Sea buckthorn

931. Name a natural product that has been
touted to help in arthritis, although significant research is
lacking.

Sea cucumber

932. Name a natural product that is a shellfish
that contains amino acids, minerals, and enzymes. It is touted
to help in arthritis.

Sea mussel

933. Name a natural product that has been
touted for autism, although scientific research regarding its
use in this area is lacking.

Secretin

934. Name a natural product that has been
touted to heighten libido but can lead to death.

Sedative solvents

935. Name a natural product that is a mineral
and has been touted to help in cancer and also in hair
growth, although significant research is lacking.

Selenium

936. Name a natural product that has been
touted for Crohn's disease, liver disease, and diarrhea,
although significant research is lacking.

Self-heal

937. Name a natural product that has been used for snakebites, although significant research is lacking, and it can cause anxiety.

Senega

938. Name a natural product that has often been used as a laxative.

Senna

939. Name an amino acid that is a component of many skin preparations.

Serine

940. Name an herb that has been touted to quell anxiety, decrease pain, and has the Western name of convolvulus mycrophyllus.

Shanka puspi

941. Name a natural product that has been touted to help in arthritis, although adverse reactions are possible including elevated liver enzymes and hepatitis.

Shark cartilage

942. Name an herb reputed to balance female hormones, help in diabetes, with the Western name of asparagus racemosus.

Shatavari

943. Name a natural product that has been used in excessive menstruation but in high doses could cause heart palpitations, abnormal thyroid functions, paralysis, and even death.

Shepherd's purse

944. Name a natural product that is a mushroom from Japan and has been touted to help in arthritis, although significant research is lacking.

Shiitake mushroom

945. Name a natural product that has been touted as an expectorant and as a diuretic, although research is lacking.

Silver linden

946. Name a natural product that is an extract from milk thistle that has been touted to help in liver disorders.

Silymarin

947. Name a natural product that is likely effective for lowering cholesterol, and no adverse effects have been reported in clinical trials.

Sitostanol

948. Name a natural product that has been touted to help with digestive disorders, although significant research is lacking.

Skirret

949. Name a natural product that has been touted to help in anxiety but in overdose could be dangerous, causing tremors, confusion, and seizures.

Skullcap

950. Name a natural product that has been

Skunk cabbage

touted for bronchitis, asthma, and whooping cough, although it can cause nausea, vomiting, and headaches in large amounts.

951. Name a natural product that has been touted to help with sore throats.                                Slippery elm

952. Name a natural product that has been touted to help menstrual bleeding and bleeding hemorrhoids but can cause gastrointestinal irritation.                Smartweed

953. Name a natural product that has been touted to help in nausea although it can cause allergic reactions.                                                  Sneezewort

954. Name a natural product that has been touted to have antiaging effects although significant research is lacking.                                         SOD (superoxide dismute)

955. Name an herb that has been used for respiratory and lung disorders and as an astringent and anti-inflammatory. Topically it has been used for hematomas, hemorrhoids, and ulcers on fingers. Long-term use may cause gastrointestinal irritation and symptoms. It may also cause hypoglycemia.                                            Solomon's seal

956. Name a natural product that has been touted to help in sinusitis, but excessive amounts could cause gastrointestinal symptoms especially swelling of the mouth, neck, and throat.                                       Sorrel

957. Name a natural product that is consumed as a food and has also been touted to help with arthritis and gout.                                            Sour cherry

958. Name a natural product that is popular in America and has been touted to help in menopause although significant research is lacking.                 Soy

959. Name a natural product that has been touted to lower high cholesterol.                                 Soybean oil

960. Name a natural product that has been touted to be a laxative although significant research is lacking.    Spanish broom

961. Name a natural product that has been used for bad breath although it should not be used by those with liver disease.                                    Spearmint

962. Name a natural product that has been touted to help in migraines although it is a toxic alkaloid and could be deadly.                                      Spigelia

963. Name a natural product that is a common food, is high in nutritional value, and was made popular by the cartoon character Popeye.

Spinach

964. Name a natural product that has been touted for gout, kidney and bladder stones, and urinary tract infections although significant research is lacking.

Spiny restharrow

965. Name a natural product that is a blue-green algae and is touted to help in weight loss, but no evidence for this claim has been found.

Spirulina

966. Name a natural product that has been used after spleenectomy, but there is concern because of the possible diseased animals from which it may have been taken.

Spleen extract

967. Name a natural product that has been touted to help with bronchitis although it can be toxic and can also interact with many prescription medications.

Spurge

968. Name a natural product that has been tried experimentally as an antibiotic although significant research is lacking.

Squalamine

969. Name a natural product that has been touted to help in PMS although effectiveness is not known.

Squawvine

970. Name a natural product that has been touted to help in congestive heart failure although it can cause heart toxicity.

Squill

971. Name a natural product that has been touted to help in bronchitis.

Star anise

972. Name a natural product that has been used to treat lice although it can cause eczema and reddening of the skin.

Stavesacre

973. Name a natural product that is over 100 times sweeter than sugar, but the question of cancer has arisen.

Stevia

974. Name a natural product that has been touted to help allergies and osteoarthritis but may cause diarrhea.

Stinging nettle

975. Name a natural product that has been touted to help in kidney stones, but effectiveness is not proven.

Stone root

976. Name a natural product that has been touted to help respiratory congestion, but significant research is lacking.

Storax

977. Name a natural product that is a common food, tastes good and is touted to have diuretic qualities.

Strawberry

978. Name a natural product that has been touted for arteriosclerosis and hypertension although side effects include nausea, vomiting, and headaches.

Strophanthus

979. Name a natural product that has been touted to boost the immune system in AIDS although effectiveness is not proven.

Suma

980. Name a natural product that has been touted for asthma and bronchitis although significant research is lacking.

Sumbul

981. Name an herb that has been used for sore throats and gastrointestinal disorders. Scientific data on its effectiveness is lacking. The oil is strongly irritating. Topically this oil can cause skin eruptions.

Summer savory

982. Name a natural product that has been touted to help suppress cough.

Sundew

983. Name a natural product that has been touted for constipation but can cause allergic reactions in those sensitive to the ragweed family.

Sunflower oil

984. Name a natural product that is possibly effective for treating osteoarthritis or rheumatoid arthritis when taken as an injection.

Superoxide dismutase

985. Name a natural product that has been touted for digestive disorders although it may cause vomiting in large amounts.

Swamp milkweed

986. Name a natural product that is possibly effective as a laxative.

Sweet almond

987. Name a natural product that has been used in malaria.

Sweet Annie

988. Name a natural product that has been used for dandruff but can cause contact dermatitis.

Sweet bay

989. Name an herb that has been used for asthma. Significant scientific research is lacking.

Sweet Cicely

990. Name a natural product that is possibly effective for leg pain, itching and swelling, and hemorrhoids due to chronic venous insufficiency.

Sweet clover

991.  Name a natural product that has been
      touted to help digestive disorders although the volatile oil is
      considered toxic.

                                                                        Sweet Gale

992.  Name a natural product that is possibly
      effective for preventing hypertension and stroke and also as
      an appetite stimulant.

                                                                        Sweet orange

993.  Name a natural product that has been
      used for urinary incontinence and urinary tract infections. It
      belongs to the same family as poison ivy and thus can cause
      skin reactions. Significant scientific data is lacking.

                                                                        Sweet sumac

994.  Name a natural product that has been
      used for headaches, nausea, and insomnia. Ironically it can
      cause headaches. It can also cause liver toxicity.

                                                                        Sweet vernal grass

995.  Name a natural product that has been
      touted to calm and relax nerves.

                                                                        Sweet violet

996.  Name a natural product that has been
      used topically for hemorrhoids. It has been used orally for
      respiratory infections, and long-term use has been associated
      with some cases of liver damage.

                                                                        Sweet woodruff

997.  Name a natural product, known as a variety
      of marigold, that is used to stimulate menses and has been
      used for worms and colic. Scientific information is lacking.
      Topically it can cause dermatitis. It can cause allergic reaction.

                                                                        Tagetes

998.  Name a natural product that has been
      touted to help in constipation, liver and gallbladder disorders,
      although sufficient reliable information is not available.

                                                                        Tamarind

999.  Name a natural product that has been
      touted to help in indigestion, gas, and
      belching.

                                                                        Tangerine peel
                                                                        (mandarin orange)

1000. Name a natural product that has
      been touted for cold sores, fever blisters, and diaper rash,
      although it is probably ineffective for these uses.

                                                                        Tannic acid

1001. Name an herb that has been used
      orally for stimulating menstrual flow. It has also been used for
      roundworm treatment in children, migraines, neuralgia,
      epilepsy, digestion, and stimulating appetite. In excessive doses
      it induces a rapid feeble pulse, severe gastroenteritis, convul-
      sions, rapid breathing, loss of consciousness, heart irregularity,
      dilated pupils, abortion, kidney, and liver damage.

                                                                        Tansy

1002. Name an herb that has been touted for
      cancer, colic, and constipation. Scientific information is lacking.
      Chronic exposure might be associated with venous occlusive

                                                                        Tansy ragwort

disease.

1003. Name a natural product that has been
touted to help with digestive disorders and to promote menstruation but can cause allergic reactions in those allergic to
the ragweed family.

Tarragon

1004. Name a natural product that has been
touted to help in blood poisoning, but toxic symptoms can
occur including confusion, staggering, and even death.

Taumelloolch

1005. Name a natural product that has been
touted to help congestive heart failure, although there is
insufficient reliable information.

Taurine

1006. Name a popular drink in America that has
an energizing effect from caffeine.

Tea

1007. Name a natural product that comes from
a small tree in Australia that has been used topically for nail
infections.

Tea tree oil

1008. Name a natural product that has been used
topically for small wounds and psoriasis, although significant
research is lacking.

Teazle

1009. Name an herb that has been reputed as an
adjunct to a conventional therapy for angina. Hepatic and
renal lesions may be possible with this herb.

Terminalia

1010. Name a vitamin that has been touted to help
diabetic neuropathy, although data is lacking.

Thiamine (vitamin B$_1$)

1011. Name an amino acid that some claim enhances
the production of antibiotics, increases the mood in those
depressed, and helps prevent fatty buildup in the liver.

Threonine

1012. Name a natural product that is possibly
effective as a male contraceptive, although it can cause gastrointestinal upset, infertility, and skin reactions.

Thunder god vine

1013. Name a natural product from the Mediterranean
that has been touted to help in sinusitis.

Thyme

1014. Name a natural product that is possibly
effective when combined with other essential oils and used
topically for alopecia.

Thyme oil

1015. Name a natural product that is possibly
effective for reducing asthma attacks in children and for
treating recurrent respiratory infections, although bovine
spongiform encephalitis is a concern due to possible contamination of the product.

Thymus extract

1016. Name a natural product that is possibly effective for fetal hypothyroidism and also thyroid cancer when it is combined with levo-thyroxine.

Tiratricol

1017. Name a natural product that has been used for centuries and is stimulating and addicting and accounts for perhaps one in every five deaths in America.

Tobacco

1018. Name a natural product that is possibly effective for inflammation of mucous membranes of the respiratory tract, although it can cause kidney irritation.

Tolu balsam

1019. Name a natural product that is actually a fruit but considered a vegetable that is high in antioxidants.

Tomato

1020. Name a natural product that has been touted to decrease nausea although it contains coumarin and could increase bleeding.

Tonka bean

1021. Name a natural product that has been used for diarrhea although it can cause nausea and vomiting.

Tormentil

1022. Name a natural product that has been touted to help topically for poison ivy, although significant research is lacking.

Touch-me-not (Jewelweed)

1023. Name a natural product that has been touted to help in diarrhea, although it can cause asthma in some individuals.

Tragacanth

1024. Name a natural product that has been touted to help in urinary tract infections although it could result in many toxic symptoms.

Trailing arbutus

1025. Name a natural product that has been used for infectious disease in immunosuppressed patients such as those with AIDS. It has been touted for many disorders: diabetes, infertility, autism, lupus, fibromyalgia, and chronic fatigue syndrome. Sufficient scientific data is lacking. It can cause fever, and there is always the concern of bovine-derived transfer factor that is produced from cows in countries where bovine spongiform encephalitis (BSE) has been reported, and might be contaminated with diseased tissue.

Transfer factor

1026. Name a natural product that has been touted for migraine headaches and poorly healing wounds but can cause blisters and burns when used topically.

Traveler's joy

1027. Name a natural product that has been touted to help in diarrhea but in large quantities can cause diarrhea.

Tree of heaven

1028. Name a natural product that has been
touted to help in arthritis.

Trypsin

1029. Name an amino acid that was popular in
the 1980s for insomnia and depression, but some of those
taking it developed eosinophilia and died. It is no longer on
the market in the United States.

Tryptophane

1030. Name a natural product that has been
touted to help in constipation, although it can cause severe
stomach pain.

Tung seed

1031. Name a natural product that has been
touted for menstrual disorders, urinary tract diseases, and
skin rashes, although significant research is lacking.

Turkey corn

1032. Name a natural product that has been
touted to be anti-inflammatory. It may work similar to COX2
inhibitors. It may also irritate the stomach.

Turmeric

1033. Name a natural product that is used in
many different areas including cosmetics and paint solvents
and has been touted to help with muscle pain, although it can
cause headache, vomiting, coma, and even death.

Turpentine oil

1034. Name a natural product that has been
touted as a cathartic tonic, although significant research is
lacking.

Turtle head

1035. Name a natural product that has been
touted for depression and ADD/ADHD but can cause nausea, fatigue, and heartburn.

Tyrosine

1036. Name a natural product that has been
used for mild inflammations of the mouth and throat. It is
often found in lozenges.

Usnea

1037. Name a natural product that has been
touted for urinary tract infections and for painful menstrual
periods.

Uva ursi

1038. Name a natural product that has been used
for diarrhea, although research is lacking.

Uzara

1039. Name an herb touted to have a calming
effect, to act as an aphrodisiac, and has the Western name of
acorus calamus.

Vacha

1040. Name a natural product that probably
works similar to modern tranquilizers and could therefore
have some addictive qualities.

Valerian

1041. Name an amino acid that can produce

Valine

hallucinations.

1042. Name a natural product that has been
touted to help in diabetes, but it may be toxic in some cases.

Vanadium

1043. Name a natural product that is a flavoring
agent and has been touted as an aphrodisiac.

Vanilla

1044. Name a natural product that has been
touted to help in sore throats, but in excessive amounts it
could cause convulsions.

Verbena

1045. Name a natural product that has been
used for gout and arthritis, but research is lacking.

Veronica

1046. Name a natural product that has been used
as a uterine stimulant to promote the onset of menses. It has
been used topically for stress and as an inhalant for anxiety.

Vetiver

1047. Name a natural product that has been
touted to enhance sexual response in women.

Viacreme

1048. Name a natural product that has been
applied topically for bug bites.

Vinegar

1049. Name a natural product that has been
touted to help in poor memory, although significant research
is lacking.

Vinpocetine

1050. Name a natural product that has been
used topically to help with wrinkles.

Vitamin A

1051. Name a vitamin that has been touted to
help in depression.

Vitamin B complex

1052. Name a vitamin that has been touted to
help in atheroclerosis, although significant research is lacking,
and has been linked to some cancers in high doses.

Vitamin C

1053. Name a vitamin that has been used to
treat rickets and has been touted to help prevent diabetes in
children, although toxicities are possible including weakness,
fatigue, kidney problems, osteoporosis, decreased growth in
children, and even pancreatitis.

Vitamin D

1054. Name a vitamin that has been touted
to help in cardiovascular disease and also Alzheimer's,
although significant research is lacking. Large doses can be
dangerous.

Vitamin E

1055. Name a vitamin that has been used to
treat hypoprothrombinemia.

Vitamin K

1056. Name a natural product that has been touted
to help in fatigue, although this claim seems unwarranted.

Vitamin O

1057. Name a natural product that has been used
for gallstones and as a tonic, although research is lacking in
regard to its effectiveness.

Wafer ash

1058. Name a natural product that has been touted
to help indigestion but is considered poisonous.

Wahoo

1059. Name a natural product that has been
touted as a laxative, although research is lacking.

Wallflower

1060. Name a natural product that has been
touted for diarrhea and ulcerative colitis although significant
research is lacking.

Water avens

1061. Name a natural product that has been
touted to help arthritis, but prolonged use could damage the
kidneys.

Watercress

1062. Name a natural product that has been
used for constipation, although research is lacking.

Water dock

1063. Name a natural product that has been
used as an expectorant and an antiflatulent, although research
is lacking in regard to its effectiveness.

Water fennel

1064. Name a natural product that has been
touted to help asthma, diarrhea, and fever, although significant
research is lacking.

Water germander

1065. Name a natural product which is
considered the most poisonous plant in North America and
is touted to help with migraine headaches and painful menstruation. It is highly toxic and ingestion can result in death.

Water hemlock

1066. Name a natural product that has been
touted for bladder and urinary tract disease, although significant research is lacking.

Water plantain

1067. Name a natural product that has been
touted to help in diabetes.

Wheat bran

1068. Name a natural product that has been
touted to help in cancer, although significant research is lacking.

Wheatgrass

1069. Name a natural product that is used for
those with lactose intolerance but can cause nausea, fatigue,
and headache in large doses.

Whey protein

1070. Name a natural product that has been

White cohosh

touted to help in menstrual disorders but is toxic.

1071. Name a natural product that is possibly
effective for inflammation of upper respiratory tract mucous
membranes and for mild inflammation of the skin.

White dead nettle flower

1072. Name a natural product that was used as a
poison in Roman times but has been touted for cholera and
hypertension.

White hellebore

1073. Name a natural product that is possibly
effective for stimulating appetite and for coughs and colds,
although it can have purgative effects in large amounts.

White horehound

1074. Name a natural product that has been
touted to help in gynecological disorders, although insufficient reliable information is available.

White lily

1075. Name a natural product that has been
touted for pulmonary congestion but can cause nerve damage with long-term use.

White mustard

1076. Name a natural product that has been
reputed to help in various infections, though it can cause gastrointestinal complaints, itching, and blood in the urine.

White sandalwood

1077. Name a natural product that is possibly
effective for mucous membrane inflammation of the upper
and lower respiratory tracts, although it can cause nausea
and vomiting.

White soapwort

1078. Name a natural product that is used as
a pain reliever and to prevent heart disease but can cause
stomach upset and nausea.

White willow

1079. Name a natural product that has been
used for urinary stones, cystitis, gout, heart disease, and to
induce menstruation. It has also been used as an aphrodisiac.
In excessive doses it can cause renal irritation or neurological
effects.

Wild carrot

1080. Name a natural product that has been
used for colds, whooping cough, bronchitis, and also in cough
syrups because of its sedative and expectorant effects.

Wild cherry

1081. Name a natural product that has been
touted to help coughs, bronchitis, and inflammation but may
cause reactions in those allergic to the ragweed family.

Wild daisy

1082. Name a natural product that has been
touted for diphtheria, influenza, septic angina, typhoid fever,
upper respiratory infections, and Crohn's disease. Topically, it
has been used for painless ulcers, inflamed nipples, and as a

Wild indigo

douche for leukorrhea (vaginal discharge). Large doses can
cause vomiting, spasms, and diarrhea.

1083. Name a natural product that has been
touted to help in asthma, although large amounts can cause
sweating, rapid heartbeat, dizziness, respiratory depression,
coma, and even death.

Wild lettuce

1084. Name a natural product that has been
used for diarrhea and painful menstruation, although significant research is lacking.

Wild mint

1085. Name a natural product that has been
used orally for skin conditions and stomach disorders. In high
doses it can cause mucous membrane irritation of the GI
tract.

Wild radish

1086. Name a natural product that has been
reputed to help in bronchitis, though insufficient scientific
data is available. It can suppress thyroid functioning.

Wild thyme

1087. Name a natural product that has been
touted to help in menstrual disorders, although there is no
significant research to back up this claim.

Wild yam

1088. Name a natural product that has been
touted for acne, although effectiveness is not proven.

Willard water

1089. Name a natural product that contains
salicylates that are also used in aspirin.

Willow bark

1090. Name a natural product that has been used
for preventing cardiovascular disease. Possible side effects
from excessive use are legion (confusion, uncoordination,
depression, seizures, anemia, arrhythmias, bleeding, and liver
damage).

Wine

1091. Name a natural product that has been
touted to help arthritis and gout, although research is lacking.

Winter cherry

1092. Name a natural product that has been used
to soothe sore throats but is probably not safe when used in
large amounts.

Wintergreen

1093. Name a natural product that has been
touted for cramps, indigestion, nausea, and flatulence,
although significant research is lacking.

Winter savory

1094. Name a natural product that has been
touted for hemorrhoids.

Witch hazel

1095. Name a natural product promoted for
reducing inflammation and edema after injuries but can cause

Wobenzyme N

GI upset. It should be used with caution by people on antico-agulant medications. There is some concern about its safety because it contains glandular material derived from animals.

1096. Name a natural product that has been used in Russia for stomach pain but can cause colic and diar-rhea.

Wood anemone

1097. Name a natural product that has been used orally for sores, venereal disorders, cancer, and tubercu-losis, although it is likely unsafe and a powerful irritant.

Woodbine

1098. Name a natural product that has been touted to help in liver disorders, although reliable informa-tion is insufficient.

Wood sage

1099. Name a natural product that has been touted to help with liver and digestive disorders but has a corrosive effect on the digestive tract.

Wood sorrel

1100. Name a natural product that has been touted to treat parasite infestations, although poisoning is possible, even leading to death.

Wormseed

1101. Name a natural product that has been touted to help in indigestion, although excessive amounts can cause hallucinations, confusion, seizures, and even death.

Wormwood

1102. Name a natural product that has been touted to lower blood glucose in diabetics, although it can cause flatulence and abdominal distention.

Xanthan gum

1103. Name a natural product that is used as a sugar substitute, although it can cause diarrhea and flatulence.

Xylitol

1104. Name a natural product that has been touted to help in wound recovery. It is related to ragweed.

Yarrow

1105. Name a natural product that has been touted to help in constipation, but it can cause spontaneous abortion in pregnant females, and excessive amounts could cause intestinal atrophy and even death.

Yellow dock

1106. Name a natural product that has been touted for urinary tract disorders, but it can cause vomiting, paralysis, and even death.

Yellow lupin

1107. Name a natural product that has been touted to help in digestive disorders.

Yellow toadflax

1108. Name a natural product that has been touted to help in tuberculosis, although significant research is lacking.

Yerba mansa

1109. Name a natural product that has been touted to help in kidney stones but can cause anxiety and liver damage.

Yerba mate

1110. Name a natural product that has been touted for bruises, insect bites, and arthritic pain.

Yerba santa

1111. Name a natural product that has been touted to help in ovarian cancer and is the source of pacli-taxel (Taxol), the FDA-approved drug for breast and ovarian cancer.

Yew

1112. Name a natural product that has been used in China for hepatitis.

Yin chen

1113. Name a natural product that has been touted as an aphrodisiac, although research is lacking.

Ylang ylang

1114. Name a natural product from the cananga odorata genuina flower that is used as a flowering agent.

Ylang ylang oil

1115. Name a popular natural product that has been used in diarrhea, vaginal candidiasis, and high choles-terol.

Yogurt

1116. Name a natural product that has been touted to help in impotence, although possible side effects are many including elevated blood pressure, hallucinations, insomnia, and many possible drug interactions.

Yohimbe

1117. Name a natural product that has been touted to lower high blood pressure but can cause gastroin-testinal irritation.

Yucca

1118. Name a natural product that has been touted to help in Alzheimer's disease, although effectiveness is not proven.

Zedoary

1119. Name a Chinese herb touted to be a weaker relative of ephedra and has stimulating properties.

Zhi shi

1120. Name a natural product that is a mineral that has been touted to help in the common cold and ADHD. Above high daily doses might increase risk of copper defi-ciency. In overdose can cause GI symptoms, irritation and corrosion of gastrointestinal tract, acute renal tubular necro-sis, and interstitial nephritis.

Zinc

# Grade—Chapter 22

Number correct _____ + bonus points _____ divided by 1000 = _____ Score

## Chapter 23

# Clinical Questions for Medical Doctors, Scientists, and Interested Others

The following questions are more clinical in nature for doctors, scientists, and those who may be interested. Please give yourself four points for each correct answer. There are six bonus questions.

| QUESTION | ANSWER |
|---|---|
| 1. A client presents in the emergency room with restlessness, headaches, a rapid and weak pulse, blurred vision, hallucinations, ataxia, and burning skin. You recall an old mnemonic for one type of poisoning: dry as a bone, hot as a hare, red as a beet, blind as a bat, and mad as a hatter. The family tells you that the client just ingested some kind of herb. What is the poisoning, and what might the herb be? | Belladonna poisoning. Nightshade, thorn-apple, jimsonweed, stingweed, devil's apple. |
| 2. An inert compound that produces a favorable physiological response in up to 35 percent of the time is what? | Placebo |
| 3. True or False:<br>Phytomedicinals (from the Greek word *phyto* that means "plants") are herbs or plant preparations that have been used for the treatment of various medical conditions. | True |
| 4. True or False:<br>Efficacy must be established in the case of an herb or food supplement. | False |
| 5. True or False:<br>The optimal dosing must be established for herbs and food supplements. | False |

6.  True or False:
    Prescription drugs are required to undergo extensive testing
    in animals first and humans later.

    True

7.  True or False:
    Saint-John's-wort (hypericum perforatum)
    is a popular first-line agent for the
    treatment of depression in Germany
    with about 3 million prescriptions written in 1990. It has
    been shown to have mild serotonin reuptake blocking prop-
    erties and may enhance GABA (y-aminobutyric acid) recep-
    tors. It is an inducer of the cytochrome P450 3A3/4 enzyme
    which is responsible for metabolizing most drugs used in
    medical practice. Therefore, drug interactions are possible.
    Finally, animal studies do not suggest reduced fertility.

    False. All the statements are
    correct except the last one.
    Animal studies do suggest
    reduced fertility.

8.  True or False:
    Omega-3 fatty acids are the building blocks of fats just as
    amino acids are the building blocks of proteins. A number of
    reports over the past 10 years have suggested that depres-
    sive disorders may be associated with deficiencies of some
    omega-3 fatty acids.

    True

9.  True or False:
    Valerian is speculated to work by
    actions on the serotonin neurotransmitter.

    False. The speculated
    mechanism of action of the
    root of the valerian plant is through
    some effect on GABA. It appears to
    inhibit the breakdown of GABA in the
    CNS. GABA is the most prevalent
    inhibitory neurotransmitter in the CNS.
    The benzodiazepine antianxiety medica-
    tions work as an indirect agonist of
    GABA.

10. True or False:
    Gingko antagonizes platelet activating
    factor but does not seem to increase
    the risk of bleeding with antiplatelet drugs and warfarin.

    False. Gingko does increase the
    risk of bleeding with
    antiplatelet drugs and warfarin.

11. True or False:
    DHEA is converted to both androgens
    and estrogens and may result in facial hair in women but loss
    of hair in men.

    True

12. True or False:
    The FDA is in charge of quality control
    of herbal preparations.

    False. No organization is in
    charge of maintaining the
    quality of an herbal product.

13. True or False:
    As a rule herbal preparations are
    more toxic than their synthetic

    False. As a rule herbal products
    are less toxic than their
    synthetic counterparts.

counterparts.

However, herbs certainly can be dangerous at times.

14. True or False:
No medicinal claims are allowed for most herbal products. The FDA requires absolute proof in rigorous scientific studies before any drug (herb or synthetic drug) can be approved for specific medicinal purposes.

True

15. Name an amino acid derived from phenylalanine that is possibly effective for improving alertness following sleep depravation but possibly ineffective for depression.

Tyrosine

16. What B vitamin is given before glucose in a patient that presents with an altered mental status secondary to alcohol in order to prevent Wernicke-Korsakoff syndrome? Thiamine (B$_1$).

Thiamin is a coenzyme in carbohydrate metabolism. Wernicke-Korsakoff syndrome is caused by thiamin deficiency secondary to the poor diet of alcoholics. The syndrome consists of ataxia, confusion, ocular abnormalities, impaired recent and anterograde amnesia.

17. True or False:
Most psychotherapeutic drugs are metabolized by the hepatic cytochrome P450 (CYP) enzyme system. It is so named because it absorbs light at a wavelength of 450 mm. The human CYP enzymes comprise several families, subfamilies, and individual members (CYP1A2, CYP2C, CYP2D6, CYP3A4). Saint-John's-wort is an inducer of the cytochrome P450 3A3/4 enzyme that metabolizes most drugs used in medical practice, including oral contraceptives, many antibiotics, calcium channel blockers, and glucocorticoids.

True

18. The P450 enzyme system of the liver metabolizes most drugs. Drugs can interact and be affected by inducing or inhibiting this system. Drugs or herbs that induce will decrease the level of other drugs. Drugs that inhibit will increase the level of other drugs. Which of the following is incorrect?
1. Grapefruit juice—inhibits CYP1A2 and CYP3A3/4
2. Cruciferous vegetables such as broccoli—a common inhibitor of the enzyme P450 enzyme system
3. Saint-John's-wort—induces CYP3A3/4

2 is incorrect. Broccoli is a common inducer, not inhibitor of the P450 enzyme system.

19. There are excellent antipsychotic medications today. However, augmentation strategies are sometimes needed. An amino acid that is a co-agonist of the NMDA receptor was recently tried. In early open trials some patients improved while others became worse when this

Glycine

amino acid was added. In some cases negative symptoms such as alogia, flat affect, anhedonia, and avolitional improved when this amino acid was added. Name this amino acid.

20. There are excellent antidepressent medications today, but sometimes depressions are refractory, and augmentation strategies are needed. Name an amino acid that is a precursor of both dopamine and norepinephrine (neurotransmitters sometimes involved in depression) that has been tried in augmentation strategies. Also, name another amino acid that is a precursor of serotonin that has been tried in resistant depressions but is no longer available in the United States because of cases of eosinophilia and death. Finally, name a precursor of a secondary-messenger system that has been tried.

1. Phenylalanine
2. Tryptophane
3. Inositol

21. Of the following matches of herbs and contraindications, which one is incorrect?

| Herb | Contraindications |
| --- | --- |
| 1. Black Cohosh | diabetes, high blood pressure medications, estrogen |
| 2. Echinacea | AIDS, TB, MS, severe allergies |
| 3. Feverfew | aspirin, coumadin, thrombotic medications |
| 4. Ginger | gallstones |
| 5. Ephedra Sinica | many drug interactions |
| 6. Garlic | nonsteroidal anti-inflammatory drugs (NSAID) |
| 7. Licorice | hepatitis, renal insufficiency, hypokalmia |
| 8. Siberian ginseng | hypotension |

8 is incorrect. Siberian ginseng is contraindicated in hypertension.

22. Which ones of the following are not accurate in their match?
   1. Angelica—angelica archangelica
   2. Black cohosh—cimicifuga racemosa
   3. Echinacea—echinacea angustifolia
   4. Feverfew—tanacetum parthenium
   5. Ginger—zingiber officinale
   6. Aloe vera—aloe barbadensis
   7. Bilberry—vaccinium myrtillus
   8. Chamomile (German)—matricaria recutita
   9. Ephedra sinica—ma-huang
   10. Garlic—allium sativum
   11. Gingko biloba—gingko biloba
   12. Golden seal—hydrastis canadensis

23 and 24 are incorrect. They should be as follows:
Saint-John's-wort—hypericum perforatum
Siberian ginseng—eleuther-ococcus senticosus

13. Grapeseed extract—vitis vinifera
14. Hawthorne—crataegus species
15. Licorice—glycyrrhiza glabra
16. Panax ginseng—ginseng
17. Saw palmetto—serenoa repens
18. Uva ursi—arctostaphylos uva-ursi
19. Gotu kola—centella asiatica
20. Green tea—camellia sinensis
21. Kava—piper methysticum
22. Milk thistle—silybum marianum
23. Saint-John's-wort—eleutherococcus senticosus
24. Siberian ginseng—hypericum perforatum
25. Valerian—valeriana officialis

23. Which of the following matches of herbs and a selected possible side effect is inaccurate?
    1. Siberian ginseng—hypertension
    2. Saint-John's-wort—photosarsitization
    3. Kava—liver failure
    4. Green tea—nervousness
    5. Uva ursi—nausea
    6. Panax ginseng—sleeplessness
    7. Licorice—excess sodium in the blood
    8. Hawthorne—tiredness
    9. Golden seal—hallucinations
    10. Gingko biloba—muscular weakness
    11. Garlic—odor on breath
    12. Ephedra sinica—tiredness
    13. Bilberry—photosensitivity
    14. Aloe vera—dermatitis
    15. Ginger—alter anticoagulant drugs
    16. Black cohosh—hypotension

12 is incorrect. Ephedra can cause anxiety, high blood pressure, glaucoma, prostate adenoma, and can be fatal especially with doses of 100 grams or more.

24. Assuming that a female patient is on fluoxetine antidepressant but is still depressed, what vitamin might help in some cases?

B$_6$ plus folic acid

25. Assuming that a bipolar II patient has improved on one of the new anticonvulsants but is still not as stable as desired, what supplement might help in some cases?

Fish oil with omega-3 fatty acids

26. Bonus Question
What is a common danger of gingko biloba in the elderly?

Gingko thins the blood. Many elderly people are already on other drugs that thin the blood such as aspirin, NSAID, or Coumadin. Spontaneous hemorrhages have occurred.

27. Bonus Question
Assuming that a diabetic is developing

1. Bilberry

some microaneurysms in his eyes and
general visual functioning is decreasing, in addition to encouraging better control of blood sugar with standard medications, what two herbs that are often low in side effects have
been added at times for augmentation effects?

2.   Grape seed extract

28.   Bonus Question
If one had parkinsonism and was on
L-dopa, what vitamin would they not
want and what vitamin might they want?

They would not want B$_6$ with
L-dopa, and they might benefit
from vitamin E, which might
slow the progression of the disease in
some cases.

29.   Bonus Question
True or False:
Depression is complex in causation. Giving a precursor of an
amine neurotransmitter that is one factor in the causation of
some depressions may not lift depression. Tyrosine, a precursor of dopamine, has been tried in depression. The following
catacholamine synthesis begins with tyrosine:
tyrosine→DOPA→dopamine→norepinephrine→epinephrine.

True

30.   Bonus Question
True or False:
Amino acids are major neurotransmitters in the central nervous system. GABA is an inhibitor neurotransmitter involved
in a calming effect, whereas the NMDA receptor of glutamate
and aspertate are excitatory.

True

31.   Bonus Question
True or False:
Alcohol is metabolized according to zero-order process. The
rate of elimination is not concentration dependent.

True

# Grade—Chapter 23

Number correct _____ + bonus points _____ multiplied by 4 = _____ Score

## Chapter 24

# Miscellaneous Questions and Answers

The following are miscellaneous questions about natural products. Please give yourself four points for each correct answer. There are two bonus questions.

| QUESTION | ANSWER |
|---|---|
| 1. True or False:<br>The Bible identifies the garden of Eden forbidden fruit as an apple. | False. The Bible never identifies the forbidden fruit. |
| 2. What herb might help some with eye disorders such as diabetic retinopathy? | Bilberry |
| 3. True or False:<br>Herbs are the primary medicine for perhaps 2/3 of the world's population of 4 billion people. | True |
| 4. True or False:<br>Most laxatives are herbal products. | True. Psyllium seed in Metamucil, cascara sagrada in Stimulax, and buckthorn in Movicol are examples. |
| 5. True or False:<br>Even today as much as 5 percent of U.S. prescription medications are still derived from plants. | False. The estimate is probably closer to 25 percent. |
| 6. True or False:<br>*Herb* refers to a plant used for medicinal purposes. | True |
| 7. True or False:<br>The basis of herbs for medicinal purposes ranges all the way from folklore to scientific studies. However, there is no firm scientific evidence for many natural products. General information has often been passed from | True |

generation to generation.

8.  True or False:                                                        True
    A drug is by definition any agent whether a pharmaceutical,
    an herb, a vitamin, a mineral, a hormone, a supplement, a bev-
    erage, an amino acid, or any other substance that is adminis-
    tered to the body to mediate or produce a biologic
    response.

9.  True or False:                                                        True
    Interest in natural products is increasing at a phenomenal
    rate. In 1992 Americans spent 4.5 billion dollars on natural
    products, and 10 years later they spend almost 20 billion.

10. True or False:                                                        False. Alcohol increases the
    Alcohol often decreases the blood                                     triglyceride level.
    level of triglycerides.

11. True or False:                                                        True
    Free radicals in the body may be involved in aging and certain
    diseases such as cancer. They are fragments of molecules pro-
    duced from oxygen and fats in cells. A free radical contains an
    unpaired electron and, as such, may combine with other mol-
    ecules to destroy an enzyme, protein, or cell.
    Antioxidants are substances that neutralize free radicals.
    Most fruits and vegetables contain significant antioxidants as
    do certain herbs and other natural products (vitamin E, coen-
    zyme Q10, peppermint, lemon balm, and bee balm).

12. Name two fruits high in lycopene that might                           Tomato
    help in aging.                                                        Watermelon

13. What is the solvent in which chemical                                 Water
    reactions of living cells take place?

14. What are substances insoluble in water                               Lipids
    with examples including triglycerides, phospholipids, and
    steroids?

15. What are a class of molecules that are                               Proteins
    polymers of amino acids with varied functions with examples
    including eggs, antibodies, fingernails, muscles, and many hor-
    mones?

16. What is the metabolic breakdown of                                  Catabolism
    substances called?

17. What is the metabolic formation of                                  Anabolism
    new substances called?

18. What acts as a catalyst for metabolic reactions?                    Enzymes

19. Name one of the most common sources of                              ATP (adenosine triphosphate)

energy for metabolic reactions.

20. What are nonprotein molecules that                     Cofactors
    assist enzymes?

21. Monosaccharides (fructose, glucose), disaccharides      Carbohydrates
    (sucrose), and polysaccharides (starch) are examples of what?

22. What are inorganic substances that are the             Minerals
    dissolved ions inside and outside the cell? They create elec-
    trochemical gradients across membranes and thus assist in
    the transport of substances entering and exiting the cell. They
    also act as cofactors in metabolic reactions.

23. What are various substances present in many            Vitamins
    foods and essential to health and growth?

24. Name two minerals that have been used by               Chromium
    diabetics to lower blood sugar but both of                Vanadium
    which carry health concerns.

25. Name a compound composed of several                    Seasilver
    vitamins, minerals, and silver that was recently removed from
    the market by the FDA.

26. Bonus Question                                          Coconut oil
    Name a natural oil that some tout helps in hypothyroidism.

27. Bonus Question                                          DGL
    Name a natural product that may help some who have irrita-
    tion of the stomach caused by aspirin or ibuprofen. However,
    it carries the risks of licorice.

## Grade—Chapter 24

Number correct _____ + bonus points _____ multiplied by 4 = _____ Score

## Chapter 25

# Questions and Answers about the Bible and Herbs

**H**erbs and supplements are popular in the Christian world today. There are some Bible verses that point to plants for medicinal purposes. For example, in Ezekiel 47:12 we find, "the leaf thereof for medicine" (KJV). However, in Old Testament days, we also did not have the many new tools and accessories we use weekly in church today—modern buildings, audiovisual tools, different apparel type than Old Testament days, or even cars to drive to church. The fallacy in the logic is to take these verses and then jump in logic to the belief that herbs are fine but modern medicine is not. This is a big jump in logic.

The New Testament is obviously not against medicine. Christ stated that those who are sick need a physician (Matt. 9:12), and Luke was the beloved physician. The Bible does not take a stand against either herbs or physicians. Logic would indicate to use the best medicine available whether it be an herb or modern-day medicine.

Many people ask what the Bible has to say about herbs and food. Here are some direct quotes and questions.

| QUESTION | ANSWER |
| --- | --- |
| 1. Name *a Bible verse* that points to the use of an herb. | Ezekiel 47:12 |
| 2. Name an interesting herb in a story of Rachel, Leah, Jacob, and sex in Genesis 30. The role of the herb in the story is cryptic. The story has more to do with the nature of man than with the exact role of the herb. Hebrew tradition has this herb as an aphrodisiac. | Mandrake |
| 3. Name *a Bible verse* that points to the need of a physician. | Matthew 9:12 |
| 4. The three wise men who visited Christ brought three gifts. Name one that has *a fragrant smell.* As an herb it has been used as a mouthwash for throat infections. | Myrrh |

Plants have been used for either foods or medicine since biblical days. Which of the following Bible references and verses in questions 4–17 do not match up? Please mark each true or false.

| QUESTION | ANSWER |
|---|---|
| 5. *Ezekiel 47:12*—"Along the bank of the river, on this side and that, will grow all kinds of trees used for food; their leaves will not wither, and their fruit will not fail. They will bear fruit every month, because their water flows from the sanctuary. Their fruit will be for food, and their leaves for medicine" (NASB). | True |
| 6. *Jeremiah 29:5*—"Build houses and dwell in them; plant gardens and eat their fruit." | True |
| 7. *Lamentations 3:15*—"He has filled me with bitterness, He has made me drink wormwood." | True |
| 8. *1 Kings 4:33*—"Also he spoke of trees, from the cedar tree of Lebanon even to the hyssop that springs out of the wall; he spoke also of animals, of birds, of creeping things, and of fish." | True |
| 9. *Numbers 11:7*—"Now the manna was like coriander seed, and its color like the color of bdellium." | True. (Incidentally, coriander has fragrance and today is used in commercial soups and for flavoring food.) |
| 10. *Song of Solomon 4:14*—"Spikenard and saffron, calamus and cinnamon, with all trees of frankincense, myrrh and aloes, with all the chief spices." | True. (Incidentally, today cinnamon is a popular spice, and myrrh is used as a fragrance in perfumes.) |
| 11. *Matthew 2:11*—"And when they had come into the house, they saw the young Child with Mary His mother, and fell down and worshiped Him. And when they had opened their treasures, they presented gifts to Him: gold, frankincense, and myrrh." | True |
| 12. *Proverbs 7:17*—"I have perfumed my bed with myrrh, aloes, and cinnamon." | True |
| 13. *Deuteronomy 32:13–14*—"He made him ride in the heights of the earth, that he might eat the produce of the fields; He made him draw honey from the rock, and oil from the flinty rock; curds from the cattle, and milk of the flock, with fat of lambs; and rams of the breed of Bashan, and goats, with the choicest wheat; and you drank wine, the blood of the grapes." | True |
| 14. *Ezekiel 4:9*—"Also take for yourself wheat, barley, beans, lentils, millet, and spelt; put them into one vessel, and make bread of them for yourself. During the | True |

number of days that you lie on your side, three hundred and
ninety days, you shall eat it."

15.   *Song of Solomon 2:5*—"Sustain me with                          True
      cakes of raisins, refresh me with apples, for I am lovesick."

16.   *Ecclesiastes 9:7*—"Go, eat your bread with                     True
      joy, and drink your wine with a merry heart; for God has
      already accepted your works."

17.   *Deuteronomy 8:7–8*—"For the LORD your                          True
      God is bringing you into a good land, a land of brooks of
      water, of fountains and springs, that flow out of valleys and
      hills; a land of wheat and barley, of vines and fig trees and
      pomegranates, a land of olive oil and honey."

18.   *John 3:16*—"Then God said, 'Let the earth        False. John 3:16 is an incorrect
      bring forth grass, the herb that yields seed,      answer. It does not match up.
      and the fruit tree that yields fruit according     John 3:16 is probably the
      to its kind, whose seed is in itself, on the       best-known verse in the Bible.
      earth'; and it was so."                            It states, "For God so loved the world
                                                         that he gave his only begotten Son, that
                                                         whoever believes in Him should not
                                                         perish but have everlasting life." It has
                                                         nothing to do with plants. The verse
                                                         listed is Genesis 1:11.

19.   Does *the Bible* promote the use of some          No. See Ephesians 5:18 ("And
      natural products in excess?                        be not drunk with wine, wherein is
                                                         excess; but be filled with the Spirit"
                                                         KJV).

20.   Do any of the above *Bible verses* indicate       No
      that we cannot use medicine?

21.   Fill in the blank:                                Medicine
      In Ezekiel 47:12 the Bible states, "Their fruit
      will be for food and their leaves for _____" (NASB).

22.   Fill in the blank:                                Wormwood
      Lamentations 3:15 states, "He has filled me with bitterness,
      He has made me drink _____."
      Name this herb that is an *aromatic bitter* in small amounts,
      that in larger amounts increases salivation, and that in excess
      causes confusion and hallucinations. One of its components is
      similar in effect to marijuana.

23.   Fill in the blank:                                Hyssop
      In 1 Kings 4:33 is found the following: "Also he spoke of
      trees, from the cedar tree of Lebanon even to the _____
      that springs out of the wall."
      This herb has been used in *upper respiratory infections*. In small

amounts it is an ingredient in many alcoholic beverages. In larger amounts it has caused seizures. Name the herb.

24. Fill in the blank:
In Numbers 11:7 is recorded, "Now the manna was like _____ seed."
This herb is high in vitamin C, iron, and minerals. It has an aromatic fragrance. It has been used for *gastrointestinal problems*. Name it.

Coriander

25. Fill in the blank:
In Proverbs 7:17 is stated, "I have perfumed my bed with myrrh, _____, and cinnamon."
This herb was used for its perfuming effects in the above reference. As an herb today it is used topically for skin irritations. Orally it has been used as a laxative. Name the herb.

Aloe

26. Fill in the blank:
Song of Solomon 4:14 states, "Spikenard and saffron, calamus and _____, with all the trees of frankincense, myrrh and aloes, with all the chief spices."
This herb is a popular spice in food and beverages. Its fragrance has made it popular as an ingredient in toothpaste, mouthwash, gargles, lotions, soaps, cosmetics, and liniments. As an herb it has been used for gas, colic, and diarrhea. It has also been used for the common cold. It is touted to have antimicrobial and antihelmintic activity. Name the herb.

Cinnamon

27. Fill in the blank:
The Bible says, "And be not drunk with _____, wherein is excess" (Eph. 5:18 KJV).
Name the herbal derivative from grapes referred to in the above reference.

Wine

28. Fill in the blank:
In Deuteronomy 8:7–8 is recorded, "For the LORD your God is bringing you into a good land, a land of brooks of water, of fountains and springs, that flow out of valleys and hills; a land of wheat and barley, of vines and fig trees and pomegranates, a land of olive oil and _____."
This food tastes great and has a wonderful fragrance. It is made by bees. It has been used to improve *wound healing* topically. Name it.

Honey

29. Tobacco, one of the most common herbs of all time, is one of the most harmful of all time. Give a Bible passage that encourages sexual purity but would also have application for taking good care of our bodies in general.

1 Corinthians 6:19–20—"Do you not know that your body is a temple of the Holy Spirit, who is in you, whom you have received from God? You are not your own; you were bought at a price. Therefore honor God with your body" (NIV).

30. True or False:
    In Deuteronomy 14 and Leviticus 11 the Israelites were told
    what to eat and what not to eat. Many animals were detailed
    in both what to eat and what not to eat. Some feel it has
    importance for us today. Fish with fins and scales were on
    the list of what to eat, and pigs were on the list not to eat.

    True

31. What herb is mentioned by name probably
    more than any other in the Bible, except perhaps wine, but it
    is associated with its fragrance rather than medicine?

    Myrrh

32. Who was the physician in biblical times
    who penned these words?
    "And they returned, and prepared spices and ointments; and
    rested the sabbath day according to the commandment."

    Luke. The words are from
    Luke 23:56 KJV.

33. A famous Bible character penned the
    following words:
    "My lover has gone down to his garden, to the bed of spices,
    to browse in the gardens and to gather lilies."

    Solomon. The words are from
    Song of Solomon 6:2 NIV.

34. Bonus Question
    A Bible character made the following statements:
    "Build houses and live in them; and plant
    gardens, and eat their produce."
    "He has filled me with bitterness, he hath
    made me drunken with wormwood."

    Jeremiah. Jeremiah made those
    comments in Jeremiah 29:5 NIV
    and Lamentations 3:15 KJV.
    Wormwood contains bitter
    compounds (absinthin and
    anabsinthin).

35. Bonus Question
    Which Bible character made the following
    comment:
    "Purge me with hyssop, and I shall be clean: wash me, and I
    shall be whiter than snow."

    David made this comment in
    Psalm 51:7 KJV. Hyssop was
    used for various infections.

36. Bonus Question
    Which Bible character recorded the
    following words of Israel, complaints that
    made God angry at Israel?
    "We remember the fish which we used to
    eat free in Egypt, the cucumbers and the
    melons and the leeks and the onions and the garlic, but now
    our appetite is gone. There is nothing at all to look at except
    this manna. Now the manna was like that of coriander seed,
    and its appearance like that of bdelium."

    Moses. These words are
    recorded in Numbers 11:5–7
    NASB. Coriander is still used as
    a culinary spice and as a
    flavoring agent in cosmetics
    and soaps.

## Grade—Chapter 25

Number correct _____ + bonus points _____ multiplied by 3 = _____ Score

# Final Tabulation and Grade

Chapter  1
Chapter  8
Chapter  9
Chapter 10
Chapter 11
Chapter 12
Chapter 13
Chapter 14
Chapter 15
Chapter 16
Chapter 17
Chapter 18
Chapter 19
Chapter 20
Chapter 21
Chapter 22
Chapter 23
Chapter 24
Chapter 25

Total Points                 Divided by 19 =              Your Total Score

# Appendices

by
Frank Minirth, MD, PhD
Virginia Neal, PhD, RN, APN, MS Psy. Pharm.
C. Alan Hopewell, PhD, MS Psy. Pharm.
John Claude Krusz, PhD, MD

As conventional medicines become more powerful, they often cause more serious side effects. Each year, eight thousand people in the United States die from bleeding caused by nonsteroidal anti-inflammatory drugs; others die from antibiotic allergies, acetaminophen overdoses, and adverse effects from other seemingly innocuous drugs. More and more consumers are unwilling to take such risks, at least not without trying natural medicines first. On the other hand, a current misconception that natural equals safe is belied by reports of deaths and serious illnesses.

Richard P. Brown, MD
Complementary and Alternative Medicine and Psychiatry
*Review of Psychiatry,* Vol. 19, 2000

Have we been fair and balanced? We hope so. Do natural products have a good? Of course they do, and even sometimes, pearls. Do psychiatric medications have a good? Of course they do, and at this time, a high advantage over herbs. Do natural products have a bad and an ugly? Of course they do, but overall less than prescription medications (See *The Physician's Desk Reference* for the bad and the ugly of prescription medications.) The difference between natural products and prescription medications is not only the amount of knowledge in regard to the two but also the effectiveness, specificity, and selectivity of the two compared. The scientific testing, purity, and knowledge is much greater with prescription medication in general. We trust we have given some of the latest knowledge possible in regard to the herbs and psychiatric medications.

The following appendices offer a deeper look into natural products. Perhaps you want more detailed information on a specific natural product. Perhaps you are a medical doctor, nurse, scientist, or interested layperson.

Appendices

A    Eight Hundred Natural Products—A Detailed Examination
B    How Natural Products Work
C    Drug-Herb Interactions
D    A List of Psychiatric Medications by Categories of Use

*Appendix A*

# Eight Hundred Natural Products—A Detailed Examination
## *What they told you and what they did not tell you*

The intention of this appendix is to provide individuals, caretakers, nurses, and physicians with interesting historical and more detailed data about the most common herbs and supplements, how they have been used, some of their health concerns, their mechanisms of actions, and examination of clinical studies regarding their efficacy. "What They Told You" is from various sources, even anecdotal, while "What They Did Not Tell You" is more scientific with an emphasis on potential side effects.

## A Brief Look at Herbs and Supplements

## What They Told You

### Abscess Root—Fevers

Orally, abscess root has been touted to reduce fevers. It has also been touted orally to reduce inflammation, stimulate sweating, as an astringent, and expectorant.

### Abuta—Acne

Orally, abuta has been touted for many ailments, including acne, asthma, dog bites, boils, burns, chills, colds, colic, diabetes, diarrhea, fertility in women, fevers, itching, sores, stimulating menstrual flow, wounds, toothaches, and as an aphrodisiac.

### Acacia—High Cholesterol

Orally, acacia is touted to reduce cholesterol levels.

In manufacturing, it is used as a pharmaceutical ingredient in making emulsions, troches, a demulcent for throat or stomach Inflammatlon, a masking agent for acrid substances (e.g., capsicum), and as a film-forming agent in peel-off skin masks.

### Acerola—Infections

Acerola is found in many multivitamin supplements since it is rich in vitamin C. It has been touted to have antioxidant and antifungal properties.

### Acidophilus

**How it has been used:** Acidophilus has been used for drug-associated diarrhea such as that seen with antibiotic use.

**Some interesting data:** It is an active bacterial culture found in yogurt. It is living bacteria that sours milk and is the most common organism in the small intestine in humans and animals.

**Historical data:** It has a long history of use in food. It is sometimes used in nondairy food products as a base.

**The usual dose:** 1 tablespoon of the liquid culture or 1 to 2 capsules after meals.

### Aconite

Aconite has been used in China for cancer pain and multiple other uses.

### Activated Charcoal—Acute Poisoning

Activated charcoal has a long use in emergency rooms in

## What They Did Not Tell You

Orally, abscess root can irritate the GI tract. It might cause sneezing and GI upset.

Insufficient reliable information is available. No adverse effects reported.

Allergy to acacia dust manifests as skin lesions and severe asthmatic attacks.

Research is lacking.

It could cause nausea, cramps, diarrhea, fatigue, and insomnia.

**Health concerns:** There is little or no control data on its use.

**Clinical studies:** Studies are lacking.

**The mechanism of action:** Acidophilus acts by making the enzyme lactase that digests milk sugar and produces lactic acid. Lactic acid helps to suppress undesirable bacteria and yeast in the gastrointestinal tract.

Aconite is extremely toxic. It can cause cardiac arrest.

Activated charcoal is often helpful in the treatment of

**What They Told You**

the management of poisoning. It has also been used for gas and to reduce blood cholesterol.

**What They Did Not Tell You**

some acute poisonings.

It is not usually used concurrently with ipecac.

### Adam's Needle—Liver and Gallbladder Disorders

Orally, Adam's needle is touted to treat liver and gallbladder disorders.

Orally, Adam's needle might cause dyspepsia and related abdominal symptoms.

### Adrenal Extract—Fatigue

Orally, adrenal extract is touted for low adrenal function; fatigue; stress; impaired resistance to illness; and for treating severe allergies, asthma, eczema, psoriasis, rheumatoid arthritis, and other inflammatory conditions.

Sublingually, adrenal extract is touted for stress-induced fatigue or exhaustion, poor stress tolerance, general fatigue, allergies, autoimmune disorders, depression, physical or emotional stress, inflammation, low blood pressure, hypoglycemia, drug and alcohol withdrawal, and discontinuing cortisone drugs.

Intravenously, adrenal extract has been used for treating adrenal cortical insufficiency, hyperkalemia, ulcerative colitis, status thymicolymphaticus, and preventing spontaneous abortion.

Orally, no adverse reactions have been reported. However, adrenal extracts are derived from raw cow, pig, or sheep adrenal glands gathered from slaughterhouses and possibly from sick or diseased animals. Products made from contaminated or diseased organs might present a human health hazard. There is also some concern that adrenal extracts produced from cows in countries where bovine spongiform encephalitis (BSE) has been reported might be contaminated with diseased tissue. Countries where BSE has been reported include Great Britain, France, The Netherlands, Portugal, Luxembourg, Ireland, Switzerland, Oman, and Belgium. However, as to date, there have been no reports of BSE transfer to humans from contaminated adrenal extract products.

Intravenously, adrenal extract can cause infection and abscess at the site of infection. In 1996, the FDA issued a nationwide alert regarding an injectable adrenal cortex extract after more than 50 cases of serious bacterial infections at injection sites were reported.

### African Wild Potato

Grown in South Africa, the African wild potato is also known as star grass or bantu tulip. It has been used to treat HIV-positive individuals. It has also been used for bladder and urinary disorders including prostate enlargement, cystitis, lung disease, TB, "yuppie flu," arthritis, and psoriasis. Applied topically, it has been used for wound healing.

Typical dose is 15 drops in a glass of water three times a day before meals.

There is insufficient reliable information available on the safety of the African wild potato. Preliminary human trials suggest it is not toxic and is possibly effective for increasing the volume of urine and improving urine flow in individuals with prostate enlargement. Reliable data is unavailable on its effectiveness or safety for other uses.

The activity of the African wild potato is thought to be due to its ability to inhibit the production of prostaglandin synthase thereby decreasing inflammatory processes. It is also believed to possibly stimulate and activate the body's T-cells thus improving the immune system.

Adverse reactions reported are possible erectile dysfunction and loss of libido. There is insufficient reliable information on its interactions with other drugs, herbs, or dietary supplements.

| What They Told You | What They Did Not Tell You |
|---|---|
| **Agar—Constipation** | |
| Agar is seaweed. It is often found in food. It is used as a laxative. Some have used it to decrease cholesterol. | Agar is usually safe for most. What they said has some truth in regard to use.<br><br>It has high thyroid content so should not be used with synthroid and other thyroid medications.<br><br>It probably works by drawing fluid into the intestines and causing swelling and thus stimulation of the intestines. |
| **Alder Buckthorn—Constipation** | |
| Orally, alder buckthorn is touted as a laxative. It has been used as a tonic and a component in the Hoxsey cancer cure. | Alder buckthorn can cause cramp-like discomfort when used orally. Chronic use can cause pseudomelanosis coli (pigment spots in intestinal mucosa) which is harmless, usually reverses with discontinuation, and is not associated with an increased risk of developing colorectal adenoma or carcinoma.<br><br>Chronic use or abuse of the bark can lead to potassium depletion, albuminuria, and hematuria. Potassium depletion can lead to disturbed heart function and muscle weakness. The fresh or improperly aged bark can cause severe vomiting due to the presence of the free anthrone, an emetic constituent. |
| **Alfalfa—PMS and Menopause** | |
| **How it has been used:** Alfalfa has been touted to help in diabetes, high cholesterol, indigestion, menopause, yeast infections, and water retention.<br><br>**Some interesting data:** Alfalfa is similar to estrogen and thus is used in menopause.<br><br>**Historical data:** It is a legume that has long been cultivated as feed for cattle and horses. | **Health concerns:** It can have gastrointestinal side effects. Also, it contains an amino acid, caravanine, which could trigger a recurrence of systemic lupus erythemations.<br><br>**Clinical studies:** Studies are lacking. |
| **Allspice (clove pepper)—Gas** | |
| Allspice is a tree of Central America, Mexico, and the West Indies. It has been used to treat indigestion, gas, toothache, and muscle pain. | High doses of allspice have been known to induce seizures. While it has been used for indigestion and gas, it can also cause nausea, vomiting, and anorexia. Allergic reactions have occurred. |
| **Aloe Vera—Skin Problems** | |
| **How it has been used:** It has been used extensively on a topical basis not only for wound healing but also for minor skin irritations and sunburn.<br><br>**Some interesting data:** It comes from a perennial plant with yellow flowers. | **Health concerns:** Several deaths have been attributed to intravenous aloe vera.<br><br>In addition, a contact dermatitis has occurred with it in topical preparations. Delayed wound healing has occurred in deep wounds. |

**What They Told You**

**Historical data:** Aloe vera has been used for centuries after its wound healing effects were first noted in the Middle East.

**The usual dose:** Applied topically to cover affected skin area.

**What They Did Not Tell You**

Finally, its use as a topical agent for many people with minor skin irritations seems common knowledge. However, it should not be used intravenously or intramuscularly. We are also skeptical of its use in constipation, ulcers, diabetes, and asthma.

**Clinical studies:** Studies are lacking.

### Alpha-lipoic Acid—Diabetic Neuropathy

Alpha-lipoic acid is a nutrient that has been used for diabetic neuropathy, to strengthen the heart, and to decrease aging.

The studies are interesting. Double-blind studies appear promising in some cases of diabetic neuropathy. The studies on the heart also may hold some encouragement. Time will tell.

### Alpinia—Stimulant

Orally, alpinia is touted as a stimulant, antiflatulent, antibacterial, antispasmodic, anti-inflammatory agent, and for fever.

Insufficient reliable information is available. No adverse effects have been reported.

### Ambrette—Pain

Orally, ambrette has been touted as a stimulant, antispasmodic, for snakebites, stomach and intestinal disorders with cramps, loss of appetite, and headaches.

In folk medicine, it is used for stomach cancer, hysteria, gonorrhea, and respiratory disorders.

Topically, the use of ambrette can cause dermal irritation.

### American Dogwood—Fatigue

Orally, American dogwood is touted for headaches and fatigue. It is also touted to increase strength; for fever, chronic diarrhea, and to stimulate appetite.

Topically, American dogwood is touted as an astringent for boils and wounds.

Historically, American dogwood was used orally as a substitute for quinine.

Reliable information is insufficient.

### American Hellebore—Hypertension

American hellebore has been used according to legend to treat hypertensive crisis.

It is extremely toxic. It can cause hypotension, arrhythmias, seizures, coma, and paralysis.

### American Ivy—Digestive Disorders

Orally, American ivy is touted for digestive disorders. It is also touted to stimulate sweating, as an astringent, and as a tonic.

Orally, ingestion of the berries, containing 2 percent oxalic acid, is considered poisonous. There is one case of a child's death following ingestion of the berries.

## What They Told You

### Amino Acids

Amino acids are even more natural than herbs. They are the raw material used by the body to manufacture human protein. There are 8 nonessential (can be manufactured in the body) amino acids (arginine, cystin, glutamic acid, glutamine, glycine, histidine, taurine, and tyrosine). There are 12 essential (must be taken in by the diet) amino acids. Amino acids are made up of carbon, oxygen, nitrogen, and hydrogen atoms. The nitrogen distinguishes protein from carbohydrates or fats.

Since amino acids are the building blocks of protein, they might help in body building.

### Andiroba—Skin Problems

Orally, andiroba bark and leaf are touted to treat fevers, herpes, as an anthelmintic, and as a tonic.

Andiroba fruit oil is taken orally for coughs.

Topically, andiroba bark and leaf are used as a wash for dermatoses, sores, ulcers, and skin troubles. It is used topically for removing ticks from the head and for skin parasites.

The seed oil is used topically to treat inflammation, arthritis, for rashes, muscle and joint aches and injuries, wounds, boils, and herpes ulcers. Seed oil is also used for mummification of human heads.

### Andrographis—Common Cold

Orally, andrographis is touted for preventing and treating the common cold, influenza, pharyngotonsillitis, allergies, and sinusitis. It has also been touted to treat HIV/AIDS.

In traditional medicine, andrographis is touted for anorexia, atherosclerosis, snake and insect bites, bronchitis, cachexia, prevention of cardiovascular disease, cholera, colic, diabetes, diarrhea, flatulence, gastritis, gonorrhea, hemorrhoids, hepatomegaly, drug-induced hepatoxicity, other hepatic disorders, myocardial ischemia, jaundice, leprosy, leptospirosis, malaria, pharyngitis, pneumonia, pruritus, pyelonephritis, rabies, skin wounds, unspecified skin diseases, syphilis, tuberculosis, tonsillitis, and ulcers. Andrographis is also used as an astringent, antiseptic, antidote, analgesic, antipyretic, anti-inflammatory, antithrombotic, expectorant, anthelmintic, laxative, and tonic.

## What They Did Not Tell You

Even amino acids can be toxic (Web MD Health, nonessential amino acids).

Large doses of arginine may cause nausea or diarrhea, and excessive tyrosine can lead to changes in blood pressure and migraine headaches.

Women taking supplements while pregnant or breast-feeding should be especially careful to avoid excessive doses. L-tryptophane caused eosinophilia and deaths in the past.

We are not aware of any studies regarding proven benefits of amino acids for body building.

Reliable information available about the safety of andiroba is insufficient. Avoid using during pregnancy or while breast-feeding.

Orally, large doses of andrographis are reported to cause gastrointestinal distress, anorexia, and emesis. Urticaria has also been reported. Preliminary evidence suggests that andrographis might inhibit male and female fertility, but this has not been demonstrated in humans. High doses of the purified andrographolide constituent (5 mg/kg three times daily) have caused headache, fatigue, rash, abnormal taste, diarrhea, itching, lymphadenopathy, and anaphylactic reactions. The andrographolide constituent can also cause dose-related increases in liver enzymes such as ALT, which return to normal when andrographolide is discontinued.

| What They Told You | What They Did Not Tell You |
|---|---|

### Androstenedione—Athletic Performance

Androstenedione is used to increase testosterone and is touted to increase athletic performance.

Androstenedione is the precursor of testosterone.

It could possibly cause various cancers and increase the risk of heart disease.

### Angelica (Dang quai)—PMS and Menopause

Angelica species comes from plants. It has been used for menopausal and premenstrual symptoms. It has also been used as a flavoring agent in many products (alcoholic beverages, ice cream, candy, etc.). It also has been used to relax smooth muscles. It has been touted to have pain-relieving effects. Finally, it has been used for allergies.

A rash has been known to occur in sunlight.

Since it might have estrogen-like activities, possible concerns could center around these activities.

### Anise

Over-the-counter compounds with anise may make it the number one herb in America for the flu. It has also been used for bronchitis, cold, liver problems, and gallbladder problems.

It has also been used for bad breath and may be present in some commercial toothpastes. It has also been used for gas, indigestion, and even impotence.

Anise can cause pulmonary edema and seizures when used in oil form. It can cause stomatitis when used as a toothpaste. It can cause hypomineralcorticism. It can cause nausea, vomiting, and anorexia.

### Annato—Wrinkles

Annato is an herb from the rain forest of Brazil. It is often found in skin-care products.

Research is lacking in effectiveness.

Contact dermatitis is possible, as with many plant products.

### Apple Cider Vinegar—Weight Loss

Apple cider vinegar has been touted for weight loss, aging, infections, high cholesterol, and osteoporosis. Topically, it has been used for acne.

Significant research is lacking in regard to its effectiveness.

Apple cider long-term can cause potassium loss and osteoporosis.

### Areca—Schizophrenia

Great quantities of areca nuts are consumed in the East. They can produce a euphoria. They have also been used in schizophrenia.

Chronic use has been associated with oral cancer, heart disease, and diabetes mellitus. Areca contains an alkaloid, arecoline, that has cholinergic effects that some think decreases psychotic symptoms.

### ArginMax—Sexual Dysfunction

ArginMax is a mixture of herbs (L-arginine, ginseng, gingko, damiana, calcium, iron, vitamins A, C, E, B-complex, zinc, niacin, and selenium) used for sexual dysfunction. L-arginine stimulates nitric oxide synthesis as Viagra does.

Research is sorely lacking for this complexity of items. The arginine may be the main ingredient.

**What They Told You**

### Arnica—Pain

Topically, arnica is used for the inflammation and immune-system stimulation associated with bruises, aches, and sprains, for mouth and throat inflammation, insect bites, and superficial phlebitis.

Historically, arnica has been used as an abortifacient.

For food uses, arnica is a flavor ingredient in alcoholic beverages, nonalcoholic beverages, frozen dairy desserts, candy, baked goods, gelatins, and puddings.

In manufacturing, arnica is used in hair tonics and antidandruff preparations. The oil is used in perfumes and other cosmetic preparations.

### Arrowroot—Diarrhea

Orally, arrowroot is used as a nutritional food for infants and convalescents and to thicken sauces in cooking. Babies cut teeth on arrowroot cookies. It is used as an aid to GI disorders and acute diarrhea and topically for irritated or inflamed mucous membranes.

### Artichoke—Indigestion

Artichoke is a vegetable that has been touted to help in indigestion, poor appetite, gallbladder problems, liver problems, arteriosclerosis, constipation, flatulence, and high blood sugar.

### Artistolochic Acid—Weight Loss

Artistolochic acid has been touted for weight loss, skin disorders, and high blood pressure.

### Arum—Colds

Orally, arum is touted for colds and inflammation of the throat. It is also used orally to stimulate sweating and as an expectorant.

**What They Did Not Tell You**

Arnica taken orally can cause irritation of mucous membranes, drowsiness, stomach pain, vomiting, diarrhea, tachycardia, shortness of breath, coma, and death.

It can cause an allergic reaction in individuals sensitive to ragweed, chrysanthemums, marigolds, daisies, and many other herbs in the same family.

Topically, arnica can cause contact dermatitis and mucous membrane irritation.

Reliable information is insufficient.

We are skeptical of the broad suggestions, but pickled or cooked artichokes are fairly innocuous except for rare allergic reactions. They are also tasty as a part of a Mediterranean-type diet.

Artistolochic acid is a known nephrotoxin from an herb. It was probably included by mistake in some "weight-loss" preparations in the early 1990s. In 1991 and 1992, about 100 women in Brussels who had taken a Chinese herbal preparation for weight loss developed renal failure with 70 requiring dialysis or kidney transplant and 18 developing urothelial cancer.

The applicable part of arum is the root. Arum can cause severe mucous membrane irritation and bleeding. This is probably due to sharp oxalate crystals present in the root. These injure the mucous membranes and may also introduce impurities into the wounds. Arum also contains cyanogenic glycosides, but the levels are probably too low to cause poisoning.

| What They Told You | What They Did Not Tell You |
|---|---|
| **Ashwaganda (withania somniferum)—All-Purpose Topic** <br> This nightshade herb has been touted for practically everything: impotence, herpes, high cholesterol, dementia, inflammation, addictions, ringworm, anxiety, ulcers, and even syphilis. | This herb illustrates the problem with many herbal products or extracts. Many are touted to be universal panaceas. They often have a minor benefit in some area, but those claiming one herb for everything are reminiscent of old-time medicine men who traveled from town to town with ill-defined, all-purpose tonics. <br><br> One of the authors was listening to the radio recently when a "doctor" touted a gastrointestinal cleansing regimen with a special natural tonic that could cure almost everything. Of course, it could only be obtained through him. And, of course, this kind of unclear marketing usually does not hold up to scientific evaluation. |
| **Asparagus—Kidney Stone Prevention** <br> Asparagus has been touted for urinary tract problems (infections, stone, etc.). Topically, it has been used for skin infections. It has even been touted for menstrual problems, AIDS, and cancer. It has been used as a laxative. | Significant research is lacking. It probably does have a diuretic effect and increases urine output, not to mention altering the "perfume" of the urine. |
| **Astragalus—Fatigue** <br> Astragalus is an herb that comes from China and has a yellow leaf. It has been touted for fatigue, loss of appetite, diarrhea, the common cold, flu, AIDS, cancer, and hepatitis. <br><br> It is usually given in powder form at 9 to 30 grams per day. | Astragalus is interesting. Certainly more research is needed. <br><br> It is an antioxidant and inhibits free radical production. It contains flavonoids, polysaccharides, multiple trace minerals, amino acids, and cumarins. Some research suggests that lower doses stimulate the immune system whereas high doses (greater than 28 grams) might suppress it. Also, there is some evidence it might have some antibiotic-like activity. <br><br> Some evidence reveals improved liver functions in chronic hepatitis. Some evidence suggests vasodilatation effects, and thus, it has been tried in angina and congestive heart failure. <br><br> Reported toxic reactions seem low overall. <br><br> It might interact with acyclovir (Zovivax) for herpes and immunosuppressants. |
| **Avocado—High Cholesterol** <br> Avocado has been touted to decrease cholesterol. Topically, it has been used to increase hair growth and help skin irritations. | Avocado might have some benefit for a small number of people in decreasing cholesterol trivially. <br><br> It can decrease the effects of warfarin, a blood thinner, and render it less effective. |

| What They Told You | What They Did Not Tell You |
|---|---|
| **B₁₂—Circadian Sleep Disturbance** | |
| $B_{12}$ has been touted for everything from depression to diabetes and heart disease. It has also been used for circadian sleep disturbance. | $B_{12}$ is probably only effective for $B_{12}$ deficiency, which may present with depression or, rarely, psychosis. |
| | It can cause edema, diarrhea, and blood clots. |
| **Barberry—Skin Infections** | |
| Barberry has been used topically for skin infections. Orally, it has been touted to slow heart rate. | Significant research is lacking for this plant product. |
| **Barley—Car Sickness** | |
| Barley sugar has been used for nausea in car sickness. | Significant controlled research studies are lacking at this point. |
| **Basil—Warts** | |
| Basil is known as a spice in pasta sauces and other foods. It is a folk remedy used for warts when applied topically. It has been used for many ailments. | It might cause cancer in large doses. Even a spice in excess can be dangerous. Moderation is a good principle not only for basil but for many other herbs as well. |
| **Bay—Ulcers** | |
| Bay has been used to treat ulcers. | Bay can cause perforation of the gastrointestinal tract. It can lower blood sugar. |
| **Bayberry—Sore Throat** | |
| Bayberry was used by the American colonists to make candles and thus was called wax myrtle or candleberry. It has been used for sore throats. | Bayberry consumption can decrease potassium and raise blood pressure. It should not be used by those with congestive heart failure, hypertension, or kidney disease. |
| **Bean Sprouts—Parkinsonism** | |
| Bean sprouts typically contain a higher content of nutrients than unsprouted beans. For example, the fava bean is considered to be one of the best sources of L-dopa, a natural precursor of dopamine in the brain. Some authors have recommended beans and bean sprouts for early treatment of Parkinson's disease. Bean sprouts also contain a higher level of protein than unsprouted beans. | Some people report having significant discomfort with intestinal gas. Others report bean products get easier to handle intestinally if they are eaten more often. Some bean enthusiasts, to reduce flatulence with bean intake, have used an over-the-counter product. |
| **Bearberry (Uva Ursi)—Urinary Tract Infection** | |
| Bearberry was used by Native Americans and was officially in the *U.S. Pharmacopoeia* until 1936 for urinary tract infections. It has been touted to have antibacterial effects and thus help in urinary tract infections. It has also been touted to reduce heavy menstrual periods by shrinking blood vessels. | Bearberry can have side effects such as nausea, abdominal cramps, and vomiting. It will not work in an acidic urine, so do not take it with cranberry juice. It should not be used in kidney disease. |
| **Bee Pollen** | |
| Bee pollen is high in nutrients and has thus been used for food. It has also been purported for impotence, ulcers, asthma, allergies, prostatitis, and altitude sickness. | Bee pollen increases blood sugar and decreases the effectiveness of insulin and oral hypoglycemics. It can also cause allergic reactions, vomiting, and diarrhea. |

| What They Told You | What They Did Not Tell You |
|---|---|
| **Beeswax—Inflammations**<br>Beeswax has been touted for anti-inflammatory effects for use in helping to prevent ulcers. It is usual for fragrance and thickening in cosmetics and as a polishing agent in other products. | Significant research is lacking in regard to beeswax's effectiveness.<br><br>Beeswax is from the honeycomb and is usually safe on the skin except for rare allergic reactions. |
| **Beet—Liver Disease**<br>Beets have been used in liver disease to help prevent fatty deposits. | Beets are usually safe in amounts consumed in food. In large amounts they can cause kidney damage.<br><br>Significant research is lacking in regard to their effectiveness in liver disorders. |
| **Belladonna—Sedative**<br>Belladonna is used primarily as a sedative, as an antispasmodic in asthma, for intestinal and bilary colic, and for motion sickness. Historically, belladonna berry juice was used by Italian women to dilate their pupils, giving them a more striking appearance. | When the leaf or root of the belladonna plant is used orally without medical supervision, it is likely unsafe. Its anticholinergic activity may cause dry mouth, decreased perspiration, dilation of pupils, blurred vision, constipation, difficulty urinating, hallucinations, fever, convulsions, and coma.<br><br>Belladonna can increase the effects of several medications including amantadine, antihistamines, tricyclic antidepressants, and phenothiazines.<br><br>It may also cause tachycardia and many complications in patients with heart disease. This herb is unsafe ingested or applied topically. |
| **Benzoin—Wounds**<br>Benzoin has been used in creams and lotions for wounds. It has also been used as an inhalant for bronchitis. | Benzoin can cause allergic reactions (including anaphylaxis) when used topically. When used orally, it can cause gastrointestinal hemorrhage. |
| **Beta-1, 3-Glucan—Cancer**<br>Beta-1, 3-glucan is a carbohydrate that is touted to help in cancer, immune problems, and various infections. It has been touted to stimulate the immune system. | Research is lacking to demonstrate its effectiveness. |
| **Beta-Sitosterol—Gallstones**<br>Orally, beta-sitosterol is promoted for coronary heart disease and hypercholesterolemia, benign prostatic hyperplasia (BPH), and prostatitis and gallstones. It is also touted for enhancing sexual activity and for preventing colon cancer. Beta-sitosterol is also used orally for boosting the immune system, preventing immune suppression and inflammation following participation in a marathon, common cold and flu, HIV/AIDS, rheumatoid arthritis, tuber- | In some patients it can cause nausea, indigestion, gas, diarrhea, or constipation.<br><br>No proven efficacy has been demonstrated for the myriad of illnesses in which it is supposed to be helpful. |

| What They Told You | What They Did Not Tell You |
|---|---|

culosis, psoriasis, allergies, cervical cancer, fibromyalgia, systemic lupus erythematosus, asthma, alopecia, bronchitis, idiopathic thrombocytopenia purpura (ITP), migraine headache, chronic fatigue syndrome, and symptoms of menopause.

### Betaine Anhydrous—Homocynstinuria

Betaine anhydrous has been used for homocynstinuria.

It probably is an effective treatment of some cases of homocynstinuria associated with increased stroke risk.

It can cause gastrointestinal upset.

### Betel Palm—Depression

Betel palm has been touted for depression. It has also been used for sore throat as a gargle.

Betel palm seems to act as an MAO inhibitor and thus, could have antidepressant effects in some. However, it can cause palpitations, dizziness, seizures, psychosis, anxiety, diarrhea, and increased asthma. As a gargle it can cause leucoplakia (precancerous lesions in the mouth).

### Beth Root—Pain

Orally, Beth root is touted for use in long, heavy menstruation and pain relief. It is also used orally as an astringent and expectorant.

Topically, Beth root is promoted for varicose veins and ulcers, hematomas, and hemorrhoidal bleeding.

Orally, ingestion of large amounts of the plant or volatile oil might produce GI irritation severe enough to cause vomiting. In pregnant women, the drastic purgative effects can cause reflex uterine contractions.

Topically, Beth root causes extreme irritation in many instances.

### Bifidobacterium Bifidum—Traveler's Diarrhea

This organism has been touted to help in restoring normal flora to the digestive tract after antibiotic treatment. It has also been used for vaginal yeast infections (douching with this organism). It has also been tried for liver disease. It has been used along with acidophilus for traveler's diarrhea.

This organism is well tolerated by most people. It can help to restore normal flora to the intestinal tract after treatment with antibiotics.

### Bilberry—Bruising

**How it has been used:** Bilberry has been used for bruising. It has also been utilized for its high value in nutrition, treatment of scurvy and urinary problems including infection and kidney stones, diabetes, diarrhea, to improve nighttime vision, and to treat eye disorders such as cataracts and macular degeneration as well as retinitis pigmentosa, varicose veins, and capillary fragility.

**Health concerns:** Little clinical research information is available for use in the treatment of various medical disorders. This supplement seems fairly innocuous for many. However, side effects are possible including constipation, bleeding if used with other blood-thinning agents, and hypoglycemia. Bilberry, like most herbs, should not be used by pregnant women or children.

**Some interesting data:** Pilots of the British Royal Air Force were given a diet including bilberry to improve their night vision on bombing raids in World War II.

**Clinical studies:** Clinical studies with human subjects involving placebo-controlled, double-blind designs not found.

## What They Told You

**Historical data:** Bilberry is also known as the European blueberry.

**The usual dose:** The dose is based on its anthocyanoside content with preparations consisting of 25 percent athocyanidin with 80 to 160 mg three times a day.

### Bioflavonoids—Pain

Bioflavonoids (citrin, eriodictyol, flavones, hesperetin, hesperidin, quercetin, rutin, etc.) have been used for pain and athletic injuries.

Quercetin has been touted for asthma.

### Biotin

Biotin has been promoted as a dietary supplement to help when weight gain is needed.

It has also been touted to help in brittle nails and to lower blood sugar.

### Birch—Urinary Tract Infections

Birch is a common tree throughout the world. It has been touted to help in urinary tract infections. Chemicals in birch (betulin and betulinic) seem to have some antiviral and anticancer effects.

### Bishop's Weed—Asthma

Orally, bishop's weed is touted for digestive disorders, asthma, angina, kidney stones, and as a diuretic.

Topically, bishop's weed has been promoted for psoriasis and vitiligo.

## What They Did Not Tell You

**The mechanism of action:** The anthocyanosides contained in bilberry extracts are thought to affect collagen metabolism by enhancing the cross-liking of fibers resulting in a stronger matrix of connective tissue such as tendons and cartilage. It may prevent release of histamine and prostaglandins, which are compounds that promote inflammation. In addition there may be some antioxidant and free radical-scavenging action.

Research is lacking.

Side effects are not known.

Few adverse reactions have been reported. A very few cases of interacting with thyroid functioning tests have been reported.

It may help in brittle nails. It does help in biotin deficiency. The effectiveness in any other conditions is not known.

Birch contains salicylate (from which came aspirin—salicylate is also found in the willow tree). Salicylate decreases the production of prostaglandins that are linked to fever and inflammation.

The essential oil (methyl salicylate) can be extremely toxic.

Orally, bishop's weed can cause nausea, vomiting, and headache. Bishop's weed can also cause allergic reactions including rhinitis and urticaria in sensitive patients. There is some concern that bishop's weed might increase liver enzymes.

The isolated constituent khellin can increase transaminase levels. However, so far this effect has not been reported for bishop's weed.

Bishop's weed might also cause photosensitivity due to the 8-MOP constituent.

## What They Told You

## What They Did Not Tell You

In some patients bishop's weed can also cause contact dermatitis. There is also concern based on preliminary evidence that bishop's weed might cause ophthalmic changes, such as pigmentary retinopathy.

Topically, bishop's weed might cause skin malignancies in patients predisposed to cancer.

### Bistort—Hepatitis C

Bistort has been used topically for bug bites, snakebites, and hemorrhoids. It has been used orally to treat irritable bowel syndrome and ulceritive colitis. Research has raised the question of interferon-like activity that has been used in hepatitis C.

Bistort can damage the liver and gastrointestinal tract.

### Bitter Melon—Diabetes Mellitus

Bitter melon has a history of being used in diabetes mellitus to lower blood sugar.

It is often given as a 500-milligram capsule (150 milligrams of a 2.5 percent extract) three times per day.

Bitter melon is probably fairly innocuous for most people. The question of gastrointestinal upset has arisen as well as the possibility of decreasing sperm production.

### Bitter Orange Peel—Dyspepsia

Orally, bitter orange peel is touted as an appetite stimulant and for dyspepsia.

Bitter orange fruit and peel are also touted orally for weight loss and nasal congestion.

The bitter orange flower and its oil are used orally for gastrointestinal (GI) disturbances, duodenal ulcers, constipation, regulating blood lipid levels, lowering blood sugar in diabetes, blood purification, functional disorders of liver and gallbladder, stimulation of the heart and circulation, frostbite, as a sedative for sleep disorders, for kidney and bladder diseases, general feebleness, anemia, imbalances of mineral metabolism, impurities of the skin, exhaustion accompanying colds, headaches, neuralgia, muscular pain, rheumatic discomfort, and hair loss.

Topically, bitter orange peel is used for inflammation of the eyelid, conjunctiva, and retina; retinal hemorrhage; bruises; phlebitis; and bed sores.

In aromatherapy, the essential oil of bitter orange is used topically and by inhalation as an analgesic.

Orally, bitter orange, which contains the adrenergic agent synephrine and N-methyltyramine, might cause hypertension and cardiovascular toxicity. Photosensitivity can also occur, especially in fair-skinned people. Frequent contact with the peel or oil can cause erythema, blisters, pustules, dermatoses leading to scab formation, and pigment spots. The ingestion of large amounts of bitter orange peel in children can cause intestinal colic, convulsions, and death.

### Bittersweet Nightshade—Eczema

Bittersweet nightshade has been touted for eczema, acne,

Bittersweet nightshade is unsafe especially when used

**What They Told You**

and warts. It has been used orally and topically.

### Black Alder—Sore Throat

Orally, black alder is touted for intestinal bleeding and pharyngitis.

Topically, it is touted for streptococcal sore throat.

### Black Cohosh—PMS and Menopause

**How it has been used:** Its main use has been for menopausal symptoms. In fact, it is probably the most widely used herb for menopausal symptoms, PMS, menopausal hot flashes, vaginal dryness, irritability, sleep problems, rheumatism, muscle pain, and depression.

**Some interesting data:** Black cohosh is sometimes confused with "blue" cohosh that is used for different problems. Black cohosh is popular in Germany for treating PMS and menopausal problems.

**Historical data:** Native Americans as well as the American colonists used black cohosh. Interestingly, it was listed as an official drug in the *U.S. Pharmacopoeia* from 1820 to 1926.

It has been used widely in Europe, and its use has grown recently in the United States (*Pharmacist's Letter/Prescriber's Letter*, p. 12).

**The usual dose:** 500–600 mg three times a day.

### Black Cohosh Root—PMS and Menopause

Black cohosh was used by Native Americans for gynecological problems—menstrual cramps, hot flashes, and PMS.

### Black Currant—Colds and Flu

Black currant berries have been used to treat colds and flu. The leaves and seed have been touted to help in arthritis, heart disease, high blood pressure, multiple sclerosis (MS), PMS, autoimmune disorders, and eczema.

**What They Did Not Tell You**

orally. It can cause headache, convulsions, and death.

Reliable information is insufficient. There are no reported adverse effects.

**Health concerns:** Not much is known about the long-term effects of black cohosh in humans. Black cohosh can upset the stomach, may affect estrogen and pituitary activity, and can increase the action of blood pressure medications. Therefore, taking black cohosh with antihypertensive drugs could lead to dangerously low blood pressure.

Women on hormone replacement therapy or pregnant women should not take black cohosh. This product also contains salicin, a precursor to salicylate, which can trigger allergic reactions in individuals sensitive to aspirin products or to products containing salicylate.

**Clinical studies:** Research is conflicting on action and therapeutic uses. Most of the studies have been done on Remifemin (which is similar in action to black cohosh) with only one controlled study reported. More studies are needed.

**The mechanism of action:** Mechanism is uncertain, and studies are conflicting on its action. Triterpine glycosides such as actein are among the most likely active agents. Information is also conflicting on whether it suppresses luteinizing hormone which is postulated as the effect on menopausal symptoms (*Pharmacists' Letter/Prescriber's Letter*, p. 11).

This herb has estrogen-like effects, and thus, estrogen dangers should be considered. It should not be used in pregnant women. Also, it may cause gastrointestinal problems in some people sensitive to the active ingredients.

The fruit may have some antibacterial effects. The seed contains GLA (gamma-linolenic acid), and omega-6 fatty acid that helps to decrease prostaglandins that play a role in increased fever. Some also feel GLA has potential

**What They Told You**

**What They Did Not Tell You**

in MS. Significant effects in this condition (MS) are doubtful.

The fruit and seed are usually safe for the most part.

### Black Haw—Menstrual Cramps

Native American females used black haw for menstrual cramps. It has also been touted for fever, headache, diarrhea, and pain.

This herb contains components such as aesculetin and scopoletin that might calm muscle spasms. It also contains salicin, which is similar to salicylate from which aspirin is made.

The leaf in particular could be potentially dangerous since it might cause water retention.

### Black Horehound—Nausea

Orally, black horehound is touted for nausea, vomiting, sedation in hysteria and hypochondria, increasing bile flow, whooping cough, and as an antispasmodic.

It is used in France for symptomatic relief of nervous disorders in adults and children, especially mild sleep disorders, and for cough.

Topically, black horehound is used as a mild astringent and for gout.

Traditionally, black horehound has been used for nervous dyspepsia. Other uses include rectal enemas against ascaridae, or intestinal worms.

Theoretically, black horehound might have additive effects when used with dopamine agonists. Some constituents of black horehound bind to dopamine D2 receptors in vitro; however, this has not yet been reported in humans. Some dopamine agonists include bromocriptine (Parlodel), levodopa (Dopar, component of Sinemet), pramipexole (Mirapex), ropinirole (Requip), and others.

### Black Root—Diuretic

Black root has been touted as a diuretic.

Black root can have many dangerous side effects (toxic to liver, central nervous system, and gastrointestinal tract) and can interact with several medications.

### Black Seed—Gas

Orally, black seed has been used for treating gastrointestinal conditions including gas, colic, diarrhea, dysentery, constipation, and hemorrhoids. It is also touted for respiratory conditions, including asthma, allergies, cough, bronchitis, emphysema, flu, and congestion. Additionally, it has been promoted for its antihypertensive, immunoprotectant, anticancer activity, and vermifuge. It is touted for women's health, including as a contraceptive, for stimulation of menstruation, and increasing milk flow.

Combined with cysteine, vitamin E, and saffron, black seed is used to decrease cisplatin-induced side effects.

Topical use of black seed oil can cause allergic contact dermatitis. Black seed may be associated with hepatotoxicity based on preliminary animal research.

**What They Told You**

Topically, black seed is touted for inflammatory conditions, including rheumatism, headache, and skin conditions.

### Black Walnut (juglans nigra)—Diarrhea

What does one do for Montezuma's revenge after traveling to Mexico? Some would recommend black walnut due to its reported antiviral, antifungal, astringent, antiseptic effects.

### Bladderwrack—Thyroid Disorders

Orally, bladderwrack is touted for thyroid disorders, iodine deficiency, lymphadenoid goiter, myxedema, obesity, arthritis, and rheumatism.

In folk medicine, bladderwrack is touted for arteriosclerosis, digestive disorders, "blood cleansing," constipation, bronchitis, emphysema, genitourinary disorders, decreased resistance to disease, anxiety, skin disorders, burns, and insect bites.

### Blessed Thistle (cnicus benedictus)—Milk Production

Blessed thistle, a member of the daisy family, has been used by breast-feeding mothers to stimulate more milk production because of the belief that its content of cnicin, a bitter alkaloid, irritates the mammary glands causing the increased milk secretion.

It has also been touted to have anti-inflammatory and gastrointestinal effects.

### Bloodroot—Plaque

Bloodroot is used topically for skin irritations. It is a major ingredient in many mouthwashes and toothpastes to reduce plaque. In dentistry it is used topically to reduce pain.

### Blue Cohosh—Gynecological Problems

Blue cohosh is related to black cohosh. It has been used to encourage menstruation and induce childbirth.

### Blue Flag—Laxative

Blue flag is related to the iris family of perennial plants. People have used it as a laxative, a diuretic, an anti-inflammatory, and for nausea.

Dosage forms include fluid extract, solid extract, tincture,

**What They Did Not Tell You**

When used in low doses, side effects have been reported to be low.

One would have to be concerned about possible genetic mutations and carcinogenic effects, especially in chronic use.

Bladderwrack can induce or exacerbate hyperthyroidism and acne. Prolonged ingestion can reduce iron absorption. High sodium content can adversely affect individuals with restricted sodium intake. Iodine can cause idiosyncratic or allergic reactions. There is one case report of heavy metal poisoning in which arsenic poisoning occurred with ingestions of a contaminated kelp product.

Blessed thistle needs research. It can have side effects such as nausea, vomiting, ulcer aggravating, and allergic reactions.

Bloodroot is probably effective topically as a dental agent for reducing plaque.

It is potentially toxic orally with many possible side effects. It could aggravate glaucoma.

This is a potentially dangerous herb. Self-medication is strongly discouraged.

Blue flag is likely unsafe when used orally. The fresh root can cause nausea, vomiting, and mucosal irritation.

Use of blue flag with other stimulant laxatives can cause potassium depletion and can irritate the GI tract.

## What They Told You

and powered root. Ten to 20 grains of powered root daily is the most common form and dosage.

### Boldo—Indigestion
Boldo comes from South America primarily and has been touted for indigestion.

It has also been promoted as a liver tonic and laxative and for irritable bowel syndrome, and anxiety.

### Boneset—Common Cold
Boneset was used by Native Americans for cold and fever. It is touted today also for aches and pain and arthritis.

### Borage—PMS
Borage is touted to help in colds, arthritis, depression, PMS, anxiety, and high blood pressure.

It is often found in potpourri. It is often found in salads and drinks in small amounts.

### Boron—Osteoporosis
Boron is a trace mineral touted for osteoporosis.

### Boswellia—Ringworm
Boswellia is often confused with myrrh, which is of the same family.

It has been used in arthritis, Crohn's disease, hepatitis, and ringworm.

### Bovine Cartilage—Poison Ivy
Bovine cartilage has been touted to help in wound healing.

It has been used topically for poison ivy, poison oak, acne, psoriasis, and hemorrhoids.

It may have anti-inflammatory effects.

### Brahmi—Asthma
Orally, brahmi is touted to aid learning.

## What They Did Not Tell You

Little is known about blue flag's pharmacological properties. Some related species can be toxic.

Boldo can be toxic to the kidneys and liver. It can cause anxiety and even seizures at high doses.

Fresh boneset can be toxic, even causing death in some instances.

When taken orally, it can be toxic to the liver.

It contains GLA (gammalinolenic acid) that may help in inflammations.

Research is lacking.

Side effects are not known.

Boswellia probably has some anti-inflammatory effects that might help in arthritis. Its claims for ringworm and Crohn's disease are interesting but unproved clinically.

It can upset the stomach.

Research is lacking.

Bovine cartilage can cause gastrointestinal upset. It can cause edema of the scrotum. It can cause allergic reactions topically.

There is lingering concern over "mad cow disease" (bovine spongiform encephalitis), a fatal disease in this species.

Insufficient reliable information is available. No adverse

## What They Told You

Traditionally, brahmi has been used orally for treating asthma, backache, hoarseness, insanity, epilepsy, rheumatism, sexual dysfunction in both men and women, as a nerve tonic, cardiotonic, and a diuretic.

### Bran—High Cholesterol
Bran is part of the coat of the seed of cereal grains such as oat or rice.

It has been used to help lower cholesterol and to help reduce postprandial blood sugar in diabetes.

### Brewer's Yeast—Diarrhea
Brewer's yeast has been used for diarrhea.

### Bromelain (pineapple)—Physical Aches and Injuries
Bromelain comes from the pineapple plant and has been used for a wide variety of problems: inflammation infections, arthritis injuries, bruising, deep vein thrombosis, varicose veins, painful menstruation, etc. In short, this herb has been used for all sorts of physical aches and injuries.

The usual dose is 80 mg per day up to 500 mg three times per day.

### Bromide—Sedative
Bromine, a chemical element, when combined with potassium to form bromide, was used often in the past as a sedative. It was also the first anticonvulsant for seizure disorders in the mid-1800s.

### Broom—Irregular Heartbeat
Broom has been touted for heart disease and circulatory problems.

## What They Did Not Tell You

effects have been reported.

Bran may help some in lowering cholesterol when combined with a low-fat diet. It also might lower postprandial blood sugar in some diabetics.

Oat bran can cause intestinal obstruction in those who have trouble chewing food or when used in excessive amounts.

Research is needed.

There is a specifically standardized product (brewer's yeast—Hansen CBS5926) that is probably effective at times for traveler's diarrhea. It is usually given at a dose of 250 to 500 mg per day starting five days before the trip. It probably has actions against organisms that cause diarrhea such as clostridium difficile and enterotoxic E. coli. It also reduces water influx into the intestine. It can cause flatulence, itching, skin eruptions, and edema.

The suggested uses of bromelain need additional research. It is probably often benign in side effects. Some side effects are allergic reactions, nausea, vomiting, diarrhea, painful and increased bleeding during menstrual periods.

One of the authors remembers one of his first patients when he entered his psychiatric residency in the early 1970s. She appeared to have classical manic symptoms. Upon taking her history, the young resident found out she had been on Miles Nervine, a bromide-containing compound that had produced her mania.

Broom is similar to the prescription drug quinidine, which has been used for irregular heartbeat. Just as quinidine should not be used in self-medication, neither

| **What They Told You** | **What They Did Not Tell You** |
|---|---|
| | should broom. |
| ### *Bryonia—Cough* | |
| Orally, bryonia is used as a laxative, emetic, diuretic, for gastrointestinal diseases, respiratory tract diseases, arthritis, liver disease, metabolic disorders, and for prophylaxis against infections. | Bryonia is likely unsafe when the root is used orally. It can cause dizziness, vomiting, convulsions, colic, bloody diarrhea, abortion, nervous excitement, and kidney damage. Large doses can cause anuria, collapse, spasms, paralysis, or death. |
| | Skin contact with fresh bryonia may cause irritation. |
| | Ingestion of 15 berries is likely to be fatal to a child. Ingestion of 40 berries is likely to be fatal for an adult. |
| ### *Buchu—Bladder and Prostate Infections* | |
| Buchu comes from Africa. It has long been used for infections of the bladder, kidneys, and prostate. It is touted to have a diuretic effect. | Research is lacking. Effectiveness is not proven. |
| | Buchu in moderation is usually safe for most people. It can cause irritation of the kidney and gastrointestinal system. It could be toxic to the liver in some. It might enhance the effects of anticoagulants. Also, the diuretic action can decrease potassium. |
| ### *Buckwheat—Varicose Veins and Hemorrhoids* | |
| Buckwheat flower is used to make buckwheat pancakes. Buckwheat is touted to help varicose veins and hemorrhoids. | A component in buckwheat (rutin) may help to strengthen veins. |
| | Buckwheat is usually safe, but as with most herbs, allergic reactions can occur. Rare anaphylactic reactions to buckwheat have resulted in death. |
| ### *Bugle—Hypothyroidism and Hyperthyroidism* | |
| Bugle has been touted for both hypothyroidism and hyperthyroidism. It has also been touted for anxiety and diabetes. | Little information could be found on bugle. |
| Bugle is sometimes in alcoholic extracts. | We are concerned with the apparent contradiction in its treating both hypothyroidism and hyperthyroidism. |
| ### *Bupleurum—Flu* | |
| Bupleurum is from China, where it is touted for the flu, the common cold, fatigue, depression, PMS, hepatitis, cancer, malaria, seizures, pain, arthritis, asthma, bronchitis, hemorrhoids, diarrhea, anxiety, many septemic infections, and for reducing cholesterol. | These claims are unfounded, and significant studies are either totally absent or lacking at best. |
| ### *Burdock—Anorexia Nervosa* | |
| Burdock has been touted for urinary tract infections, acne, colds, and cancer. It has even been touted for anorexia nervosa. It might lower blood sugar in large amounts in | Burdock is touted for much and proven for little. |
| | In research and in theory the leaf and flower of burdock |

**What They Told You**

some people.

In Europe it is a food flavoring in many food preparations, and in Asia it is eaten as a food.

**What They Did Not Tell You**

seem to have some antibacterial (gram positive and gram negative) and antitumor activity. But there is a long distance from research to proven results.

The effectiveness of this herb is not proven.

As with most herbs it should not be used by pregnant women as it can cause uterine contractions.

As with many claims, those for anorexia nervosa seem to be unproved and unsubstantiated.

### Burnet—Varicose Veins

Burnet has been touted for ulcerative colitis, diarrhea, uterine bleeding, varicose veins, and hemorrhoids.

Topically it has been used for skin eruptions.

Effectiveness of burnet is not known in significant human research.

It is probably usually safe, but this is not known for sure.

### Burning Bush Root—Digestive Disorders

Orally, burning bush root is touted for digestive and urogenital disorders and to promote hair growth.

Topically, burning bush root is touted for eczema, impetigo, and scabies.

In Chinese medicine (China and Korea), the root is applied topically for arthritis, fever, hepatitis, skin inflammation, thread fungus, uterine hemorrhages, to calm children crying as a result of a nervous state, and as a sedative and tonic.

In folk medicine, burning bush root is touted as a diuretic and spasmolytic.

Historically, burning bush root was used for desiccation, epilepsy, hysteria, worm infestations, and to promote menstruation.

In India, burning bush root is used for amenorrhea and birth control.

Topically, skin contact can cause phototoxicity.

### Butcher's Broom—Varicose Veins

Butcher's broom comes from Europe, Africa, and Asia. It has been used for varicose veins, hemorrhoids, and inflammation. One of the more interesting suggestions is for preventive protection against the poison of snakebites because of a component butcher's broom contains, namely spartein.

Few side effects have been reported, but research is needed.

| What They Told You | What They Did Not Tell You |
|---|---|
| **Butterbur—Migraine Headaches**<br>Butterbur is an herb that has been touted for migraine headaches, cough, irritable bowel syndrome, and arthritis. | Reported side effects seem to be few. However, when UPAs (unsaturated pyrrolizidine alkaloids) are added, veno-occulsive disease can occur with enlarged liver, reduced urine, and distended abdomen. |
| **Buttercup—Arthritis**<br>Orally, buttercup is touted for arthritis, blisters, bronchitis, chronic skin complaints, and nerve pain. | Orally, ingestion of buttercup can cause severe irritation of the gastrointestinal tract, with colic and diarrhea. Irritation of the urinary tract can also occur.<br><br>Topically, skin contact can cause blisters and burns which are difficult to heal. Buttercup can also cause phototoxic skin reactions. |
| **Cabbage—Gastritis**<br>Cabbage has been used for gastrointestinal problems. | Significant research is lacking in regard to its effectiveness.<br><br>Cabbage can decrease the effectiveness of some medications (warfarin, phenacetin, acetaminophen, oxazepam, and others). |
| **Cacao (chocolate)**<br>Cacao is an herb that has been used for many, many years for flavoring in food and drinks. It has been touted for its stimulating effects. | Cacao can interact with MAOI antidepressants and theophylline for asthma. It is dangerous for those hypersensitive to chocolate. |
| **Cade Oil—Itching**<br>Topically, cade oil is touted for itching, psoriasis, eczema and seborrhea, parasitic skin conditions, as an antiseptic in wound dressings, and in analgesic and antipruritic preparations.<br><br>Historically, cade oil has been used for treating various skin disorders, scalp conditions, hair loss, and cancers. | Cade oil contains a constituent called creosol. Creosol is a mild to moderate irritant. Topically, cade oil may cause eye irritation. |
| **Caffeine—Mental Alertness**<br>Caffeine has been tried by millions for a variety of reasons (morning drink, stimulant, migraines, mental alertness, enhancing athletic performance, weight loss, asthma, and even Parkinson's disease prevention). | Caffeine does increase mental alertness in many. It is in various other medication combinations for migraines and other forms of pain.<br><br>Caffeine may best illustrate indirectly the principle that many herbs are safe for many in small amounts, but they can be dangerous. The potential side effects of caffeine are many (anxiety, insomnia, gastric irritation, rapid heartbeat, headache, ringing in the ears, arrhythmias of the heart, fibrocystic breast disease possibly, and substance dependency, to name a few). |

**What They Told You**

**What They Did Not Tell You**

Caffeine can interact with many medications (aspirin, minor tranquilizers, asthma medications, cimetidine, clozaril, amphetamines, diabetic medications, antabuse, estrogen, lithium, oral contraceptives, some antibiotics such as Levaquin and Tequin, Lamisil, and Calan, to name just a few).

### Calamine—Itching Skin

Calamine lotion has long been used topically to calm itching skin and bug bites.

Research is lacking, but it has a long accepted history.

Contact dermatitis is possible.

### Calamus—Digestive Disorders

Orally, calamus is touted for digestive disorders including ulcers, gastritis, and flatulence, and to stimulate appetite and digestion. Some people use calamus to induce sweating. Others chew it to remove the smell of tobacco.

Historically, calamus has been used orally as a sedative and for acute and chronic dyspepsia, gastritis, gastric ulcer, anorexia, rheumatoid arthritis, strokes, and topically for skin diseases.

Native Americans of the Cree tribe chewed the root for its stimulant, euphoric, and hallucinogenic effects.

Calamus oil may contain beta-isoasarone, a known carcinogen associated with kidney damage, tremors, and convulsions.

### Calcium—Antacid

Calcium has been tried for replacement purposes, as an antacid, for osteoporosis, to reduce the risk of colorectal cancer, and PMS.

Calcium is certainly indicated at times for various reasons. It has helped some as an antacid. It might help some in osteoporosis, but this is not known for sure.

Calcium can cause gastrointestinal upset and possibly even GI hemorrhage (calcium chloride).

It can interact with many medications (diuretics, thyroid medications, Cipro antibiotic, estrogen, and adendronate).

### Calcium L-Glucarate—Cancer Prevention

L-glucarate is a chemical in the body that has been touted to possibly help in cancer prevention and retardation. It is touted to work by several mechanisms: antioxidant activity against free radicals that may play a role in cancer and the inhibition of the enzyme beta-glucuronidase that is possibly involved in less reduction of toxins involved in cancer.

There are many more direct and proven ways to decrease the risk of cancer—stop smoking, stop alcohol use, avoid known environmental risks such as radiation and asbestos and dangerous chemicals, decrease obesity, add high-fiber diet, etc.

The question remains whether the reduction of free radicals by such agents as L-glucarate, glutathione, coenzyme Q10, lipoic acid, and vitamins E and C will help.

## What They Told You

### Calendula—Skin Infections

Calendula has been used topically for reported antifungal, antibacterial, antiviral, and anti-inflammatory actions for skin problems—burns, dermatitis, warts, bunions, bee stings, eczema, hemorrhoids, varicose veins, etc.

### Camphor—Itching

Camphor is used topically to relieve pain (hemorrhoids, cold sores, warts, bug bites, minor burns, and itching. It has been used orally to induce vomiting, for gas, and in respiratory tract disease.

### Canada Balsam—Hemorrhoids

Topically, Canada balsam is touted for hemorrhoids and as an antiseptic.

In dentistry, Canada balsam is used in root canal sealers and dentifrices.

Historically, Canada balsam has been used for burns, sores, cuts, tumors, heart and chest pains, cancer, mucous membrane inflammation, colds, coughs, warts, wounds, urogenital complaints, and as a pain reliever.

### Capsaicin (topical)—Arthritic Pain

Capsaicin is the active ingredient from hot peppers. It has been used topically (in cream form) for arthritic pain.

### Capsicum

Capsicum is a plant of the pepper family and is used as a condiment under several names including cayenne, chili pepper, paprika, and Tobasco. Medically, it has been used primarily as a digestion aid, as an antigas preparation, to improve circulation, and to reduce blood clotting tendencies. It has been used for muscle aches, skin problems, headaches, and to lower blood pressure. Topically, it has been used for the pain of shingles, arthritis, peripheral neuropathy, fibromyalgia, and to relieve muscle spasms. Capsicum is the main ingredient in pepper sprays used for self-defense.

Typical dosage orally is 30 to 120 mg three times a day. Capsicum cream comes in 0.025 to 0.075 percent capsicum concentrations and is applied to affected areas 3 to 4 times daily.

## What They Did Not Tell You

Research is lacking.

Camphor induces a local vasoconstriction which provides pain relief and help with itching.

Too much camphor (even through skin absorption) can be toxic. Side effects include vomiting, headache, confusion, dizziness, restlessness, hallucinations, convulsions, coma, and death.

There is insufficient reliable information available about the effectiveness of Canada balsam. No adverse effects reported.

Capaicin has an effect on substance P which has to do with the mediation of pain.

Capsicum is considered generally safe when used in the usual amounts in food and topical preparations for short-term use. Long-term use can cause hepatic or renal damage. Data is insufficient to support its use in fibromyalgia and neuropathy.

Capsicum is thought to work by depleting substance P in nerve fibers, therefore reducing pain. Capsicum is highly irritating to the eyes and mucous membranes. It should not be used near the eyes or on sensitive skin. Use may lead to prolonged bleeding times, GI irritation, excessive sweating, and allergic reactions.

There are multiple interactions with other herbs and supplements such as increasing the effects of cocaine, enhancing the effects of Siberian ginseng, increasing the sedative effects of kava, valerian, chamomile, and Saint-John's-wort. Multiple interactions with medications have

**What They Told You**

**What They Did Not Tell You**

been reported including ACE inhibitors, antihypertensive drugs, barbiturates, theophylline, cocaine, antacids, aspirin, and antiplatelet drugs.

Capsicum is likely unsafe in children and during pregnancy and/or lactation. It is likely safe if consumed in the amounts generally found in foods. Insufficient reliable information is lacking on its overall safety when used orally or topically.

### Caraway—Gas

Caraway fruit and seeds have been used to help to reduce gas since ancient times. It is commonly found on rye bread.

For the most part, effectiveness is probably good, as is safety.

### Cardamom—Gas and Bad Breath

Cardamom has been used for its antiflatulence properties. It is a possible antiseptic herb with an aromatic smell that has been used for bad breath, mouth inflammation, and sore throat. It has also been used to stimulate the central nervous system in fatigue. Also, it has been used in upper respiratory problems—bronchitis and colds. Finally, it has been used in GI problems (indigestion) and liver problems.

Research points that cardamom is perhaps effective for flatulence.

Warnings have been given to those with gallbladder problems. Gallstone colic has been reported. Allergic reactions are always possible.

It is usually safe for most people.

### Carob—Indigestion

The carob fruit has been used for indigestion. It has been touted as a chocolate substitute.

Carob comes with strong recommendations from herbalists, but there is insufficient scientific information for known effectiveness. It appears to be usually safe and unlikely of drug interactions.

### Cascara Sagrada

Cascara is an herb present in many laxatives in health food stores.

Cascara probably is a strong laxative for constipation but not without potential dangers—becoming dependent on it for bowel movement if used for long periods of time, potential complications in gastrointestinal problems such as irritable bowel syndrome, Crohn's disease, colitis, and abdominal pain.

Cascara should not be used with certain heart medication that could result in potassium depletion.

### Cassia—Gas

Orally, cassia has been touted for gas (flatulence), muscle and GI spasms, preventing nausea and vomiting, diarrhea, infections, the common cold, and loss of appetite. It has also been touted for impotence, enuresis, rheumatic conditions, testicle hernia, menopausal symptoms, amenor-

Topically, allergic skin reactions and dermal and membrane irritation have been reported.

**What They Told You**

rhea, and as an abortifacient. Cassia is also touted for angina, kidney disorders, hypertension, cramps, and cancer.

Topically, cassia is used in suntan lotions, nasal sprays, mouthwashes, gargles, toothpaste, and as a counterirritant in liniments.

### Castor Oil—Laxative
Castor oil has long been used as a laxative. It has been used externally for various skin problems.

### Cat's Claw (uncaria tomentora)—Common Cold
This herb is from South America. It is touted to enhance the immune system and thus has been used for arthritis and the common cold.

### Catnip
Catnip comes from a plant found in the United States and has been touted to help in anxiety, migraine, and the common cold. Topically, it has been used for hemorrhoids.

### Catuaba—Aphrodisiac
Orally, catuaba is touted as an aphrodisiac, for male sexual impotence, agitation, exhaustion and fatigue, insomnia related to hypertension, nervousness, neurasthenia, poor memory or forgetfulness, as a tonic, and for skin cancer.

### Cayenne Pepper—Arteriosclerosis
Cayenne pepper is the fruit of a tropical plant.

It has been touted to help in reducing the likelihood of arteriosclerosis by reducing blood cholesterol and triglyceride levels, as well as decreasing symptoms of postherpetic neuralgia, various pain disorders, diabetic neuropathy, cluster headaches, psoriasis, and arthritis.

The topical form (topical capsaicin) is the form used in arthritis, psoriasis, diabetic neuropathy, and postherpetic neuralgia. The creams contain .075 percent capsaicin and are often used 3 to 4 times a day.

**What They Did Not Tell You**

Castor oil is strong (causing both peristalsis and fluid absorption) and with continued use, loss of bowel tone can occur.

As with many herbs castor oil should not be used in pregnancy or in children. The question of a contraceptive activity has also come up.

Cautions are often given against taking cat's claw with insulin, other hormones, vaccines, immunostimulants, skin problems, chronophilia, organ transplants, or pregnancy.

Some species (such as uncaria guianensis) are toxic.

Side effects of catnip include uterine stimulation, headache, malaise, nausea, vomiting, and dangerous interactions with alcohol and sedatives.

Reliable information is insufficient.

One of the authors recalls an incident many years ago when his wife accidentally used cayenne pepper in the main dish of a meat preparation. "I must admit we all felt no pain for a while other than that from the pepper itself!"

No, seriously, cayenne is an often modest additive to food preparations and is usually considered safe. The pain-relieving effects seem particularly interesting. Further research should be interesting. The question of skin cancer from repeated topical exposure has been raised.

| What They Told You | What They Did Not Tell You |
|---|---|
| **Cedar—Warts** | |
| Cedar has been used topically for warts and orally for respiratory infections. | Research is lacking.<br><br>Cedar can cause nausea, vomiting, diarrhea, seizures, and death. |
| **Celery—High Blood Pressure** | |
| Celery is eaten worldwide and has been touted to lower blood pressure and lower seizure threshold. It has been touted to thin the blood. It has also been touted to have antifungal effects. Finally it has been touted in oil form to lower blood sugar. | Celery can cause uterine contractions. It could cause depression possibly by the same mechanism it might lower blood pressure—by lowering circulatory dopamine, norepinephrine, and epinephrine. It could conceivably cause bleeding. And, of course, allergic reactions are possible. |
| **Centaury—ADHD** | |
| Centaury is often used in small amounts for flavoring in beer and various food preparations. It has been touted for gastrointestinal discomfort, high blood sugar, high blood pressure, internal parasites, kidney stones, and ADHD. | Interesting is that it has been touted for so much but, as far too often with herbs, proven for nothing. Information is largely anecdotal. |
| **Cereus—Angina** | |
| Cereus has been touted to help in angina. | Research is lacking.<br><br>Cereus might interact with heart medications such as digoxin. |
| **Cetyl Myristoleate—Arthritis** | |
| Orally, cetyl myristoleate is touted for rheumatoid arthritis, osteoarthritis, systemic lupus erythematosus, multiple sclerosis, ankylosing spondylitis, Reiter's syndrome, Behcet's syndrome, Sjogren's syndrome, psoriasis, fibromyalgia, emphysema, benign prostate hyperplasia (BPH), silicone breast disease, leukemia and other cancers, and relief of various types of back pain. | Reliable information is insufficient. |
| **Chamomile—Insomnia** | |
| This is an herb from Germany. It is touted to have several interesting properties: sedation and calming; anti-inflammatory (like the nonsteroidal anti-inflammatory drugs); antiallergic response; antispasmotic with help for gas; and many more—skin problems, bruises, respiratory problems, and gallbladder problems.<br><br>The usual dose is 350 mg capsules 3 times per day. Individuals may gargle with chamomile tea for gum disease. It is often applied directly to inflamed joints. Herbal teas are popular, and this is probably number one in the world. | Chamomile is similar to ragweed, and thus it could be allergenic in some people. Also, it has a coumarin-like compound and thus could thin blood and should not be used with other drugs (aspirin, gingko biloba, nonsteroidal anti-inflammatory drugs, etc.) that thin blood.<br><br>Chamomile is known to result in abortions and should not be used during pregnancy and lactation. Asthmatics should also not use this herb. Cross effects may result from allergy to sunflowers, ragweed, or members of the aster family (echinacea, feverfew, milk thistle). Burning of the face, eyes, and mucous membranes may occur with topical use. |

| What They Told You | What They Did Not Tell You |
|---|---|
| | Chamomile may increase the effects of alcohol and may interfere with the actions of anticoagulants. Chamomile may increase the effects of other sedatives. Overall this herb is probably safe for most people. |
| | This herb illustrates what makes a lot of herbs so popular—broad results claims for a variety of problems. The general safety and centuries of use make them popular and deserving of research. |

### Chanca Piedra—Kidney Stones

| | |
|---|---|
| This is a rain-forest herb. It has been touted to have antiviral and antibacterial effects. It has also been touted as a diuretic that helps with kidney stones. | Research is lacking. |
| | Possible side effects are not known. |

### Chaparral

| | |
|---|---|
| Chaparral has been touted to help heal skin lesions, acne, and for arthritis and allergies. Reportedly, it promotes hair growth and has been historically used as a tonic and "blood purifier." In addition, chaparral has been used for arthritis, cancer, tuberculosis, and weight loss. | Chaparral has been listed in a recent publication sold in several local stores as a product that has "no side effects." In reality, chaparral is likely unsafe and should be avoided. Incidences of serious poisonings, hepatitis, kidney, and liver damage have been reported when chaparral was taken orally. It is currently being investigated by the FDA. |
| Typical dosage is unknown. | |
| It is often found in herbal teas. | |

### Chasteberry—PMS

| | |
|---|---|
| This herb has long been used for treatment of PMS and other menstrual conditions (menstrual irregularities and breast pain). It has also been touted for acne. | This herb probably works on the pituitary gland and thus explains its possible hormonal effects (decreased prolactin, increased progesterone, increased follicle-stimulating hormone, increased luteinizing hormone, increased testosterone. Hormonal changes can be good or bad. The bad possibilities include depression, problems with oral contraceptives and hormone-replacement therapy, and finally conceivably even cancer. However, having said this, the herb often seems safe for many. |

### Chaulmoogra Oil—Leprosy

| | |
|---|---|
| Chaulmoogra oil has been used topically for centuries in the past for leprosy and other infections of the skin. | This had a valuable use in the past, but it has long been surpassed with more effective medicines. |

### Cherry—Gout

| | |
|---|---|
| This delicious fruit has been touted to help in colds, cough, gout, and even in fish poisoning. | Research is lacking, but cherry has been part of common cold remedies for years. |

### Chickweed—Weight Loss

| | |
|---|---|
| Chickweed has been used as a diuretic, for weight loss, for appetite suppression, for cellulite reduction, and as an anti-inflammatory. | Chickweed's use is based purely on folklore. |

**What They Told You**

**What They Did Not Tell You**

### Chicle

In manufacturing, chicle is an ingredient in hair preparations and a gum base in chewing gum. It was introduced to the United States by Santa Anna when a prisoner of the Republic of Texas.

No reported adverse effects reported.

### Chicory—Rapid Heart Rate

Chicory is an herb that has been used for indigestion and lack of appetite. It has also been touted for liver and heart problems. Finally, it has also been touted for bacterial infections, high blood sugar, and high cholesterol.

It is rich in beta-carotene.

Three to 5 grams of powdered chicory root daily is the amount often taken.

Chicory is interesting. In mice it seemed to have liver protective effects. It contains insulin that might help the immune system. It is believed to slow the heart rate in some due to a digitalis-like compound. It might have a mild sedative effect due to a constituent (lactucopicrin) and thus, it might counter coffee's stimulating effects. This accounts for its being added to some canned brands of coffee.

It is apparently safe for most people and low on drug interactions.

### Chinese Cucumber—Diabetes

Orally, Chinese cucumber seed is used for coughs, reducing fever, swelling, tumors, and diabetes.

Reliable information is insufficient.

### Chive—Intestinal Worms

Chives have been touted to rid infected individuals of worms.

Chives are a common flavoring agent in foods.

Significant research is lacking.

### Chlorella—Fibromyalgia

Chlorella is an algae that is touted as a complete food rich in vitamins, minerals, protein, and carbohydrates.

It has been touted to protect against ultraviolet radiation.

It has been touted for fibromyalgia and to help improve the immune system.

Research is lacking.

It can cause gastrointestinal upset. Allergic reactions are possible. Infection is possible.

### Chlorophyll—Wound Healing

Orally, chlorophyll is touted for reducing colostomy odor, bad breath, constipation, detoxification, and wound healing.

Intravenously, chlorophyll is touted for treating chronic relapsing pancreatitis.

### Chocolate—Stimulant

Chocolate comes from the cocoa bean. It is high in antioxidants. Its caffeine acts as a stimulant. It has also been touted to calm the stomach.

Chocolate has a long history of folk use and is generally accepted on that basis.

## What They Told You

### Choline—Bipolar Disorder

**How it has been used:** Choline has mood-stabilizing possibilities and has been used for liver disease including chronic hepatitis and cirrhosis as well as for memory loss and dementia.

**Some interesting data:** It may help in rapid-cycling bipolar disorder.

**Historical data:** Choline has traditionally been considered a B vitamin; however there is some controversy about whether it can be synthesized by the human body (Natural Medicines Comprehensive Database, Therapeutic Research, 1995–2001).

**The usual dose:** The usual dose is 25 mg/kg/day bid.

## What They Did Not Tell You

**Health concerns:** At best, choline is a weak mood stabilizer. If it does have any mood-stabilizing qualities, it is when it is "combined with lithium" (*Psychopharmacology Update*, 1999, College of Medicine, Houston).

It may cause a fish smell. Diarrhea at high doses has been reported.

It may require lithium to be effective.

**Clinical studies:** Choline is likely effective in treating nutrition-associated hepatic dysfunction, according to a study published in the *Journal of the American Diet Association* in 1997.

**The mechanism of action:** Choline is a vitamin-B-complex cofactor. It is a precursor to acetylcholine and a methyl donor for the synthesis of several other compounds necessary for the function of nerve tissue.

### Chondroitin Sulfate—Osteoarthritis

Chondroitin is the connective tissue found in joints. It has been touted for osteoarthritis.

More research is needed.

### Chromium—Antidepressant

**How it has been used:** Chromium is commonly used as a supplement for diabetes mellitus to decrease glucose in the blood. It has also been utilized as an appetite suppressant. It has been touted to have an antidepressant effect and has also been used for PMS.

**Some interesting data:** Hypoglycemic effects were discovered when patients in the ICU were given intravenous feedings containing chromium. Another interesting discovery in the medical literature stems from the fact that patients with Type 2 diabetes lose more chromium in the urine than nondiabetics.

**Historical data:** Chromium is a trace mineral often reported to lower cholesterol, improve artery function, and help lower blood sugar in diabetics.

**The usual dose:** 400 to 500 micrograms two times a day.

**Health concerns:** Indigestion has occurred in individuals taking chromium, and there are case reports in the medical literature of renal failure with high doses (*American Family Physician*, 1 September 2000, Vol. 62, No. 5, p. 1055). There is some question of cancer at high dosages. Obviously, it is usually benign for most at low dosages.

**Clinical studies:** In one US study of 180 patients with Type 2 diabetes, a placebo group and two groups of patients taking differing amounts of chromium (100 micrograms twice a day vs. 500 micrograms twice a day) resulted in significant improvements in glycosylated hemoglobin (HbA1c) at 2 months. Both groups treated with chromium had improved glucose levels in 4 months when compared with the placebo group. Another study involving 17 patients demonstrated that diets low in chromium may decrease glucose tolerance in individuals with borderline diabetes. Some studies have not demonstrated that chromium has any beneficial effect on blood glucose levels in humans (*American Family Physician*, 1 September 2000, Vol. 62, No. 5, p. 1054).

**What They Told You**

**What They Did Not Tell You**

Studies seem to indicate that chromium reduces body fat even without exercise.

Also, in human and animal studies it lowered cholesterol. Some studies have reported weight loss at 400 to 600 mg/day. Some studies suggest that it improved mood.

**The mechanism of action:** Chromium is thought to act by counteracting insulin resistance and increasing insulin-receptor sensitivity. "Researchers theorize that chromium picolinate may sensitize insulin-sensitive glucoreceptors in the brain, resulting in appetite suppression, activation of the sympathetic nervous system to stimulate thermogenesis, and down-regulation of insulin secretion" (Natural Medicines Comprehensive Database, Therapeutic Research Monograph, Chromium, 2001, pp. 1–2).

### Chrysanthemum—Prostate Cancer

This herb has been touted for prostate cancer.

Preliminary research is interesting in prostate cancer, but significant research is certainly lacking.

Chrysanthemum could cause an allergic reaction. It could interact with heart medications.

### Chuchuhuasi—Low Sex Drive

This is a rain-forest herb that is touted to stimulate the sex drive.

Research is lacking.

Side effects are not known.

### Cinnamon—Bronchitis

Cinnamon is a popular spice. It has been used for its reported antiseptic qualities. It has also been used for gastrointestinal problems and menstrual irregularities.

Cinnamon is usually benign. Allergic reactions are always possible. Overall cinnamon is a neat spice for many.

### Clary Sage—PMS

Clary is often added to beverages, foods, and even soaps because of its fragrance.

Clary is usually safe in the small amounts found in foods.

Its efficiency is not known.

It has been touted for digestive disorders and kidney disease. It has been used to aid in the removal of splinters from the skin. It has been used as a sedative and for PMS.

Higher doses can cause dizziness, drowsiness, and headaches.

### Cleavers (lady's bedstraw)—Laxative

Cleavers is a mild laxative for many people. It is a relative of coffee but caffeine-free.

Cleavers is usually a gentle laxative. Caution has been given to diabetics in regard to using this herb.

It has also been used for high blood pressure.

## What They Told You

### Clematis—Migraine Headache

Clematis has been used in the past for migraine headaches.

### Clivers—Enlarged Lymph Nodes

Orally, clivers is used as a diuretic, a mild astringent, for dysuria, lymphadenitis, psoriasis, and specifically for enlarged lymph nodes.

Topically, clivers is used for ulcers, festering glands, breast lumps, and skin rashes.

### Clove—Toothache and Bad Breath

Clove has been used for centuries for its local ability to dull pain as in toothache. It also has been used topically for athlete's foot and bunions. It has been used for bad breath and is found in many mouthwashes. It has even been reported to protect the retina from macular degeneration.

### Clown's Mustard Plant—Irritable Bowel Syndrome

Orally, clown's mustard plant is touted for gastrointestinal conditions such as dyspepsia, irritable bowel syndrome (IBS), gastritis, and bloating. It is also touted for gout, musculoskeletal aches and pains (rheumatism), tachycardia, asthma, bronchitis, and edema (dropsy).

### CMO (cerasomal-cis-9-cetylmyristolcate)—Rheumatoid Arthritis

This fatty acid has been touted to help in arthritis.

### Cod Liver Oil—Hypertension

Orally, cod liver oil is touted for hyperlipidemia, hypertriglyceridemia, hypertension, coronary heart disease, osteoarthritis, and systemic lupus erythematosus (SLE).

Topically, cod liver oil is touted to accelerate wound healing.

### Codonopsis—Fatigue

This herb has been touted to help in fatigue. It has been touted to have a stimulating effect on the nervous system through chemicals called atractylenoids. It has been said to take several months to work.

## What They Did Not Tell You

Clematis can irritate the gastrointestinal mucous membranes. It has caused confusion, seizures, and death.

Reliable information is insufficient.

Clove is certainly interesting. It can be irritating topically. It can cause bronchospasms and pulmonary edema in allergic reactions.

Orally, clown's mustard plant can cause nausea and diarrhea in some patients. Some patients might be hypersensitive to clown's mustard plant.

Research is lacking.

Orally, cod liver oil can have a fishy taste and might cause belching, nosebleeds, halitosis, and heartburn. High doses can cause nausea and loose stools. Long-term cod liver oil supplementation is associated with an increased risk of cutaneous malignant melanoma in women. There is one case of lipoid pneumonia as a result of long-term cod liver oil use. There is also some concern about vitamin A and vitamin D toxicity in people using cod liver oil long-term.

Significant research is lacking.

**What They Told You**

**What They Did Not Tell You**

### Coenzyme A—Fatigue

This enzyme is touted to increase energy and boost the immune system.

Significant research is lacking.

### Coenzyme Q10—CHF (Congestive Heart Failure)

Coenzyme Q10 is an antioxidant similar to vitamin E. It has been touted to help in heart disease, angina, and hypertension. It has been touted to help in AIDS. It has also been touted to lower blood sugar.

Coenzyme Q10 is interesting. No doubt research will focus on its possible role in heart disease protection.

Apparently it is usually safe for most people. It might elevate liver functions in high doses. Gastrointestinal distress is possible.

### Coffee—Fatigue

Who does not know about coffee, the most-used herb of all time? It is a stimulant and thus helps in sleepiness.

As a stimulant coffee can cause difficulty falling asleep, restlessness, irritability, and rapid heartbeat. However, it is usually safe for most people and enjoyed worldwide.

### Cola—Fatigue

Cola was made famous by its use in the past in Coca-Cola. It is used for fatigue.

Cola contains caffeine and theobomine—central nervous system stimulants.

Although used safely by many, it can cause anxiety, restlessness, rapid heartbeat, tremors, delirium, irregular heartbeat, ringing in the ears, and even seizures.

It can interact with many drugs such as: Tylenol, aspirin, several minor tranquilizers, heart medications, Tagamet, amphetamines, some antipsychotics, oral hypoglycemics, Antabuse, estrogen, ergotamine, ephedra, MAOIs, birth control pills, theophylline, and many more.

### Coleus Forskohlii

Coleus forskohlii comes from a plant grown along mountain slopes in India, Nepal, Thailand, and Sri Lanka. It is touted to help in high blood pressure, angina, eczema, psoriasis, and asthma.

It has also been touted for weight-loss programs, hypothyroidism, and depression.

It is often given at 50 mg 3 times per day.

This herb may work by enzyme changes in the body (an increase in cyclic adenosine monophosphate), which then activates many other enzymes in diverse cellular functions such as relaxation of arteries, relaxation of smooth muscles, inhibition of most cell degranulation, and histamine release.

If the above pharmacology is correct, then caution would be in order for antihypertensives or antiasthmatics.

Double-blind tests are needed.

### CollagenPlus—Weight Loss

CollagenPlus has been described as a wellness product that helps with weight loss and improving health. It contains a combination of conjugated linoleic acid, collagen protein, pyruval glycine, L-carnitine, chromium polynicoti-

More comprehensive studies are needed to answer questions concerning the health benefits of CollagenPlus as well as identify any significant dangers.

| **What They Told You** | **What They Did Not Tell You** |
|---|---|

nate, vitamin C, aloe vera, and garcinia cambogia. This combination has been recommended to decrease buildup of fat, produce lean muscles, burn fat and calories, prevent conversion of carbohydrates to fat, improve the flow of nutrients into the cells, and increase cellular metabolism—all of this with no side effects!

Usual dosage is 1–2 tablespoons mixed with 8 ounces of water on an empty stomach in the morning and at bedtime.

### Colloidal Silver—Topical Fungal Infections

Colloidal silver has been touted topically for fungal infections, acne, burns, bacterial infections, and sore throat.

Significant research is lacking in regard to effectiveness.

Orally it has been touted for bacterial, fungal, and yeast infections.

In regard to potential side effects, it can lead to an irreversible bluish skin color when used topically or orally.

It can also cause renal damage and neurological damage.

### Colostrum—Irritable Bowel Syndrome

Colostrum is the first food from the mother's breast. It transfers immunity to her baby. It also contains growth factors that help in the development of the digestive tract and give strength and stamina.

Several huge questions arise in regard to colostrum. First, does it really work, or does the reality of the benefit of colostrum from the mother to the newborn baby transfer to the theory of cow's colostrum having benefits in the adult today? Does it carry any danger itself such as mad cow disease? Is it pure? Is its benefit destroyed by the packaging process?

Colostrum is touted to have many health benefits: in infections, in irritable bowel syndrome, in antiaging, and in bodybuilding, to mention only a few.

Hopefully, it will prove to be of some benefit, and it seems that side effect probability is overall low.

### Coltsfoot—Cough

Coltsfoot has long been used as a cough suppressant.

Coltsfoot can seriously damage the liver, and the flower buds may be carcinogenic.

### Comfrey—Diuretic

Comfrey leaves have been used as a healing herb since 400 BC. Native Americans used it for several ailments. It has been used for respiratory ailments, arthritis, fractures, and to aid in regrowth of new tissue. It has been called the "knitter and healer herb."

Comfrey is possibly safe when used externally on unbroken skin for less than 10 days. Oral ingestion is unsafe and can be highly toxic. Prickly comfrey is more toxic than the common version of comfrey, although both may be labeled the same.

Comfrey is for external use only. Ointments are commonly made with 5–20 percent comfrey.

### Common Stonecrop—Hypertension

Orally, common stonecrop is touted for coughs and hypertension. Topically, common stonecrop is used for wounds, burns, hemorrhoids, warts, eczema, and mouth ulcers.

Reliable information is insufficient about the safety of common stonecrop. Avoid using during pregnancy or while breast-feeding.

## What They Told You

### Conjugated Linoleic Acid (CLA)—Obesity

CLA has been touted for obesity, lowering cholesterol, lowering blood sugar, and in cancer prevention.

Dosages of 2–4 grams per day have been used.

### Copper—Copper Deficiency

Copper has been touted for various inflammations and for osteoporosis.

It has been used to treat anemia due to copper deficiency.

### Coral—Base for New Bone Growth

Coral has been used as a base in surgery (as orthopedic and facial) for new bone growth.

### Cordyceps—Increase Energy

Orally, cordyceps is touted for strengthening the immune system, for reducing the effects of aging, promoting longevity, treating lethargy, and improving liver function in people with hepatitis B. It is also touted to treat coughs, chronic bronchitis, respiratory disorders, kidney disorders, frequent nocturia, male sexual dysfunction, anemia, heart arrhythmias, high cholesterol, liver disorders, dizziness, weakness, tinnitus, wasting, and opium addiction. It is also touted as a stimulant, a tonic, and an adaptogen which is used to increase energy, enhance stamina, and reduce fatigue.

### Coriander—Loss of Appetite

Coriander has been used for loss of appetite, gas, and diarrhea. It has been touted to lower blood sugar and blood lipids. It has been used as a fungicide and a bactericide. It has been used for stomachache and nausea. In folk medicine it was used for worms and joint pain.

It has a fragrance and has often been used in soaps and for flavoring tobacco. It is often used in small amounts as a flavoring in foods.

## What They Did Not Tell You

CLA is certainly interesting. It might lower weight and cholesterol in some. More research is needed.

It usually seems to be safe for most, although gastrointestinal upset and fatigue have been reported. It does not seem to interact with other medication.

Copper is effective for copper deficiency. Otherwise, research is lacking.

It can cause gastrointestinal upset, liver failure, and renal failure. As little as one gram of copper can result in renal failure and death.

This use is probably effective for many.

Reliable information is insufficient.

Coriander has vitamin C, calcium, and magnesium, potassium, and iron. It contains a nice smelling volatile oil, linalool.

The blood-sugar-lowering and blood-lipid-lowering effects were in mice. Interesting, but there is a big jump from mice to humans.

It probably does help some in loss of appetite and upset stomach.

It is of the carrot family. Interactions are few. It seems to be safe in smaller amounts, but true safety is not known. It could interact with medications that lower lipids or blood sugar.

## What They Told You

### Corkwood—Motion Sickness

Corkwood contains scopolamine (which is now commercially available) that has been used to prevent the nausea and vomiting of motion sickness.

### Corn Cockle—Warts

Historically, corn cockle seeds were used for treating cancers, hard tumors, warts, hard swelling of the uterus, and to induce inflammation of the conjunctiva and cornea. The root was used historically for exanthemata (acute skin eruptions signifying a viral or coccal infection) and hemorrhoids. Various plant parts have also been used as a diuretic, expectorant, menstrual stimulant, poison, vermifuge, and for jaundice.

### Corn Silk—Diuretic

Corn silk has long been used for its diuretic effects. Thus, it has been used in PMS, urinary tract infections, and a variety of other conditions.

### Cosamin—Osteoarthritis

Cosamin has been touted for osteoarthritis.

### Couch Grass—Urinary Tract Infections

Couch grass has been touted for UTIs, renal stones, and prostatitis because of its diuretic-like properties.

### Country Mallow—Weight Loss

In herbal combinations country mallow is used orally for weight loss to burn fat, to increase energy, for impotence, sinus, allergy, throat diseases, asthma and bronchitis, and to promote a strong skeletal system.

In combination with ginger, country mallow root is used orally for intermittent fever.

In combination with milk and sugar, country mallow root is used for urinary urgency and leukorrhea.

Traditionally, country mallow is used orally to treat bronchial asthma, colds, flu, chills, lack of perspiration, headaches, nasal congestion, cough and wheezing, urinary infections, and edema. It is also traditionally used orally for heart disease, facial paralysis, healing chronic tissue inflam-

## What They Did Not Tell You

Corkwood inhibits acetylcholine and causes rapid heartbeat, confusion, anxiety, dizziness, and blurred vision.

Oral use can cause GI irritation, severe muscle pain and twitching, depression, and coma. Acute poisoning symptoms include: diarrhea, salivation, vertigo, vomiting, paralysis, and respiratory depression. Repeated poisoning by small doses is referred to as "githagism."

Allergic reactions are possible. It is conceivable that it could trigger uterine contractions, so it, as most herbs, should not be used by pregnant females.

The potential risk of transmission of bovine spongiform encephalopathy (BSE, mad cow disease) is raising patients' concern about products containing chondroitin. Chondroitin is produced from bovine trachea. In some cases manufacturing methods might lead to contamination with other diseased animal tissues.

Significant research is lacking.

The country mallow ephedrine constituent can cause dizziness, motor restlessness, irritability, insomnia, headache, anorexia, nausea, vomiting, flushing, tingling, difficulty urinating, tachycardia, and heart palpitations when taken orally.

Use of botanical sources of ephedrine such as country mallow have been associated with muscle conditions including myalgia, cardiomyopathy, rhabdomyolysis, eosinophilia myalgia syndrome, and hypersensitivity myocarditis. Botanical sources of ephedrine such as country mallow have also been associated with kidney stones, acute hepatitis, psychosis, and sudden death. The country mallow constituent ephedrine can also cause a drastic increase in blood pressure, cardiac arrhythmias, heart failure, asphyxia, and hyperthermia.

**What They Told You**

mation, sciatica, insanity, neuralgia, nerve inflammation, chronic rheumatism, and emaciation. Country mallow is also traditionally used orally as a stimulant, analgesic, diuretic, tonic, aphrodisiac, and before and after cancer chemotherapy to aid recovery. Country mallow is traditionally used topically for numbness, nerve pain, muscle cramps, skin disorders, tumors, joint diseases, wounds, ulcers, and as a massage oil.

**What They Did Not Tell You**

### Cowslip—Anxiety

Cowslip has been touted for anxiety, insomnia, upper respiratory infections, and sinusitis.

Cowslip could possibly cause hypotension followed by hypertension.

It might interact with drugs for hypertension, anxiety, and some antibiotics (Vibramycin).

### Cramp Bark—Muscle Spasms

Cramp bark has been touted for muscle spasms and pain.

Significant research is lacking.

Side effects are not known.

### Cranberry—Urinary Tract Infections

**How it has been used:** Cranberry has been used for bladder infections, cystitis, kidney inflammation, urinary tract infections, and gout.

Cranberry has been used for decades if not centuries in an attempt to help in urinary tract infections.

**Some interesting data:** The plant is bushy with tough leaves and bright red berries. The berries are plentiful around Thanksgiving and Christmas holidays.

**Historical data:** It grows mostly in eastern North America but can be found from Tennessee to Alaska.

**The usual dose:** Eight to sixteen ounces daily of cranberry juice have been suggested by some to treat urinary tract infections. Others have suggested that a main problem with cranberry juice is the large amount (16 ounces per day) needed to help with urinary tract infections.

**Health concerns:** Most cranberry juice is high in sugar.

**Clinical studies:** More serious studies are needed.

**The mechanism of action:** It was originally thought that cranberry juice helped by increasing acid in the urine, making it less desirable for bacteria; however it is now believed that cranberry's main action is to prevent bacteria from anchoring to the wall of the bladder. Without anchoring, the bacteria cannot cause infection.

### Creatine—Alzheimer's

Creatine has been used in Alzheimer's disease and other neurodegenerative diseases such as Huntington's disease, Parkinson's disease, and amyotrophic lateral sclerosis.

Creatine is also a supplement that is currently popular

Creatine is certainly interesting in regards to possibly helping in Alzheimer's dementia. It increases brain levels of creatine and phosphocreatine. It inhibits activation of the mitochondrial permeability transition which may be neuroprotective since mitochondrial dysfunction and

## What They Told You

among athletes and is used to increase athletic performance. It is naturally found in many tissues throughout the body and is found in steak. It is currently allowed by The International Olympic Committee and other sports organizations.

### Cucumber—High Blood Pressure
Cucumber has been used for years for its reported diuretic effect.

### Cudweed—Mouth and Throat Diseases
Topically, cudweed is touted as a gargle or rinse for diseases of the mouth or throat.

### Cyanacobalanin (Vitamin $B_{12}$)—Pernicious Anemia
Vitamin $B_{12}$ is touted for treating pernicious anemia.

It has been touted for depression.

### Cypress—Colds
Cypress branches have been used topically (as an ointment) for colds.

### Daffodil—HIV
Daffodil has been used topically to aid in wound healing and for joint pain.

Orally, some have even suggested it might have anti-HIV and anticancer activity.

## What They Did Not Tell You

oxidative stress are thought to have roles in neurodegenerative disease and aging.

The studies are highly conflicted as to whether it increases athletic performance. It probably does not for most.

While it has been safe for many, it does not appear safe for all. Serious adverse side effects have been reported. It certainly should not be used by those with kidney disease, diabetes mellitus, and those on ACE inhibitors, antihypertensive medications, or NSAI medications such as Motrin.

Significant research is lacking.

Topically, cudweed can cause an allergic reaction in individuals sensitive to the asteraceae/compositae family. Members of this family include ragweed, chrysanthemums, marigolds, daisies, and many other herbs.

Vitamin $B_{12}$ is effective in pernicious anemia but not in most depressions.

Many drugs (alcohol, antibiotics, Colestid, Glucophage, Tagamet, Zantac, Pepcid, Prevacid, Prilosec, Protonix, Aciphex, oral contraceptives, K-Dur, and nicotine to name a few) can contribute to $B_{12}$ depletion.

Vitamin $B_{12}$ can cause diarrhea, itching, thrombosis, and anaphylaxis.

One of the authors grew up near a swamp where there were many large cypress trees many years ago. Even then any use of cypress other than for beauty was most unlikely. Its effectiveness is not known.

Chewing daffodil can cause shivering, vomiting, diarrhea, fainting, and paralysis.

| What They Told You | What They Did Not Tell You |
|---|---|
| **Daisy—Pain** | |
| Daisy has been touted for antimicrobial and antifungal effects. It has also been touted for pain, arthritis, and gastrointestinal upset. | Significant research is lacking. |
| **Damiana (Turenura Diffusa)—Aphrodisiac** | |
| Damiana, a Mexican herb, is touted to greatly enhance the sex drive. | Signficant research is lacking. One chemical present in damiana is similar to cyanide. |
| **Dandelion—Hepatitis** | |
| Dandelion is a common plant. It has been used in liver disease and is touted to have a diuretic effect. It has also been used in diabetes and premenstrual syndrome.<br><br>The fluid extract is usually 4 to 10 milliliters 3 times per day. The capsule is often 515 mg three times daily. | Gastric upset is possible, as are other conceivable side effects. Dangerous interactions with other medicines (antihypertensives, diuretics, insulin, lithium, oral hypoglycemics). One concern is that dandelions are often treated with herbicides. |
| **Danshen—Cardiovascular Diseases** | |
| Orally, danshen is touted for circulation problems, ischemic stroke, angina pectoris, and other cardiovascular diseases. It is also touted for menstrual problems, chronic hepatitis, abdominal masses, insomnia due to palpitations and tight chest, acne, psoriasis, eczema, and other skin conditions. Danshen is also touted orally to relieve bruising and to aid in wound healing. | Orally, danshen can cause pruritus, upset stomach, and reduced appetite. |
| **Da Qing Ye—Hepatitis** | |
| In Chinese medicine, da qing ye is touted to treat acute parotitis, upper respiratory infection, encephalitis, hepatitis, lung abscess, dysentery, acute gastroenteritis, and HIV. In combination with seven other herbs (PC-SPES), da qing ye is touted to treat prostate cancer. | Orally, da qing ye can cause nausea and vomiting. Intramuscularly, da qing ye can cause blood in the urine. |
| **Deanol—Attention Deficit Disorder** | |
| Orally, deanol is touted for treating attention deficit disorder (ADD), enhancing memory and mood, boosting cognitive function, treating Alzheimer's disease, increasing intelligence and physical energy, improving athletic performance, preventing aging or liver spots, improving red blood cell function, improving muscle reflexes and increasing oxygen efficiency, extending life span, treating autism, and treating tardive dyskinesia. | Orally, deanol can cause constipation, urticaria, headache, drowsiness, insomnia, overstimulation, vivid dreams, confusion, depression, blood pressure elevation, hypomania, an increase in schizophrenia symptoms, and orofacial and respiratory tardive dyskinesia. |
| **Deer Velvet—Morphine Tolerance** | |
| See HGH.<br><br>In addition to the information under HGH, some evidence suggests that deer velvet might inhibit the development of tolerance to repeated doses of morphine. | Significant research is lacking.<br><br>Since it contains some sex hormones, individuals with breast or cervical cancer should avoid this hormone. |

| What They Told You | What They Did Not Tell You |
|---|---|
| **Devil's Claw—Arthritis** | |
| Devil's claw has been touted for arthritis and upper respiratory infections. | Significant research is lacking. |
| Others claim it has hypoglycemic effects and helps in loss of appetite. | Devil's claw should not be used with medications for diabetes mellitus, acid reflux, blood thinners, heart problems, and high blood pressure. |
| | It can cause uterine contractions. |
| **DGL—Ulcers** | |
| DGL has been touted to be beneficial in ulcer treatment. | DGL is derived from licorice but touted not to cause blood pressure elevations. |
| | Only time will tell how effective and safe it might be. It has most often been studied in contrast to Tagamet and Zantac. We scarcely doubt it could begin to compare to new drugs like Nexium. |
| **D-Glucarate—Cancer** | |
| D-glucarate is a nutrient that has been used in the fight against cancer. It is touted to help remove toxins and carcinogens from the body. D-glucarate is found in many fruits and vegetables and can be bought as a supplement. | Significant research is lacking. |
| **DHEA—Depression** | |
| **How it has been used:** Antidepressant effects, to slow or reverse aging, increase strength, improve energy, increase muscle mass, and to slow the progression of degenerative brain disorders, as well as treating erectile dysfunction. | **Health concerns:** DHEA taken orally can cause acne, hair loss, voice deepening, hirsutism, and liver dysfunction. The possible benefits may not outweigh the dangers. Problems with "insulin resistance, hypertension, reduced HDL or good cholesterol, increased male and female hormones" have been reported (*Psychopharmacology Update*, 1999, Baylor College of Medicine, Houston). |
| **Interesting data:** DHEA is manufactured from constituents of wild yam extract. Ingesting wild yam cannot be converted to DHEA by the body; therefore taking wild yam will not increase DHEA levels in humans. Individuals interested in taking DHEA should avoid wild yam products labeled as "natural DHEA" (Natural Medicines Comprehensive Database, Therapeutic Research, 1995-2001). | "There is some evidence that its long-term use can cause oily skin, acne, the growth of body hair, a deepening voice, and possibly aggressive or psychotic behavior" (*The Harvard Medical Letter*, Vol. 16, No. 3, September 1999). |
| **Historical data:** It has been used for its mood-lifting effects. It is a hormone secreted by the adrenal glands that is needed for the synthesis of testosterone and estrogen. | **Clinical studies:** Most studies were small and lasted from a few weeks to six months. Further studies are needed to establish safety profile and appropriate uses. |
| **The usual dose:** 25 to 50 mg per day have commonly been used. | **The mechanism of action:** DHEA is produced in the adrenal glands and liver of humans where it is then metabolized to androstenedione, the major human precursor to androgens (male hormone) and estrogens (female hormone). DHEA is also produced in the central |

**What They Told You**

**What They Did Not Tell You**

nervous system and is concentrated in the limbic regions and may function as an excitatory neuroregulator.

### Diets

Ninety percent of Americans feel overweight, 50 percent are overweight with a BMI of greater than 25, and 30 percent are obese with a BMI of greater than 30.

Thus diets are popular. In fact, 20 percent of Americans are in a weight-loss program in any given year, and weight loss is a 10-billion-dollar business annually.

Additional diet programs may include diets that restrict food or nutrient components or supplement nutrients such as low-sodium, fat-restricted, low-cholesterol, low-saturated-fat, protein-restricted, high-fiber, high-potassium, or high-calcium diets. These diets are useful in the management of certain medical conditions.

There are hundreds of diet plans currently on the market, all the way from A to Z, from zone types, blood types, to body types. Names such as Hollywood, Grapefruit, Mayo Clinic, Sugar Buster, Vegetarian, Scarsdale, Vinegar, Mediterranean, Grape Seed, and the Soup Diet, to name but a few.

But do the diets really work? They probably do not over 90 percent of the time. Then the question is why do they not work? Perhaps because weight comes from a complex set of factors—genetics, early environment, defense mechanisms, and current stress, to name just a few. However, diets can work and a good nutritionist can help.

Many diets come and go. At times, for example, the Adkins Diet (high protein, low carbohydrate) has been one of the best known for weight loss. Does it work? *The Medical Letter* (12 June 2000), one of the most respected medical journals in the world, responded this way, "In the first week to 10 days of such a diet, ketosis increases water loss, which can cause rapid weight loss. With rehydration, the initial weight loss tends to disappear."

Perhaps the most prudent approach to dieting and weight loss and maintenance is to practice good dietary habits that include eating fresh rather than preserved, packaged, or convenience foods. Include plenty of vegetables and fruit, raw when possible to preserve the nutritional value. Select whole-grain rather than processed breads and flour products. Eat fish, poultry, and legumes for protein and cut down on red meat. Lower fat-containing foods and use polyunsaturated fats and vegetables rather than saturated ones. Cut down on simple sugar products.

### Dill—Gas

Dill has been used for gas.

Significant research is lacking.

### DIM—Cancer

DIM is a plant nutrient derived from cruciferous vegetables such as broccoli, cabbage, and cauliflower. It is touted to decrease cancer in women by altering the ratio of the

Significant research is lacking.

| What They Told You | What They Did Not Tell You |
|---|---|
| different types of estrogen and by doing so to decrease the risk of cancer. | |

### DMAE (Dimethylsulfoxide)—Pain

| | |
|---|---|
| DMAE is made from wood. It is touted topically for pain, aching muscles, and arthritis. | Significant research is lacking. |

### DMG (Dimethlglycine)—High Cholesterol

| | |
|---|---|
| DMG has been touted to lower serum lipids and to boost the immune system. It has also been touted to be helpful for those with seizure. | Signficant research is lacking.<br><br>Side effects are not known. |

### Dong Quai—PMS

| | |
|---|---|
| This herb comes from China and has been touted to help in women's issues: PMS, menopause, and uterine cramps. It contains estrogen-like compounds. It has been touted to increase sex drive in females. | Dong quai has estrogen-like compounds and, thus, conceivably similar side effects. The argument has always been whether these natural estrogens (dong quai, chasteberry, black cohosh, red clover, and evening primrose) are safer than synthetic manufactured estrogens. |

### Dopamine

| | |
|---|---|
| See Monoamine Precursors. | |

### Dragon's Blood—Diarrhea

| | |
|---|---|
| Orally, dragon's blood is touted for diarrhea, digestive disorders, and as a coloring agent.<br><br>Topically, dragon's blood is used as an astringent. | Reliable information is insufficient. |

### Dwarf Elder—Arthritis

| | |
|---|---|
| Orally, dwarf elder is touted for arthritis, weight reduction, and as a diuretic. | Orally, ingestion of large quantities of any plant part of dwarf elder may cause vomiting, bloody diarrhea, cyanosis, dizziness, headache, and unconsciousness. Death has been reported. Cyanide poisoning can be caused by any plant part of dwarf elder. Sambunigrine, a cyanogenic glycoside, is present in the plant. |

### Echinacea—Common Cold

| | |
|---|---|
| **How it has been used:** It has been used most for the common cold. In addition, it has been used for breast pain, other upper respiratory illnesses, infection, immune system depression, cancer, gonorrhea, and psoriasis.<br><br>**Some interesting data:** Echinacea species are flowering herbs found in midwestern North America from Saskatchewan to Texas. It receives its name from a Greek word meaning "sea urchin" (Murray, p. 92).<br><br>**Historical data:** It is the most-used plant among Native | **Health concerns:** Megadoses of echinacea might interfere with the work of the immune system. Some people have experienced allergic reactions, nausea, vomiting, chills, or fever. Individuals suffering from autoimmune disorders (such as systemic lupus or multiple sclerosis) should not take echinacea. Certain species of echinacea could contain very small amounts of pyrrolizidine alkaloids, which, at higher levels, has been linked to a lethal toxicity of the liver. Studies have revealed damage to the reproductive cells in animals and thus should not be used by young females. |

**What They Told You**

Americans. It has been called the "herbal equivalent of vitamin C" (Duke, p. 90).

**The usual dose:** Twice daily dosage of 500 mg capsules.

**What They Did Not Tell You**

**Clinical studies:** Numerous studies of the effectiveness of echinacea to boost the immune system have been reported, but "few are of good quality" (*American Family Physician*, October 1998, p. 1136).

In a double-blind Germany study, flu-like symptoms were significantly reduced with echinacea versus placebo in about three days. In other studies upper respiratory symptoms seemed significantly reduced with echinacea. The German Commission E recommends that echinacea use should not exceed eight successive weeks and that it not be taken with IDS, TB, MS or collagen-vascular diseases.

**The mechanism of action:** Active compounds in echinacea include cichoric acid, polysaccharides, flavonoids, echinacosides, and essential oils. Studies suggest echinacosides are responsible for its anti-inflammatory, antiviral, and immunostimulating properties through the stimulating of T-lymphocyte proliferation and interferon production and the mobilization of other phagocytic leukocytes. Anti-inflammatory properties appear to be due to inhibition of the pro-inflammatory enzyme, hyaluronidase (a mechanism much like cortisone) (*Pharmacist's Letter/Prescriber's Letter*, 2000, p. 7). "Studies show an increase in phagocytosis, lymphocyte activity, cellular respiratory activity and activity against tumor cells but direct bactericidal and bacteriostatic properties have not been demonstrated" (*American Family Physician*, October 1998, p. 1137).

### Elderberry or Elder—Common Cold

Elderberry wine is well known, but elderberry has also been used for the common cold and fever. It has been said to have insulin-like properties. It also may have diuretic-like properties.

The bark and leaves are toxic. Hypersensitivity reactions are possible.

### Elecampane—Hookworm

Elecampane has been touted for hookworm and roundworms.

Elecampane should not be used with medications for diabetes mellitus, high blood pressure, or anxiety.

Large doses can cause gastrointestinal upset and even paralysis.

### Emu Oil—Topically for Stretch Marks

Emu oil has been touted topically for poison ivy, rashes, hemorrhoids, wounds, insect bites, arthritis, joint pains, burns, stretch marks, acne, psoriasis, wrinkles, and damaged hair.

Significant research is lacking.

## What They Told You

It has been touted to lower cholesterol and for headaches and URIs.

### English Ivy—Bronchitis
English ivy has been touted for bronchitis.

### EPA (eicosapentaenoic acid)—Schizophrenia
This is another name for omega-3 fatty acid. It has been touted for schizophrenia, bipolar disorder, and cystic fibrosis.

### Ephedra—Weight Loss
**How it has been used:** Ephedra has primarily been used in many weight-loss herb preparations. Other key uses reported are for asthma, hay fever, and the common cold.

Ephedra is frequently marketed in combination with caffeine products for weight loss. Ephedra found in dietary supplements is usually either a formulation of powdered stems and aerial portions or a dried extract.

Ephedrine and pseudoephedrine can directly and indirectly stimulate the sympathetic nervous system, increasing systolic and diastolic blood pressure, increasing heart rate, causing peripheral vasoconstriction, bronchodilation, and central nervous system stimulation. Ephedrine shows antitussive, bacteriostatic, and anti-inflammatory activity in animals. Ephedrine can have diuretic, hypoglycemic, and hyperglycemic effects. It can stimulate uterine contraction and theoretically can be catabolized to mutagenic nitrosamines. Ephedrine causes relaxation of the smooth muscle in the gastrointestinal tract, urinary retention by relaxing the detrusor muscle, and diminishes contraction of the bladder sphincter.

**Some interesting data:** Ephedra is a branching shrub found in dry areas of the world including regions of China, Asia, America, Pakistan, and India. Ma huang is a form of ephedra obtained from the stems and branches of the shrub.

**Historical data:** Use of ephedra dates back to around 2800 BC. Its early use was for severe night sweats. Practitioners of Western medicine became interested in ephedra in the 1920s when ephedrine was developed and used for treatment of the common cold and allergies. In

## What They Did Not Tell You

Effectiveness of English ivy is not known.

Allergic reactions are possible.

More research still needs to be done. Some preliminary research is interesting.

It can thin the blood.

**Health concerns:** Ephedra can cause CVA (stroke), MI (heart attack), agitation, and psychosis.

"Ephedrine-containing herbal products have been associated with adverse cardiovascular events, seizures, and even death" (*American Family Physician,* 1 March 1999, Vol. 59, p. 1239). Ephedra will increase blood flow to the heart, brain, and muscles at the expense of the kidneys and gastrointestinal tract. It causes constriction of the vessels supplying blood to the skin, mucus membranes, and viscera.

The Food and Drug Administration (FDA) has recommended that individuals with heart disease, high blood pressure, thyroid disease, diabetes, or difficulty urinating due to enlargement of the prostate not take ephedra products. Individuals taking medication to lower blood pressure or treat depression are also cautioned against taking ephedra (Murray, p. 114).

Irritability, anxiety, and hyperactivity are also common side effects of its use.

Chronic use of ephedra (ma huang) can cause rapid development of tolerance and dependence (*Pharmacist's Letter/Prescriber's Letter,* 2000, p. 23).

Ephedra taken orally can cause dizziness, motor restlessness, anxiety, irritability, insomnia, headache, anorexia, nausea, vomiting, flushing, tingling, difficulty urinating, tachycardia, heart palpitations, hyperthermia, drastic increase in blood pressure, heart failure, asphyxia, and death.

## What They Told You

1997, the FDA proposed a ban on supplements with more than 8 mg of ephedrine, setting the maximum daily dose of 24 mg. In March 2000, the FDA withdrew the provisions of the 1997 proposal, stating the original ruling was based on unreliable evidence of adverse effects (*Pharmacist's Letter/Prescriber's Letter,* 2000, pp. 23–24).

**The usual dose:** Dosages depend on the alkaloid content. If the alkaloid content is 1 to 3 percent, the dose would be 12.5 to 25 mg of ephedra taken 2 to 3 times daily. If the preparation is 10 percent alkaloid, the dose would be 125 to 250 mg three times daily.

## What They Did Not Tell You

Several strokes have recently been attributed to ephedra, with at least one case resulting in a complete right hemispherectomy in a young male army officer. Reports associate the use of botanical sources of ephedrine, including ephedra, with myopathies, including myalgia, cardiomyopathy, rhabdomyolysis, eosinophilia-myalgia syndrome, and hypersensitivity myocarditis. Botanical sources of ephedrine have also been associated with nephrolithiasis, acute hepatitis, psychosis, and sudden death.

Reports filed with the FDA have involved adverse effects such as jitteriness, insomnia, addiction, chest tightness, hypertension, cardiac arrest, brain hemorrhage, seizures, stroke, and at least 39 fatalities with pressure to remove ephedra from many preparations.

Combining ephedra with caffeine, caffeine-containing herbs, coffee, cola nut, maté, or guarana increases the risk of adverse effects. Possibly, coadministration of ephedra with digitalis might cause cardiac arrhythmias. Theoretically, concomitant use of Elavil might reduce the hypertensive effects of the ephedrine contained in ephedra. Amitriptyline blocks the hypertensive effects of ephedrine.

Ephedra can raise blood glucose levels and interfere with diabetes drug therapy. Possibly, concomitant use of ephedra and ergot alkaloids may cause hypertension, due to the ephedrine contained in ephedra. Concomitant use of ephedra with MAOIs may increase the risk of hypertension and possible subarachnoid hemorrhage.

Theoretically, concomitant use of ephedra and urinary acidifying drugs may reduce the ephedrine-related effects of ephedra. Ephedra might also cause false-positive urine amphetamine or methamphetamine test results. Ephedra may induce or exacerbate angina due to its cardiac stimulant effects. Use of ephedra is contraindicated with anorexia due to the purported appetite suppressant effects of ephedra. Bulimic patients might also be at increased risk for the adverse effects of ephedra due to inadequate nutritional status. Large doses of ephedra could cause or exacerbate anxiety due to its CNS stimulant effects. Ephedra might exacerbate urinary retention in patients with benign prostatic hypertrophy (BPH) due to its effects on the detrusor muscle. Use in cases of cerebral insufficiency is contraindicated as ephedra might further decrease cerebral

| What They Told You | What They Did Not Tell You |
|---|---|
| | blood flow due to its vasoconstrictive effects. Ephedra may interfere with blood sugar control and exacerbate high blood pressure and circulatory problems in people with diabetes. Ephedra may exacerbate tremor and may exacerbate narrow-angle (angleclosure) glaucoma by causing mydriasis. |
| | Ephedra may cause tachycardia, arrhythmias, or induce angina in patients with heart disease due to its cardiac stimulant effects. Contraindicated, Ephedra may stimulate the thyroid and exacerbate hyperthyroid symptoms. Ephedra may exacerbate hypertension, can cause kidney stones, and could exacerbate the symptoms of pheochromocytoma. |
| | **Clinical studies:** Double-blind, placebo-controlled studies revealed superiority of ephedrine-caffeine combinations over placebo. In studies when patients had lower side effects, the dosages were started low or increased gradually. However, we feel the potential for danger usually outweighs the benefits. |
| | **The mechanism of action:** Its basic action is that of epinephrine (adrenaline). Ephedra acts as an agonist on the beta2 adrenergic receptors. Unlike epinephrine, it can be absorbed orally, has a longer action, and has a profound effect on the brain and CNS. The muscles of the airway (trachea, bronchial tree) and the uterus are relaxed. Forms of ephedra-like drugs have been used to stop premature labor and treat chronic asthma. |

*Epinephrine*
See Monoamine Precursors.

*Ergot—Ob-Gyn Hemorrhage*

| Ergot has been used in ob-gyn conditions. | Ergot can cause gastrointestinal symptoms, altered heart rate, edema, numbness, and angina. It can be poisonous in chronic use and may even cause death. |
|---|---|

*Esberitox—Common Cold*

| Esberitox has been touted for use in the common cold, the flu, and in ear infections. | Reliable information is insufficient. |
|---|---|

*Essiac—Cancer*

| Essiac is touted for treating cancer. | Reliable information is insufficient. |
|---|---|

*Eucalyptus—Decongestant*

| Eucalyptus has been known for much other than being the tallest tree in the world. It has been used for upper | The oil is toxic and could be lethal. |
|---|---|

## What They Told You

respiratory infections (an ingredient in Vick's VapoRub), asthma, arthritis, various infections, and even for bad breath.

### Euphrasia (See Eyebright)

Euphrasia is a flowering plant with the nickname "eyebright." It has been used for bloodshot eyes, eye fatigue, styes, inflammatory disorders of the skin, and impotence.

Lotions and poultices have been made; however, reliable dosage amounts are unavailable.

### Evening Primrose Oil—PMS

**How it has been used:** The main use over the years has been for PMS. Evening primrose oil is probably the number one supplement for PMS.

Some people also use this in the hope of reducing the risk of cardiovascular disease by supposedly lowering serum cholesterol and triglycerides and decreasing platelet aggregation. Women have used this preparation for decreasing symptoms of PMS, breast pain, and potentially lowering incidence of cystic breast disease. Other uses include treatment for rheumatoid arthritis, multiple sclerosis, atopic dermatitis, and diabetic neuropathy.

**Some interesting data:** This product may easily deteriorate. One way to check for freshness is to open a capsule and taste or smell the material. A bitter or rancid smell means it has degraded and should be discarded.

**Historical data:** It has been used in some cultures to shorten the duration of childbirth.

**The usual dose:** The dose of three to four grams has been recommended by some.

## What They Did Not Tell You

Eucalyptus should not be used concurrently with insulin, oral hypoglycemic agents, barbiturates, or amphetamines.

External use only is certainly best with this one.

Efficacy concerning the use of euphrasia has not been documented. More research is needed.

**Health concerns:** Mild gastrointestinal problems have been reported including indigestion, nausea, softening of stools, and headaches. Individuals taking phenothiazine drugs with EPO may lower seizure threshold. It may increase the risk of temporal lobe epilepsy. Pregnant women should avoid EPO as it may increase the risk of prenatal complications.

Some products did not contain EPO but instead contained substituted hydrogenated oil. Checking the reputation of the manufacturer is recommended.

**Clinical studies:** Recent reviews of the literature have concluded that the studies of primrose oil have been small and poorly designed. Compelling evidence that it is better than placebo seems to be lacking.

**The mechanism of action:** Action is ascribed to the oil containing high concentrations of cis-linoleic and cis-gammalinolenic acid that resemble "essential fatty acids" because only limited amounts are made and some people seem to benefit from adding oils of this type to their diet. These fats are incorporated into cell membranes or converted to Type 1 prostaglandins which, in turn, diminishes the production of Type 2 prostaglandins. Type 2 prostaglandins increase inflammation and pain, platelet aggregation, and blood vessel reactivity. These actions may be instrumental in possible benefits in arthritis, thrombosis, PMS, and atopic dermatitis. A deficiency in these fatty acid products may account for the problems seen in atopic dermatitis. It is also thought that individuals who have problems with diabetes, high alcohol consumption, high-fat diets, and vitamin deficiencies have some possible enzymatic

## What They Told You

## What They Did Not Tell You

insufficiency required for converting linoleic acid to gammalinolenic acid.

### Eyebright—Red Eyes

This herb comes from North America and is touted to help make eyes more bright in hay fever, insomnia, hangover from alcohol, and conjunctivitis. It contains glycoside, touted to have a strengthening effect on the capillaries of the eye.

We could find no significant research. It seems only folklore backs up the use of eyebright and possible benefit.

### False Unicorn Root—Menstrual Problems

This herb has been touted for menstrual problems and menopause. Reportedly, it has a uterine stimulant effect.

The effectiveness of false unicorn root is not proven.

It usually does not interact with other drugs and usually seems to be safe for many. It can cause nausea and can irritate the gastrointestinal tract.

### Fennel—Bad Breath

Fennel is touted to help in bad breath. It has been popular with both chefs (served with fish) and herbalists as well. It was listed in the *U.S. Pharmacopoeia* until 1970. It has largely been used to relieve gas and help digestion.

Fennel is usually safe. Of course it, as the vast majority of herbs, should not be used by pregnant or nursing women. Rare allergic reactions have been reported.

It is usually safe and may help with gas and bad breath.

### Fenugreek—Diabetes Mellitus

Fenugreek has been touted to lower blood sugar in both Type 1 and Type 2 diabetes mellitus.

Often fenugreek is used in conjunction with gymnema, bitter melon, chromium, and vanadyl in an attempt to lower blood sugar.

Fenugreek is often innocuous, but one danger certainly lies in possible hypoglycemic reactions when used with insulin or other hypoglycemic medications. It can also thin the blood and therefore could conceivably be dangerous when used with other blood-thinning agents.

### Feverfew—Migraine Headaches

**How it has been used:** Feverfew has been used to prevent and treat migraine headaches, treat rheumatoid arthritis, reduce fever, chills, colds, hay fever, sinus headache, and to stimulate menstruation. Topically, it has been used for toothaches and as a general antiseptic and insecticide. The major use has been for migraines.

**Some interesting data:** Feverfew is an herb with a powerful, distinctive smell that has been described as "fresh-like." It is known as "Bachelor's Button" and has been used since the Middle Ages. In Latin, *feverfew* means "driver of the fevers." In ancient Greece, feverfew was used by physicians to enhance contractions of the uterus during childbirth.

**Health concerns:** Some people have experienced mouth sores, skin rashes, and oral inflammation upon ingestion. Other reports describe a "post-feverfew syndrome" when people stop taking the herb which included nervousness, insomnia, joint pain, or stiffness (*Pharmacist Letter*, p. 9). It should not be used during pregnancy, by nursing mothers, or in young children. Bleeding time can be increased; therefore, individuals taking anticoagulants should be carefully monitored for bleeding. Overall, side effects do not seem to be reported often, and it has been used when individuals are unable to obtain relief on standard prescription medications or when there were too many side effects on standard medications.

**Clinical studies:** A double-blind study was done in

**What They Told You**

**Historical data:** In the first century AD, Greek physicians recommended the herb for "all inflammations and hot swellings" (Ritchason, p. 87). Early settlers introduced the plant to North America, and it is found in the wild and in gardens all over the US and Canada.

**The usual dose:** 25 mg 2 times daily up to 380 mg 3 times a day.

**What They Did Not Tell You**

London for migraines. Numbers of patients participating were small, and conclusions were unclear. A larger double-blind study was done at the University of Nottingham in the 1970s involving 72 patients who were randomly assigned to receive either one capsule daily of feverfew or a placebo. Treatment with feverfew was associated with reduction of headaches and lessening of severity in those who had headaches (Murray, p. 118). Several other studies having double-blind, placebo-controlled trials found similar results. Further studies need to be done to document its usefulness in treating headaches and other disorders.

**The mechanism of action:** Although its mechanism of action is poorly understood, several sources remark that feverfew may act more like the nonsteroidal anti-inflammatory agents (NSAIDs) by hindering the body's release of prostaglandins. Feverfew may also have some effect on platelets, deterring the thickening or clotting of blood.

### Fiber—High Cholesterol
Many foods and food parts have fiber (oat bran, whole-grain cereals, rice, vegetables, fruit, mucilages, pectin, cellulose, flaxseed, beans, hemicellulose, etc.). Fiber supplements are also available.

Fiber can help to lower cholesterol in some.

Some fiber, along with a low-fat diet, does lower cholesterol in some people to some degree.

### Figwort—Acne
Figwort has been used topically for various skin disorders (acne, itching, contact dermatitis, and psoriasis).

Figwort may have some antiprotozoacidal and anti-inflammatory activity topically, but significant research is lacking.

It is related to foxglove from which the famous heart medicine digitalis was initially derived. Some have dared to use it orally for cardiac purposes, but since it can cause heart block, this is extremely unwise.

### Fir—URIs
Fir has been touted for URIs and arthritic pain.

Significant research is lacking.

### Fireweed—Inflammation
In folk medicine fireweed is touted for inflammation, fevers, tumors, wounds, as an astringent, and as a tonic.

Reliable information is insufficient.

### Fish Oils
Fish oils contain the long-chain omega-3 fatty acids eicosapentaenoic acid (EPA) and docosahexaenoic acid (DHA).

Fish oils may have a mood-stabilizing effect in some and may lower blood lipids in some.

## What They Told You

Fish oils are often used for hypertension, hyperlipidemia (high cholesterol), coronary heart disease, bipolar disorder, rheumatoid arthritis, psoriasis, atopic dermatitis, ulcerative colitis, Bechet's syndrome, and Raynaud's disease. Fish oils seem to be most effective for hypertriglyceridemia, with several clinical trials showing reduction of triglyceride levels by 20 percent to 50 percent. Fish oils may be effective in reducing mortality after myocardial infarction; may reduce mildly elevated blood pressure; may help with depression; may be useful in cases of transplant, cancer, and diabetes, attention-deficit disorder; and may be useful with inflammatory diseases. Fish oils appear to work as the long-chain omega-3 fatty acids complete with arachnoid acid and has anti-inflammatory effects due to the inhibition of leukotriene synthesis.

## What They Did Not Tell You

Fish oils appear to be ineffective when taken with evening primrose oil for the prevention of preeclampsia, preterm labor, and intrauterine growth retardation.

Fish oils have a fishy taste, may result in a bodily fishy odor, may result in belching, halitosis, heartburn, and nosebleeds. High doses have been associated with nausea and loose stools.

Fish oils may interact with anticoagulant or antiplatelet drugs, resulting in excessive bleeding. These agents can include Saint-John's-wort, gingko, ginseng, aspirin, clopidogrel (Plavix), dalteparin (Fragmin), dipyridamole (Persantine), enoxparin (Lovenox), heparin, ticlopidine (Ticlid), warfarin (Coumadin), and others. Fish oils may also normalize EKG readings in some patients with ventricular ectopic beats and may decrease the ventricular ectopic beats. Fish oils may also decrease pulmonary function in aspirin-sensitive individuals, may lower blood mean arterial pressure and increase the risk of bleeding with cirrhosis, may interfere with glucose control, and may interact with additive effects with hypertensive agents for the treatment of hypertension.

### Flavonoids—Aging
Flavonoids are antioxidants and as antioxidants are touted to have antiaging effects.

Research is lacking.

### Flaxseed—Bipolar Disorder
Flaxseed has been used because if its source of omega-3 fatty acids that have been used in mood stabilization. It can also have a laxative-like effect and helps in regularity of bowel movements.

Flaxseed may have a mood-stabilizing effect in some and lower blood lipids in some.

There can be rare cases of induction of mania.

### Flaxseed Oil—Bipolar Disorder
Flaxseed oil contains rich sources of omega-3 fatty acids. It has been used in attempts to decrease cholesterol, reduce high blood pressure, decrease PMS, decrease arthritis, and decrease psoriasis. It has been used to stabilize manic-depressive disorder. It has been touted to protect against stroke and heart attack. It has been used for perimenopausal symptoms.

Omega-3 fatty acids have been reported to precipitate manic behavior in some bipolar individuals. Thus, while it could conceivably have some antidepressant effect and some antimanic effects, it could also conceivably precipitate a manic attack in bipolar individuals.

### Folic Acid—Pernicious Anemia
Folic acid is used for pernicious anemia along with $B_{12}$. It has also been used in alcoholism, ulcerative colitis, and other folic acid deficiency states. It is given to pregnant females to prevent neural tube defects.

Small doses of folic acid are usually safe and may very well be unsafe in large doses.

Studies have not backed up the claim that it helps to prevent heart disease.

**What They Told You**

**What They Did Not Tell You**

*Folic Acid + B₆—Depression*

**How it has been used:** It has been mainly recommended for use in combination to elevate mood. Other uses include prevention of cervical dysplasia, a precancerous condition in women, and neural tube defect in the fetus. It has also been used to protect against heart attacks, cancer, and arterial disease as well as to treat depression.

**Some interesting data:** Folic acid has been used in pregnant females to prevent neural tube defects. Of course, it has been used in anemia. It was recently tried as a preventative in heart disease, but one of the most recent studies implicated an antidepressant effect in women on an SSRI (Prozac).

**Historical data:** It has been used to treat acute poisoning from mushrooms of the genus Gyromitra.

**The usual dose:** $B_6$—5 to 200 mg per day; folic acid—400 mcg per day.

**Health concerns:** High doses of folic acid (above 1000 mcg/day) may alter sleep patterns, increase vivid dreaming, increase hyperactivity, and deplete levels of zinc. Large doses of $B_6$ (pyridoxine) greater than 2 grams a day can cause neurotoxicity resulting in sensory ataxia and breast tenderness.

**Clinical studies:** Folic acid is necessary for red blood cell formation and healthy cell division. Vitamin $B_6$ is important in healthy metabolism and nerve function. Supplementation with folic acid improved response to Prozac in women but not in men. Subjects were randomized and received 500 micrograms per day of folic acid or placebo for 10 weeks. Response and recovery rates were significantly increased in women who were supplemented with folic acid. Drug side effects were lower in both men and women receiving folic acid and Prozac (*Psychiatry Drug Alerts,* Vol. XIV, p.1). It has been known to exacerbate seizure and psychotic behavior.

**The mechanism of action:** $B_6$ is involved in food metabolism and release of energy. It is essential for amino acid metabolism and formation of blood proteins and antibodies. $B_6$ also helps with regulation of electrolytic balance.

More basic information is needed on how folic acid and $B_6$ actually act chemically.

*Fool's Parsley—Gastrointestinal Complaints*

Orally, fool's parsley is touted for gastrointestinal complaints in children, infantile cholera, summer diarrhea, and convulsions.

Orally, there are reports that fool's parsley caused deaths when it was mistaken for garden parsley. However, there is some evidence that the botanical to blame was actually spotted hemlock. Nevertheless, caution is warranted.

*Foxglove*

Foxglove is the original herb from which one of the most famous heart medicines of all time came (digitalis purpurea).

Potentially dangerous side effects are possible. The new digitalis preparations are far better and should only be used under the supervision of a medical doctor.

*Fructo-Oligosaccharides*

Orally, fructo-oligosaccharides are touted for prebiotic activity, specifically for bifidobacteria in the GI tract. Fructo-oligosaccharides are also touted for reducing serum cholesterol and increasing fecal mass.

Orally, the use of FOS can cause flatulence in amounts exceeding 10 grams, excessive flatus at 30 grams per day, GI sounds and bloating at 40 grams per day, and abdominal cramps and diarrhea at 50 grams per day.

## What They Told You

### Fumitory—Biliary Colic
Fumitory has been used in biliary colic, in skin infections, and in constipation.

### GABA—Anxiety
The amino acid GABA has been touted to help in anxiety.

### Galantamine
Galantamine is another "smart drug" extracted from flowers such as the snowdrop, the daffodil, and the spider lily. It has a long history of use for neuromuscular ailments including nerve inflammation and nerve pain. A prescription product of galantamine is available under the trade name Reminyl for the treatment of Alzheimer's disease. Galantamine is a substance that inhibits the biochemical action of acetylcholinesterase, an enzyme that destroys acetylcholine. Acetylcholine is a neurotransmitter (carrier of nerve impulses across gaps between neurons).

Acetylcholine is crucial to the formation of memory in the brain. Molecules of acetylcholine act on two kinds of neuronal receptors: nicotinic receptors and muscarinic receptors. Nicotinic receptors tend to decrease in number and sensitivity with age. Activating the nicotinic receptors makes them more responsive to acetylcholine, allowing them to be "turned up," thus enhancing cognitive function. Galantamine has reportedly been used for jet lag, fatigue, male erectile impotence, and dementia including Alzheimer's disease.

## What They Did Not Tell You

Fumitory might help in biliary disorders, but more significant research needs to be done.

It can certainly be dangerous in large doses, even causing convulsions and death. It can interact with heart medications.

GABA (y-amino butyric acid) is one of the more important neurotransmitters in the central nervous system. It has an inhibitory effect and thus is important in producing a calming effect. Minor tranquilizers such as Valium, Librium, Xanax, and Sexax bind to specific receptors that are separate from but adjacent to the GABA receptors and thereby potentiate the bind of GABA to its own receptors. The binding of GABA to its receptors results in increased chloride ion conduction, cell membrane hyperpolarization, and decreased initiation of action potentials and a calming effect.

The question is whether giving GABA direct as an amino acid by mouth would produce the same results. Other questions also arise. Would it be potentially addicting as the minor tranquilizers can be?

Side effects include, among others, chest pain, flatulence, incontinence, mild nausea, diarrhea, decreased appetite, weight loss, dizziness, vomiting, anorexia, and seizures. Care should be given in prescribing to patients with a history of pulmonary conditions (such as severe asthma or obstructive pulmonary disease), moderately impaired hepatic function, or moderately impaired renal function.

Galantamine is an example of both a supplement available over the counter and the prescription drug Reminyl often given by a neurologist or psychiatrist. This drug demonstrates that either a supplement or prescription medicine can have side effects. One difference here is knowledge—knowledge of the physician, knowledge of side effects, and knowledge of when to use or not use the drug.

## What They Told You

Dosage varies from 4 mg 2 times daily to 12 mg 3 times daily. The usual dose is 8 to 12 mg 2 times a day.

### Gamma Linolenic Acid (GLA)—Rheumatoid Arthritis
Orally, gamma linolenic acid (GLA) is touted for rheumatoid arthritis, oral mucoceles (mucous polyps), hyperlipidemia, systemic sclerosis, diabetic neuropathy, and to hasten the response to tamoxifen in people with breast cancer.

### Gamma Oryzanol—Menopause
Orally, gamma oryzanol is touted for hypercholesterolemia and dyslipidemia, increasing testosterone and human growth hormone levels, improving strength during resistance exercise training, and for treating symptoms associated with menopause and aging.

### Ganoderma—Anxiety
Ganoderma is an herb (fungus) that has been touted for multiple uses (anxiety, insomnia, respiratory infections, AIDS, and cancer).

In Asian pharmacies it is often sold under the name reishi.

### Garcinia (Citrin and Brindal Berry)—Obesity
Garcinia has been touted for weight loss.

### Garlic—High Blood Pressure
How it has been used: Garlic has been used for hypertension, headaches, cough, earache, arteriosclerosis, hysteria, vaginitis, various inflammations and infectious conditions, TB, ringworm, snakebite, diarrhea, athlete's foot, and worms. Orally, garlic is used for reducing high blood pressure, prevention of coronary heart disease by improving lipid levels, preventing age-related vascular changes and atherosclerosis, reducing reinfarction and mortality rate post-myocardial infarction, and for treating earaches and menstrual disorders. Garlic is also used orally for treatment of Helicobacter pylon infection (ulcers) and cancer prevention. Other uses include immune system stimulation, treatment of diabetes, arthritis, allergies, traveler's diarrhea, colds, flu, and prevention and treatment of bacterial and fungal infections. An aged garlic extract has been used orally for enhancing circulation, fighting stress and fatigue, and maintaining healthy liver function. Topically, garlic oil is used for tinea pedis,

## What They Did Not Tell You

Orally, GLA might prolong bleeding time.

Reliable information is insufficient.

Significant research is lacking.

Ganoderma can have multiple side effects (skin eruptions, itching, dizziness, and diarrhea, to name a few).

Significant research is lacking.

It is safe for most people.

Health concerns: Garlic appears to be nontoxic at recommended dosages but has caused irritation to the gastrointestinal tract. Large doses can cause dizziness, excess gas, headache, and sweating. Garlic may interact with and/or magnify the effectiveness of drugs metabolized by the liver, including Xanax, Elavil, Tegretol, corticosteroids, Desipramine, Valium, Tofranil, and Coumadin. You will have a garlicky scent on your breath and skin. There is an "odorless" form, but that issue is questionable.

Clinical studies: The result of a meta-analysis in the past suggested garlic could significantly reduce total cholesterol levels. However, recent rigorous studies have failed to substantiate garlic's value as a lipid-lowering agent. Other studies have suggested a mild, short-term lowering of blood pressure and an increase in serum insulin levels. Improved diabetes control in animal studies has been documented. However, its use in diabetic

**What They Told You**

tinea corporis, tinea cruris, and onychomycosis. Intravaginally, garlic is used alone or in combination with yogurt for vaginitis. In traditional Chinese medicine, garlic is used for diarrhea, amoebic and bacterial dysentery, tuberculosis, bloody urine, diphtheria, whooping cough, scalp ringworm, hypersensitive teeth, and vaginal trichomoniasis. Garlic has also been traditionally used to treat colds, flu symptoms, fever, coughs, headache, stomach ache, sinus congestion, athlete's foot, gout, rheumatism, hemorrhoids, asthma, bronchitis, shortness of breath, arteriosclerosis, low blood pressure, hypoglycemia, hyperglycemia, cancer, old ulcers, snakebites, and as an aphrodisiac.

In foods and beverages, fresh garlic, garlic powder, and garlic oil are used as flavor components.

**Some interesting data:** Garlic has had many usages for many years. Today it is often tried for hypertension, high cholesterol, and high blood sugar.

**Historical data:** Records of use of garlic date back to 5000 years ago. Hippocrates and Aristotle noted many uses for garlic. Pasteur noted some antibiotic activity in 1858. Albert Schweitzer used it in Africa for treatment of dysentery, and it was used as an antiseptic to prevent gangrene in World War I and II (Murray, p. 122).

**Usual dose:** 1 tablet of 400 mg daily.

**What They Did Not Tell You**

patients has not been sufficiently evaluated (*American Family Physician,* 1 October 1998, Vol. 58, No. 5, p. 1137).

In diabetic rats, s-allylcysteine sulfoxide (an active ingredient of garlic), improved the diabetic condition by lowering the blood glucose (*American Family Physician,* 1 September 2000, Vol. 62, No. 5, p. 1055). Finally, garlic has been demonstrated at least as having "mild, short-term, antihypertensive effects" (*American Family Physician,* October 1998, p. 1137).

Also, the German Commission E considers garlic effective for "preventing age-related vascular changes" (*Pharmacist's Letter,* the updated therapeutic use of herbs, p. 10, 2000).

A recent federal study shows that garlic can seriously interfere with drugs used to treat the AIDS virus. In addition, it has been known for some time that garlic taken orally can have dose-related effects such as halitosis, mouth and gastrointestinal burning or irritation, heartburn, flatulence, nausea, vomiting, and diarrhea. The use of garlic may also make changes to intestinal flora, and prolonged bleeding time may occur with high dietary consumption. Some cases of asthma have been reported, along with possible allergies to pollen. Eczema, blisters, and scarring have been reported in some cases following prolonged topical exposure.

**Mechanism of action:** Allicin, an active ingredient in garlic, may interfere with the creation of carcinogenic nitrosamines in the stomach (Duke, p. 107). Another possible mechanism of action may be to act directly to increase the secretion of insulin from beta cells, or it may enhance the release of insulin from its bound state. The only study using humans did not show glucose-lowering effects of garlic when compared with placebo (*American Family Physician,* 1 September 2000, Vol. 62, No. 5, p. 1055).

### Gentian—Gas

Gentian is a related species to gentiana. It is touted to help in digestive disorders and flatulence.

Gentian contains gentianine that may have anti-inflammatory activity. Another constituent (gentian) could interfere with both H-2 antagonists and proton pump inhibitors used for gastroesophageal reflux disease. It could also interfere with some antibiotics such as doxycyclone.

It can cause gastrointestinal irritation.

**What They Told You**

**What They Did Not Tell You**

It definitely should be avoided by pregnant females.

One major danger of this herb is that it often grows next to hellebore, which is highly toxic.

### Gentiana—Hepatitis

Gentiana is another herb from China. It is used to treat disorders of the liver.

Research is nonexistent as far as we could find.

### Germanium—Pain

Germanium is a mineral touted to help in pain, osteoporosis, fatigue, AIDS, cancer, high blood pressure, and cataracts.

Significant research is lacking.

Side effects include anemia, renal tubular degeneration, weakness, neuropathy, and death.

### Ginger Root—GI Distress

**How it has been used:** Ginger root has been used for motion sickness, nausea, and vomiting.

**Some interesting data:** Ginger has been used as a flavoring and as an ingredient in digestive, laxative, antiflatulent, and antacid preparations. It may reduce GI distress and vestibular disturbance during SSRI withdrawal. It has been used for nausea and dizziness associated with Buspar.

**Historical data:** Ginger has typically been grown in warmer climates including India, Jamaica, and China.

**The usual dose:** 500 mg bid to 1000 mg tid. For travel, the usual dose is 500 mg 30 minutes before travel and then qid when traveling.

**Health concerns:** Some patients taking ginger have experienced abdominal discomfort, dermatitis, CNS depression, and cardiac arrhythmias.

**Clinical studies:** Little control data exists. When used orally in small amounts, ginger has generally been recognized as safe. Some studies have reported improvement in morning sickness in pregnancy; however, its safety for use during pregnancy has not been established.

**The mechanism of action:** Active constituents of ginger are gingerols, which seem to have a variety of pharmacological applications including analgesic, antipyretic, and sedative properties. Ginger may help reduce nausea and vomiting by increasing gastrointestinal motility. Some 5HT receptor activity may be present.

### Gingko Biloba—Dementia

Gingko has been used in dementia, SSRI sexual dysfunction, prevention of cognitive decline, and in combination with antipsychotics for schizophrenia.

The usual dose is 60–120 mg 2 times per day.

Gingko increases the risk of bleeding and is contraindicated with aspirin, nonsteroidial anti-inflammatory drugs, and surgery. The actual benefits in dementia appear modest at best. In a study reported August 21, 2002, LAMA showed no beneficial effect on memory and related memory functions in healthy adults.

### Ginseng—Aphrodisiac

**How it has been used:** Ginseng has been used mainly to improve mood, enhance energy, reduce stress, and as a male aphrodisiac. The increased sex drive may be the most interesting aspect.

**Some interesting data:** Ginseng is one of the best-

**Health concerns:** There are "more than 20 ginsenosides each with different pharmacological activity" (*Psychopharmacology Update,* Efficacy and Safety of herbal products as psychotherapeutic agents, November 2000). Probably only 25 percent of commercial products labeled as ginseng actually contain ginseng.

## What They Told You

known herbs in Chinese medicine. There are a number of varieties including American ginseng, Himalayan ginseng, Oriental ginseng, and Siberian ginseng. The underground roots of the ginseng plant, which sometimes takes the shape of the human form, are utilized for health purposes. Panax ginseng has been used in depression, to enhance memory, fight fatigue, protect against physical and emotional stress, and for antiaging properties. Siberian ginseng, used for mental fatigue, has been touted to have less menstrual side effects. Siberian ginseng has been used as a general energizing tonic, antistress agent, immunostimulant, anti-inflammatory, and for colds and flu.

**Historical data:** Russian and Chinese athletes have used ginseng to increase endurance and energy levels. The Chinese have used it to help the elderly endure the long winters and have also used it as an aphrodisiac for males.

**The usual dose:** 500 mg once a day, I gram dried root per portion of vegetable soup, I tablespoon of fresh roots, or ½ teaspoon of dried roots. Doses of 500 mg 3 times per day for a week have been recommended.

## What They Did Not Tell You

Some data suggests that it may have several side effects:
1. Decreased blood glucose.
2. Inhabitation of platelet aggregation; therefore it should not be used with anticoagulants.
3. An estrogen effect with vaginal bleeding and swollen breasts.
4. Cortocosteroid-like pharmacological activity.
5. Mania, insomnia, and headache (one case when taken with an MAOI—phenelzine).
6. High doses can result in severe headaches.
7. Skin rashes have occurred.
8. Estrogen-dependent malignancies could be worsened with ginseng.
9. Infant death, increased heart rate, edema, and insomnia have also been reported (*Pharmacist's Letter/Prescriber's Letter,* 2000, p. 18).
10. Paradoxical effects on blood pressure in that low doses increase blood pressure and higher doses tend to produce a lowering of blood pressure.
11. Several studies show ginseng products to be adulterated, mislabeled, or contaminated.
12. Nervousness, high blood pressure, nosebleeds, mania, menstrual irregularities, and hot flashes are all possible side effects of ginseng.
13. Additional products added, such as Ephedrine and caffeine, to increase energy (*Pharmacist's Letter/Prescriber's Letter,* 2000, p. 18).
14. Serum cortisol (stress chemical) levels are elevated in nondiabetic individuals (Murray, p. 271).

**Clinical studies:** Double-blind, repeated placebo-controlled studies seem to be lacking. It has been called a dose of immortality. There are "anecdotal reports of antidepressant action" (*Psychopharmacology Update,* 2000, Baylor College of Medicine). There is one case at least of mania when ginseng was added to an MAOI antidepressant (phenelzine). It is usually a stimulating herb that is used in many herbal mixtures. Panax ginseng has been used for a sexual stimulant. In one placebo-controlled study from Korea "at 300 mg/day for 3 months better sexual performance was reported." This study needs replication (*Review of Psychiatry,* Vol. 19, 2000). If this proves to be true and overall the above side effects appear low, then this drug might prove interesting when sex drive is low with antidepressant medication (SSRIs). This would be an interesting area of research.

**The mechanism of action:** Many complex chemicals in ginseng can cause CNS depression and CNS stimulation.

**What They Told You**

**What They Did Not Tell You**

It is thought to act on the adrenal gland as well as modifying brain-wave tracings and to affect the hypothalamo-pituitary-adrenal axis, promoting secretion of ACTH (a hormone produced by the adrenal gland). In addition, claims are made that ginseng has some glycogen-sparing effects during exercise.

### Globe Flower—Scurvy
Orally, globe flower is touted for scurvy.

Orally, ingestion of globe flower can cause severe irritation of the gastrointestinal tract, with colic and diarrhea. Irritation of the urinary tract can also occur.

Topically, skin contact can cause blisters and burns that are difficult to heal.

### Glucomannan (Konjae mannan)—Weight Loss
This herb comes from Asia (Indonesia and Japan). It has been touted for weight loss and as a laxative also.

It is touted to expand many, many times when exposed to liquid and thus create a sense of fullness and a decreased desire to eat and thus weight loss eventually.

No significant research is present, but interesting!

### Glucosamine-Chondroitin—Osteoarthritis
**How it has been used:** Glucosamine-chondroitin has been used for cartilage building in the treatment of osteoarthritis. Chondroitin alone has been used for osteoporosis, ischemic heart disease, and hyperlipidemia.

**Some interesting data:** Glucosomine-chondroitin is mostly derived from marine exoskeletons although it can be produced synthetically.

**Historical data:** It was originally derived from marine exoskeletons.

**The usual dose:** The usual dose is 500 mg 3 times a day.

**Health concerns:** Glucosamine can cause mild GI upsets such as gas, bloating, and cramps. Allergic reactions have also occurred in people allergic to shellfish; therefore, individuals allergic to shellfish should use glucosamine with caution. Theoretically, glucosamine might worsen diabetes by increasing insulin resistance in Type 2 diabetes.

**Clinical studies:** The National Institutes of Health are currently sponsoring a 16-week clinical trial of glucosamine alone and chondroitin alone including a placebo group and a combined glucosamine-chondroitin group. We do have many clients come in and claim that glucosamine-chondroitin has helped their joint problems. Controlled studies are needed. Overall, it seems fairly innocuous and may help at times.

**The mechanism of action:** Glucosamine is required for the synthesis of the body's tendons, ligaments, cartilage, synovial fluid as well as blood vessels, heart valves, and structures of the eye. Glucosamine stimulates chondrocyte metabolism in cartilage. Glucosamine may desensitize cell membranes to the effects of insulin.

| What They Told You | What They Did Not Tell You |
|---|---|
| **Glutathione—Aging**<br>Glutathione is an antioxidant and as such is touted to have antiaging effects. | Significant research is lacking. |
| **Goat Rue—High Blood Sugar**<br>Goat rue has been touted to lower blood sugar in diabetes. | Effectiveness of goat rue is not known.<br><br>It can be toxic in some. Anxiety and headache are just two possible side effects. |
| **Goldenrod—Urinary Tract Infections**<br>Goldenrod has been used for urinary tract infections. | It probably does have some bacteriostatic and anti-inflammatory effects. Also, it does have a diuretic effect.<br><br>Allergic reactions are possible.<br><br>It might interfere with diuretic therapy. |
| **Goldenseal (berberine)—Infections**<br>Goldenseal is touted to have antibiotic-like activities. It was used by Native Americans to fight various infections. It has been used to lower blood sugar in Type 2 Diabetes.<br><br>Supplements of 465 mg 2–3 times a day are often recommended. | Side effects are possible: increased blood pressure, convulsions, respiratory failure, hypoglycemia, increased uterine contractions, and death to name a few. |
| **Gossypol—Male Contraceptive**<br>Gossypol has been used as a male contraceptive. | Gossypol might decrease sperm production, but the side effects can be horrible for some—heart failure and paralysis, just to name a couple. |
| **Gotu Kola—Wound Healing**<br>Gotu kola has been used for years for wound healing. It has also been touted for treating cellulite, varicose veins, and scleroderma. In short, it has been used for years as a skin and tissue rejuvenator.<br><br>The usual dose is 60 to 120 mg daily. | The question of skin cancer from repeated topical exposure has been raised. |
| **Goutweed—Gout**<br>Orally, goutweed is used for gout and rheumatic disease. It is also used for hemorrhoids, kidney, bladder, and intestinal disorders. | Reliable information is insufficient. No adverse effects have been reported. |
| **Grains of Paradise—Stimulant**<br>Orally, grains of paradise fruit and seeds have been touted as a stimulant. | Theoretically, may cause GI and lower urinary tract irritation when taken orally. |

**What They Told You**

**What They Did Not Tell You**

### Grape Juice (red)—Asthrosclerotic Heart Disease

Red grape juice has been touted to have protective effects on the heart similar to but less than red wine.

Many studies have demonstrated cardioprotective effects of moderate intake of various types of alcohol. Red wine may be the most protective.

But what about those with a potential for alcoholism or who do not wish to drink an alcoholic beverage? It seems that red grape juice, just like red wine, contains polyphenols that cause synthesis of endothelin (ET–1) to decrease. Since ET–1 is a potent vasoconstrictor and plays a role in endothelial dysfunction and early fatty-streak formation, its decrease would logically have some heart protective effects.

### Grape Seed Extract—Antiaging

**How it has been used:** This extract has mostly been used in an attempt to slow aging. Claims have been made that grape seed extract will improve circulation, counter-act the aging process, treat cancer, help night blindness, stop wrinkles, and relieve ADHD symptoms.

**Some interesting data:** The alpha-hydroxy acid in the grapes has been used to remove dead skin cells from the face, which appeared to improve the appearance of the complexion.

**Historical data:** Grapes were first stomped and made into wine over 5000 years ago, and various forms of grapes have been used for a wide range of ailments including just about every illness known to man.

**The usual dose:** 75 to 300 mg daily for 3 weeks, then a daily maintenance dose of 40 to 100 mg per day has been tried by some people.

**Health concerns:** Double-blind clinical studies on the use of grape seed extract in treating or preventing various disease processes are insufficient.

**Clinical studies:** Some studies involving laboratory procedures of instrumental data utilizing spectrophoto-metrical measurements on tissue, as well as in vitro studies on rat and human tissue, indicate some growing basic research interest in the polyphenols and antioxidant effects of proanthocyanidins ingredients in grapes. Serious studies await being done.

**The mechanism of action:** Active ingredients are antioxidant bioflavonoids called proanthocyanidins. These antioxidants are believed to scavenge free radicals (*Pharmacist's Letter/Prescriber's Letter*, 2000, p. 19). It has long been proposed that free radicals in the body have to do with aging and even cancer. It seems doubtful that grape seed extract alone will significantly deter the aging process.

### Grapefruit

Grapefruit is often used for reducing cholesterol and reversing atherosclerosis; as a supplemental source of potassium, vitamin C, and fiber; for reducing hematocrit; as an anticancer agent; and as an aid in weight reduction. In combination with cyclosporine, grapefruit is used for treating psoriasis.

Grapefruit is a good dietary source of potassium, vitamin C, pectin, and other nutrients. Grapefruit juice contains furanocournanns, including bergamottin and dihydroxy-bergamottin, which inhibit cytochrome P450 3A4

Grapefruit juice inhibits hepatic and gut wall CYP3A4. Grapefruit juice increases bioavailability and plasma con-centrations of numerous drugs. Human research indi-cates that blended grapefruit segments, and an extract of grapefruit core and peel, also inhibit CYP3A4.

Evidence suggests that grapefruit juice inhibits p-glyco-protein counter-transport activity. This is thought to reduce the absorption of some drugs by pumping them back into the gut. Grapefruit affects absorption of some drugs affected by p-glycoprotein activity. However, the clinical effect of grapefruit on drugs affected by p-glyco-

## What They Told You

(CYP3A4) (3769,5070,507 1). In addition, bergamottin inhibits CYPs 1A2, 2A6, 2C9, 2C19, 2D6, and 2E1 (5072). Grapefruit juice also contains naringin, naringenin, limonin, and obacunone, which are known to inhibit human hepatic microsomes. Grapefruit pectin, which is found in whole fruit but not juice, can reduce cholesterol and promote regression of atherosclerosis. Studies suggest grapefruit can affect blood components. Some evidence suggests the constituent, naringin, might induce red cell aggregation. Consuming one half to one grapefruit per day can reduce an individual's hematocrit level. An analysis of grapefruit's anticancer effects suggests that consumption could reduce the risk of pancreatic cancer.

## What They Did Not Tell You

protein activity requires further investigation. It may be necessary to withhold grapefruit juice for 3 days to avoid interactions with felodipine and nisoldipine.

Grapefruit can reduce hematocrit. Concomitant use of grapefruit with red yeast increases the serum levels of lovastatin, a constituent of red yeast.

Some studies suggest that grapefruit juice increases the maximum blood levels and duration of effect of midazolam (Versed) and triazolam (Halcion); other studies suggest there is no effect. Grapefruit juice increases the maximum blood levels and duration of effect of diazepam (Valium). Grapefruit juice increases absorption and plasma concentrations of buspirone. Some studies suggest grapefruit juice decreases caffeine clearance, possibly increasing the effects or adverse effects.

Grapefruit juice increases absorption and plasma concentrations of anilodipine (Norvasc), nifedipine (Procardia, Adalat), nisoldipine (Sular), felodipine (Plendil), nimodipine (Nimotop), nicardipine (Cardura), diltiazem (Cardizem), and verapamil (Calan, Isoptin, Verelan). The hemodynamic response to felodipine (Plendil) plus grapefruit juice may be influenced by altered autonomic regulation. Grapefruit juice increases absorption and plasma concentrations of carbamazepine. Grapefruit juice is reported to increase the bioavailability of a single dose of carvediolol by 16 percent.

Grapefruit juice increases absorption and plasma concentrations of cisapride. Clornipramine. Cyclosporine, 1 7-beta-estradiol, ethinylestradiol, lovastatin (Mevacor), sinivastatin (Zoeor), and atorvastatin (Lipitor).

Grapefruit juice impairs itraconazole absorption. Concomitant use of grapefruit juice and losartan may reduce losartan effectiveness, but this requires further study.

Grapefruit juice decreases quinidine clearance and prolongs the half-life by about 20 percent. Grapefruit juice increases absorption and plasma concentrations of terfenadine Grapefruit juice may interact with warfarin (Coumadin).

_**Gravel Root—Kidney Stones**_

Research is lacking, and side effects are not known.

## What They Told You

Gravel root has been touted for BPH and kidney stones.

### Green Tea—Cancer Prevention

Green tea is consumed a lot in China. It is touted to have cancer prevention qualities possibly through its inhibition of nitrosamines in cured bacon and ham.

It has also been used extensively for cavity prevention through possible antibacterial actions.

Orally, green tea is used to improve cognitive performance, treat stomach disorders, vomiting, diarrhea, and headaches. It is used as a diuretic and in combination products for weight loss.

Green tea has been used in Crohn's disease to maintain remission, to reduce the risk of prostate cancer, colon cancer, to protect against heart disease, to protect against dental caries, to prevent kidney stones, and green tea bags are used as a wash to soothe sunburn, as a poultice for bags under the eyes, as a compress for headache or tired eyes, and to stop the bleeding of tooth sockets.

Green tea may also reduce oxidative DNA damage, lipid peroxidation, and free radical generation; and might reduce mutagenic activity in smokers. Green tea has also been used for weight loss. Early evidence indicates that a green tea extract rich in ECG can increase calorie and fat metabolism, but caffeine could also contribute to these effects. The impact of ECG and green tea on weight loss remains to be determined. For diarrhea, tannins in green tea can produce antidiarrheal effects. Green tea contains a significant amount of caffeine.

## What They Did Not Tell You

Green tea in moderation is usually not toxic.

One fallacy in the logic is that certainly most cancers are not caused by nitrates.

Consumption of more than 300 mg caffeine, which is equivalent to approximately 5 cups of green tea per day, has been associated with significant adverse effects. Caffeine found in green tea crosses the placenta, producing fetal blood concentrations similar to maternal levels. Although controversial, some evidence suggests that high doses of caffeine might be associated with premature delivery, low birth weight, and loss of the fetus. Some sources suggest keeping caffeine consumption below 200 mg per day, and excessive use of green tea in pregnancy should be avoided.

It is also likely unsafe when taken orally by infants because it has been associated with impaired iron metabolism and microcytic anemia. This may be caused by tannins in green tea which bind and prevent iron absorption in the gastrointestinal tract. Children are also more susceptible to the adverse effects of caffeine present in green tea.

Consumption of green tea may cause irritability and increased bowel activity in nursing infants. Large doses or excessive intake of green tea should be avoided during lactation.

Orally, green tea can cause gastrointestinal upset and constipation. There is one report of liver dysfunction with the excessive use of green tea. High doses of the caffeine constituent of green tea can cause headache, diuresis, anxiety, nervousness, insomnia, restlessness, agitation, tremor, irritability, tachyarrhythmias, palpitations, premature heartbeat, quickened respiration, heartburn, loss of appetite, nausea, vomiting, diarrhea, dizziness, ringing in the ears, elevated blood sugar, elevated cholesterol, hepatotoxicity, delirium, and convulsions. The chronic use of caffeine, especially in large amounts, can sometimes produce tolerance, habituation, and psychological dependence. The abrupt discontinuation of caffeine can result in physical withdrawal symptoms, including headaches, irritation, nervousness, anxiety, and dizziness. Some evidence shows caffeine is associated with fibrocystic breast disease in women; however, this is controversial and has been disputed. The adverse effects

**What They Told You**

**What They Did Not Tell You**

of caffeine from green tea can be more severe in children than adults. In infants, green tea ingestion has been associated with impaired iron metabolism.

Concomitant use interacts with the caffeine in green tea and can increase the effects and risk of adverse effects. Natural products that contain caffeine include coffee, black tea, guarana, mate, and cola. Concomitant use of ephedra (ma huang) interacts with the caffeine in green tea and can potentiate the stimulant effects and risk of adverse effects. The concomitant use of iron and green tea can impair iron metabolism in infants and children, resulting in a high incidence of microcytic anemia.

Theoretically, concomitant use may inhibit the hemodynamic effects of adenosine. Possibly, green tea could increase the risk of bleeding when used concomitantly with anticoagulants. Green tea is reported to have antiplatelet activity; however, this interaction has not been reported in humans.

Theoretically, green tea might interact with and inhibit antipsychotic medications such as fluphenazine (Permitil, Prolixin), chlorpromazine (Thorazine), haloperidol (Haldol), prochlorperazine (Compazine), thioridazine (Mellaril), and trifluoperazine (Stelazine). Possibly, concomitant administration of clozapine (Clozaril) could cause acute exacerbation of psychotic symptoms due to the caffeine in green tea. Caffeine can increase the effects and toxicity of clozapine due to inhibition of clozapine metabolism; cases of death due to agranulocytosis are associated with clozapine toxicity, and careful blood monitoring is needed with this medication.

Concomitant use with beta-adrenergic agonists can increase the cardiac effect of beta-adrenergic agonist drugs due to the caffeine in green tea. Beta-adrenergic agonists include albuterol (Proventil, Ventolin), metaproterenol (Alupent), terbutaline (Brethine), and isoproterenol (Isuprel). Concomitant use might reduce the sedative effects of benzodiazepines due to the caffeine components. Concomitant use of Disulfiram (Antabuse) could increase the risk of adverse effects of caffeine in green tea. Disulfiram decreases the clearance and increases the half-life of caffeine. Oral contraceptives can decrease caffeine clearance by 40–65 percent.

Phenytoin enhances metabolism and excretion of caffeine. Verapamil can increase plasma caffeine levels by 25

## What They Told You

## What They Did Not Tell You

percent (14). Consumption of large amounts of green tea is reported to antagonize the effects of warfarin.

The caffeine in green tea can prolong bleeding time and increase bleeding time, can increase urine creatine levels, and might have hyperglycemic effects.

### Ground Ivy—Sinusitis

Ground ivy has been touted for sinusitis.

No significant research as to its effectiveness is known.

It can have side effects—anorexia, congestion, edema, and turning blue, to name a few.

### Guarana—Stimulant

Guarana, an herb from South America, is considered to be the richest source of caffeine in the world (much higher than coffee). It has been used for its stimulating effects.

Orally, guarana is used for weight loss, to enhance athletic performance, and to reduce fatigue. In folk medicine, guarana has been used as a stimulant, tonic, aphrodisiac, diuretic, and astringent. It has also been used to prevent malaria and dysentery and for chronic diarrhea, fever, heart problems, headache, rheumatism, lumbago, and heat stress. It is also used as a flavoring in candy and beverages.

Guarana can be stimulating, addicting, and even dangerous. Guarana contains high caffeine and, like coffee, can increase blood pressure, heart palpitations, rapid heartbeat, headache, anxiety, restlessness, insomnia, tremors, and even seizures.

Overdose of guarana can cause painful urination, abdominal spasms, and vomiting. The caffeine constituents in guarana can cause insomnia, nervousness, restlessness, agitation, gastric irritation, nausea, vomiting, diuresis, fast heartbeat, arrhythmias, increased respiratory rate, muscle spasms, tinnitus, headache, delirium, and convulsions. The adverse effects of caffeine can be more severe in children. The chronic use of caffeine, especially in large amounts, can sometimes produce tolerance, habituation, and psychological dependence. Abrupt discontinuation can sometimes result in physical withdrawal symptoms, including irritability, anxiety, headaches, and dizziness.

The combining of ephedra with guarana increases the risk of adverse effects, due to the caffeine contained in guarana. Associated jitteriness, hypertension, seizures, temporary loss of consciousness, a report of ischemic stroke and hospitalization requiring life support with the use of a combination ephedra and guarana has been reported.

Concomitant use of guarana and caffeine-containing herbs/supplements constitutes therapeutic duplication (due to the caffeine contained in guarana) which increases the risk of caffeine-related adverse effects. Other natural products which contain caffeine include black tea, cocoa, coffee, cola nut, green tea, and mate. Concomitant use of ephedra (ma huang) can increase

**What They Told You**

**What They Did Not Tell You**

the risk of stimulatory adverse effects, due to the caffeine contained in guarana.

Possibly, concomitant use may increase the pain-relieving activity of acetaminophen as well as aspirin, due to the caffeine contained in guarana. Caffeine increases the pain-relieving activity of acetaminophen and aspirin by up to 40 percent. Theoretically, concomitant use may reduce the sedative and anxiolytic effects of benzodiazepines, due to the caffeine contained in guarana. Possibly, concomitant use could increase the cardiac inotropic effects of beta agonists, due to the caffeine contained in guarana. Beta-adrenergic agonists include albuterol (Proventil, Ventolm), metaproterenot (Alupent), terbutaline (Brethine), and isoproterenol (Isuprel). Concomitant use of cimetidine (Tagamet) may increase serum caffeine concentrations and the risk of adverse effects, due to the caffeine contained in guarana. Cimetidine decreases the rate of caffeine clearance by 30–50 percent. Coadministration of clozapine (Clozaril) might acutely exacerbate psychotic symptoms, due to the caffeine contained in guarana. Caffeine can increase the effects and toxicity of clozapine as caffeine doses of 400–1000 mg per day inhibit clozapine metabolism. Concomitant use of any CNS stimulants may increase the risk of stimulant adverse effects, due to the caffeine contained in guarana. CNS stimulants include nicotine, cocaine, sympathomimetic amines, and amphetamines. Theoretically, concomitant use of coffee and diabetes drugs may interfere with blood glucose control, due to the caffeine contained in guarana. This is based in the claim that caffeine could have hyperglycemic effects. Disulfiram decreases the rate of caffeine clearance, and concomitant use may increase serum caffeine concentrations and the risk of adverse effects, due to the caffeine contained in guarana.

Estrogen inhibits caffeine metabolism, and concomitant use might increase serum caffeine concentrations and the risk of adverse effects, due to the caffeine contained in guarana. Possibly, concomitant use may increase the GI absorption of ergotamine, due to the caffeine contained in guarana, as caffeine increases the GI absorption of ergotamine.

Theoretically, abrupt guarana withdrawal may increase serum lithium levels, due to the caffeine contained in guarana. Concomitant intake of large amounts of guarana with MAOIs could precipitate a hypertensive crisis, due to the caffeine contained in guarana.

**What They Told You**

**What They Did Not Tell You**

Use of oral contraceptives might increase serum caffeine concentrations and the risk of adverse effects, due to the caffeine contained in guarana, as oral contraceptives decrease the rate of caffeine clearance by 40–65 percent.

Concomitant use of caffeine and phenylpropanolaniine can cause an additive increase in blood pressure and increase serum caffeine concentrations, and concomitant use could cause an additive increase in blood pressure and serum caffeine concentrations, due to the caffeine contained in guarana.

Concomitant use of Quinolones might increase serum caffeine concentrations and the risk of adverse effects, due to the caffeine contained in guarana. Quinolones decrease caffeine clearance. Quinolones (also referred to as fluoroquinolones) include ciprofloxacin (Cipro), enoxacin (Penetrex), gatifloxacin (Tequin), levofloxacin (Levaquin), lomefloxacin (Maxaquin), moxifloxacin (Avelox), norfloxacin (Noroxin), ofloxacin (Floxin), sparfloxacin (Zagam), and trovafloxacin (Trovan). Possibly, concomitant use could increase serum caffeine and riluzole concentrations and the risk of adverse effects of both caffeine and riluzole, due to the caffeine contained in guarana. Caffeine and riluzole are both metabolized by cytocbrome P450 1 A2, and concomitant use may reduce metabolism of one or both agents. Terbinafme decreases the rate of caffeine clearance, and concomitant use of terbinafme (Lamisil) may increase serum caffeine concentrations and the risk of adverse effects, due to the caffeine contained in guarana. Large amounts of caffeine might inhibit theophylline metabolism, and concomitant use could increase serum theophylline concentrations and the risk of adverse effects, due to the caffeine contained in guarana.

Verapamil increases plasma caffeine concentrations by 25 percent, and concomitant use might increase plasma caffeine concentrations and the risk of adverse effects, due to the caffeine contained in guarana.

Grapefruit juice interacts with the caffeine in guarana and can increase caffeine levels as well as the risk of adverse effects.

Guarana could prolong bleeding time and increase bleeding lab test results, due to its caffeine content. It could increase blood pressure and blood pressure read-

**What They Told You**

**What They Did Not Tell You**

ings. Guarana may also influence lab tests such as serum urate test results determined by the Bittner method, increase urine catecholamine concentrations and test results, increase urine creatine concentrations and test results, interfere with dipyridamole thallium imaging studies, increase urine 5-hydroxyindoleacetic acid concentrations and test results, and increase urine vanillyl-mandelic acid (VMA) concentrations and test results.

Guarana may cause false-positive diagnosis of uroblastoma, when diagnosis is based on tests of urine VMA or catecholamine concentrations, and may cause false-positive diagnosis of pheochromocytoma, when diagnosis is based on tests of urine VMA.

The caffeine in guarana can aggravate gastric duodenal ulcers, can aggravate depression and anxiety disorder, may aggravate some kidney disease, and can induce cardiac arrhythmias in sensitive individuals.

---

### Guar Gum—Diabetes Mellitus
Guar gum has been touted to lower blood sugar and cholesterol.

Research is inadequate.

---

### Gugulipid (guggal gum)—High Cholesterol
This herb comes from a tree native to Arabia and India.

In placebo-controlled studies this herb has significantly lowered cholesterol and triglyceride levels. Side effects appear to be low.

The dosage is often at 25 mg of guggulsterone 3 times per day. For a 5 percent guggulsterone content extract the usual dose is 500 mg 3 times per day.

The above sounds good, but research is still limited.

---

### Gum Arabic—Dental Plaque
Gum arabic is touted for dental care.

Significant research is lacking into its effectiveness.

It has been used intravenously and can be extremely toxic to the liver or kidneys. Certainly, the chewing gum is better than other forms.

---

### Gymnema—Diabetes Mellitus
Gymnema is touted to possibly be the best herbal treatment for diabetes mellitus. It is relatively new to America and came from a vine in Asian forests. It has been touted for both Type 1 and Type 2 diabetes mellitus.

One danger with almost anyone with diabetes on insulin or other hypoglycemic medication is that of lowering the blood sugar too much.

---

### Hamamelis Virginiana (devil's claw)—Skin Infections
This herb is native to North America and has been used for skin problems—burns, bug bites, dermatitis, wounds, and hemorrhoids.

Significant research is lacking.

**What They Told You**

**What They Did Not Tell You**

*Harpagophytum Procumbers—Arthritis*
This herb comes from Africa. It has been touted to help in arthritis because of anti-inflammatory and analgesic effects.

This herb can have side effects: ulcers, undesirable interactions with medication for diabetes, high blood pressure, and heart disease.

*Hartstongue—Urinary Tract Diseases*
Orally, hartstongue is touted to treat digestive disorders and urinary tract diseases.

Reliable information is insufficient.

*Hawthorn—Congestive Heart Failure*
Hawthorn comes from a spring tree in Europe.

It has been used mostly for its reported benefits to the heart in cardiovascular insufficiency, artheorosclerosic heart disease, high blood pressure, and irregular heart rhythm. It not only reportedly helps in mild congestive heart failure but also gives subjects a subjective sense of well-being.

Hawthorne should not be used with digitalis unless closely monitored by a physician since the two could potentially interact.

Reported side effects include: rash, nausea, fatigue, unusual perspiration, and a lowering of blood pressure.

*Hay Flower—Arthritis*
Topically, hay flower is touted as heat therapy for degenerative disorders, including arthritis. It is used as a bath additive for musculoskeletal and joint disorders.

In folk medicine, hay flower has been used as a bath additive for rheumatic conditions, lumbago, chilblains, and neurasthenia. It has also been touted as an inhalant for inflammatory conditions of the respiratory tract.

Topically, rare skin reactions and hay fever have occurred with the use of hay flower.

*Hemlock—Anxiety*
Hemlock has been used as a sedative.

Hemlock is unsafe. It can cause salivation, sweating, cardiovascular collapse, and death.

*Hemlock Spruce—Cough*
Orally, hemlock spruce is touted for coughs, the common cold, bronchitis, fever, inflammation of the mouth and pharynx, muscular and nerve pain, arthritis, and as an antibacterial.

Topically, hemlock spruce is touted for inflammation of the respiratory tract, arthritis pain, nerve pain, and for feelings of tension. It is also touted topically as a counterirritant and to improve circulation.

In folk medicine, it is touted orally for tuberculosis and topically as a bath additive for individuals who are mentally ill.

Reliable information is insufficient.

| What They Told You | What They Did Not Tell You |
|---|---|
| *Hempnettle—Bronchitis*<br>Orally, hempnettle is touted for mild respiratory tract inflammation, cough, and bronchitis.<br><br>Traditionally, it has been touted for pulmonary afflictions and as a diuretic. | Reliable information is insufficient. No adverse effects have been reported. |
| *Henbane—Spasms of the Gastrointestinal Tract*<br>Henbane has been touted for spasms of the gastrointestinal tract. | It contains a poisonous alkaloid and can cause death. |
| *Henna—Skin Conditions*<br>Orally, henna is touted for gastrointestinal ulcers.<br><br>Topically, henna is touted for dandruff, eczema, scabies, fungal infections, and ulcers. It is also used topically for applying decorative henna "tattoos."<br><br>Traditionally, henna has been used for amebic dysentery, cancer, enlarged spleen, headache, jaundice, and skin conditions. | Orally, henna can cause an upset stomach, possibly due to tannin content.<br><br>Topically, henna can cause contact dermatitis, including redness, itching, burning, swelling, scaling, fissuring, papules, blisters, and scarring.<br><br>There are reports of occupational exposure associated with immediate-type hypersensitivity involving urticaria, rhinitis, wheezing, and bronchial asthma.<br><br>In infants with glucose 6-phosphate dehydrogenase (G6PD) deficiency, topical henna use has been associated with hemolysis, anemia, reticulocytosis, and indirect hyperbilirubinemia.<br><br>Prolonged use on hair may turn the hair orange-red, unless mixed with other dyes to get different shades. |
| *Herbs and Surgery*<br>Generally, the use of supplements and herbs in patients undergoing a surgical procedure is not addressed. Basically, the message given is that dietary herbs and supplements are important for optimal health to ensure that your body gets the substances it needs for well-being and balance. Various ingredients support your need for energy and performance. They are "natural" and "not harmful," implying their overall safety. | The public's enormous enthusiasm for herbal products has led to morbidity and mortality for patients undergoing surgical procedures including serious complications such as "myocardial infarction, stroke, bleeding, inadequate oral anticoagulation, prolonged or inadequate anesthesia, organ transplant rejection, and interference with medications indispensable for patient care" (*Jama*, 11 July 2001, Vol. 286, No. 2).<br><br>The article identifies 8 of the most commonly used products that pose serious complications during and following surgical procedures. Echinacea has been associated with allergic reactions and decreased effectiveness of immunosuppressants. Ephedra: ma huang increased risks of decreasing blood supply to the heart, stroke, increased heart rate, increased blood pressure, and |

**What They Told You**

**What They Did Not Tell You**

heart irregularities. Garlic, ginger, gingko, and ginseng increased incidences of bleeding.

Kava increased the sedative effect of anesthetics. Saint-John's-wort caused an induction of the cytochrome P450 enzyme systems, thus affecting the levels of a number of medications often used before, during, and after surgery such as cyclosporin, warfarin, steroids, protease inhibitors, benzodiazepines, and digoxin (*Jama,* 11 July 2001, Vol. 286, No. 2).

### HGH (human growth hormone)—Aging

HGH is indeed a hormone of pituitary gland origin. It is available by prescription and is FDA approved to stimulate skeletal growth in pediatric patients with growth hormone deficiency as in Turner's Syndrome. However, precursors of HGH and derivatives of HGH are currently sold over-the-counter as supplements touted for antiaging effects.

Supplement preparations might contain "over-the-counter Human Growth Hormone (HGH) releasing amino acids (Arginine, Ornithine, Carnitine), a homeopathic preparation of HGH, Bovine Colostrum, and Deer Velvet." Other supplements offer "Insulin-like Growth Factor—a mixture of Insulin-like Growth Factor I, Insulin-like Growth Factor II, Transforming Growth Factor Alpha, Transforming Growth Factor Beta, Epidermal Growth Factor, Vascular Endothelial Growth Factor, Nerve Growth Factor, Fibroblastic Growth Factor, Interloukins, Bone Morphogenetic Protein 4, and Related co-factors."

These supplements are touted in many and various aspects for antiaging. They are touted to increase muscle mass, reduce fat, increase energy, increase sexual performance, increase cardiac function, improve the immune system, increase athletic performance, lower blood sugar, lower cholesterol, create younger looking skin, increase hair growth, remove wrinkles, improve vision, and increase memory.

Prescription HGH has raised the question of a small number of possible associations with leukemia. Infrequent side effects include headaches, muscle pain, weakness, hyperglycemia, edema, joint pain, and carpal tunnel syndrome. Rare side effects of gynocomartia and pancreatitia have occurred. With chronic, excessive use rare cases of acromegally have occurred.

The theory behind HGH is that HGH declines with age. We produce 500 micrograms at age 20 years, 200 micrograms at 40 years, and only 25 micrograms at 80 years.

The effectiveness and safety of the supplement forms are not known.

### Hibiscus—Spasms

Hibiscus has been used as a stimulant and as an anitspasmodic. It has been used to flavor coffee.

Significant research is lacking.

### HMB (Beta-Hydroxy-Beta-Methylbutyrate)—Hypertension

Orally, HMB is touted for increasing the benefits from weight training and exercise, for cardiovascular disease,

Reliable information is insufficient.

## What They Told You

hypercholesterolemia, and hypertension. In combination with arginine and glutamine, HMB is also touted orally for treating weight loss in people with AIDS.

### Hops—Insomnia
Hops have been touted for years to decrease anxiety and improve sleep.

500 mg is often given at bedtime.

### Horehound—High Blood Sugar
Horehound has been touted to lower blood sugar and help in upper respiratory infections.

### Horse Chestnut—Varicose Veins
Horse chestnut has been used for varicose veins. It is indigenous to the Balkan countries. Because of its antioxidant and capillary-toughening action, it has been touted to help not only in varicose veins but also for cellulite and wrinkles and even hemorrhoids.

Most of the supplements contain around 20 percent.

### Horseradish—Sinus Congestion
Horseradish has been used for upper respiratory infections and allergies.

### Horsetail—Beauty Aid and Osteoporosis
Horsetail, believe it or not, is touted as a beauty aid—good for the hair, skin, and nails. It is rich in natural abrasives and has been used for scouring purposes in kitchens. It has been touted to help in a variety of problems—cystitis, inflammations, bladder and kidney stones, urinary tract infections, and wounds.

Horsetail has also been used in osteoporosis.

### 5-HTP (5-hydroxy tryptophane)—Depression
This is a precursor of serotonin. It has been used in depression. At least 10 cases of eosinophilia-myalgia have occurred worldwide.

### Huperzine A—Alzheimer's
Orally, huperzine A is touted for Alzheimer's disease, memory and learning enhancement, age-related memory impairment, increasing alertness and energy, protection

## What They Did Not Tell You

Hops have a long-accepted reputation for their calming effects on the central nervous system.

Significant research is lacking. It should not be used with migraine medications, diabetic medications, or antiarrhythmias.

Pure forms of horse chestnut may be toxic to the kidneys, liver, and gastrointestinal tract. The seeds especially can be toxic and have even caused death.

The taste of horseradish can be horrible for some. It is strong and should not be used for those with ulcers.

Horsetail can have side effects—nicotine-like poisoning especially when given to children, heart disease intensification, and kidney disease intensification.

Horsetail contains nicotine, and therefore nicotine toxicity could occur with symptoms of weakness, dizziness, fever, weight loss, cold extremities, and even death. Horsetail can also have potentially dangerous interactions when used with stimulants, diuretics, some cardiac medications, and theophylline for asthma.

Orally, huperzine A can cause nausea, sweating, blurred vision, hyperactivity, anorexia, decreased heart rate, and fasciculations. Adverse effects that have been reported with other acetylcholine inhibitors and theoretically

**What They Told You**

from neurotoxic agents including organophosphate nerve gases, glutamate toxicity, and for treating myasthenia gravis.

**What They Did Not Tell You**

might occur with huperzine A, include vomiting, diarrhea, cramping, hypersalivation, increased urination/incontinence, and bradycardia.

### Hydrangea—Urinary Tract Infections

Hydrangea has been touted for urinary tract infections.

It can cause dizziness.

Effectiveness is not known.

### Hyssop

Hyssop has been used for high blood pressure, upper respiratory infections, gallbladder problems, gastrointestinal problems (such as gas and colic), urinary tract infections, and as an anti-inflammatory.

Hyssop in small amounts is generally safe. It is often added in small amounts to alcoholic beverages. In larger amounts it has caused seizures.

Hyssop could cause abortion in pregnant females, nausea, diarrhea, and seizures.

### Iberis Amara—Irritable Bowel Syndrome

Iberis amara, an herb from Spain, has been touted to calm the various symptoms of irritable bowel syndrome. It has also been called clown's mustard, wild candytuft, and bitter candytuft.

Research is needed.

Iberis amara contains glycosides and flavonoids among other components.

### Iberogast—Indigestion

Iberogast is touted for nonulcer dyspepsia, gastroesophageal reflux disease, irritable bowel syndrome, and drug-induced dyspepsia.

Reliable information is insufficient.

### Iceland Moss—HIV

Iceland moss has been touted for upper respiratory infections. It has even been touted to possibly help in HIV infections. It is touted to have antimicrobial, antiviral, and anticancer actions. It is used as a flavoring agent in beer and as an emergency food source in Iceland.

Research is lacking.

Iceland moss can irritate the gastrointestinal tract. Allergic reactions are always possible.

It appears to be low in drug interactions for most, but the fiber in it can impair absorption of oral drugs.

It can potentially have lead contamination.

### Ignatius Bean—Faintness

Orally, ignatius bean is touted for faintness; as a bitter or tonic; and as an agent to invigorate, refresh, or restore body function.

Orally, 30–50 mg ignatius bean (5 mg strychnine) can cause restlessness, feelings of anxiety, heightening of sense perception, enhanced reflexes, equilibrium disorders, painful neck and back stiffness, followed later by twitching, tonic spasms of jaw and neck muscles, painful convulsions of the entire body triggered by visual or tactile stimulation with possible opisthotonos, muscle hypertonicity, and agitation. Dyspnea may follow spasm of respiratory muscles. Seizures occur within 15 minutes

| What They Told You | What They Did Not Tell You |
|---|---|
| | of ingestion (or 5 minutes of inhalation) and may result in hyperthermia, metabolic and respiratory acidosis, rhabdomyolysis, and myoglobinuric renal failure. 1–2 grams ignatius bean (50 mg strychnine) can be fatal; most deaths occur 3–6 hours postingestion from respiratory and subsequent cardiac arrest, anoxic brain damage, or multiple organ failure secondary to hyperthermia. Strychnine accumulates with extended administration, particularly in individuals with liver damage. Chronic use of subconvulsive amounts can cause death after a period of weeks. |

### Indian Almond—Cardiovascular Conditions

Orally, terminalia arjuna is touted for cardiovascular conditions, including ischemic heart disease and angina, hypertension, and hyperlipidemia. It is also touted as a diuretic, for earaches, dysentery, venereal and urogenital disease, and as an aphrodisiac.

No reported adverse effects in humans.

In animal studies, terminalia chebula has caused hepatic and renal lesions.

Orally, terminalia belerica and terminalia chebula are touted for hyperlipidemia and digestive disorders, including both diarrhea and constipation, and indigestion. They have also been touted for HIV infection. Terminalia belerica is also touted as a hepatoprotectant and for respiratory conditions, including respiratory tract infections, cough, and sore throat. Terminalia chebula is also touted for dysentery.

Topically, terminalia belerica and terminalia chebula are touted as a lotion for sore eyes. Terminalia chebula is also touted as a mouthwash and gargle.

Intravaginally, terminalia chebula is touted as a douche for treating vaginitis.

In traditional Ayurvedic medicine, terminalia belerica has been touted as a "health-harmonizer" in combination with terminalia chebula and emblica officinalis. This combination is also touted to lower cholesterol and to prevent necrosis of cardiac tissue. It has also been touted to balance the three humors, kapha, pitta, and vata. It has also been touted for asthma, bile duct disorders, scorpion stings, and for poisonings.

### Indian Frankincense

Indian frankincense comes from the bark of several boswellia tree species. Orally, it has been used for arthritis, rheumatism, syphilis, painful menstruation, stomach troubles, and as a diuretic. Other uses include using the oil

Indian frankincense is likely safe when consumed in amounts found in food. There is insufficient reliable information of its effectiveness. Some preliminary studies show antiarthritis and anti-inflammatory effects.

**What They Told You**

in soaps, cosmetics, foods, and beverages.
Usual dose is 350 mg three times daily. No typical dosage for topical application has been determined.

### Indian Gooseberry—Pain

Orally, Indian gooseberry is touted for lowering cholesterol, treating atherosclerosis, treating cancer, dyspepsia, eye problems, joint pain, diarrhea, dysentery, organ restoration, and as an anti-inflammatory and antimicrobial. It is also used orally for obesity.

### Indian Long Pepper—Pain

In folk medicine, Indian long pepper was used orally to treat headache, toothache, asthma, beriberi, bronchitis, mucous membrane inflammation, PMS, and many other diseases.

### Indian Physic—Cough

Orally, Indian physic is used for digestive disorders and as an emetic.

### Indian Snakeroot—Hypertension

Indian snakeroot has been touted for hypertension, schizophrenia, snakebites, fever, constipation, and epilepsy.

### Indigo—Liver Toxicity

Indigo has been touted to help in liver toxicities, diabetes mellitus, upper respiratory infections, and cancer.

### Indium—Antiaging

Indium is a trace element and has been touted as "a fountain of youth" with a broad array of benefits (antiaging, for cancer, depression, weight loss, improved health, enhanced athletic performance, diabetes, glaucoma to name just a few). It has been touted as "the missing trace mineral."

**What They Did Not Tell You**

The principal constituent of Indian frankincense is the resin that contains boswellic acid, which has anti-inflammatory properties.

No known interactions with other herbs, supplements, drugs, or foods.

Reliable information is insufficient about the safety of Indian gooseberry when used in amounts greater than those found in foods. No interactions are known to occur, and there is no known reason to expect a clinically significant interaction.

Reliable information is insufficient about the effectiveness of Indian long pepper. Concomitant administration speeds absorption and slows elimination of phenytoin (Dilantin).

Reliable information is insufficient about the safety of Indian physic. Avoid using during pregnancy or while breast-feeding.

Indian snakeroot may lower blood pressure a little in some people because of reducing catacholamine.

The possible side effects are many (vomiting, diarrhea, drowsiness, fatigue, sexual dysfunction, hypertension, hypotension, and bradycardia). After discontinuation of use, depression may last several months.

Many drug interactions are possible.

There are different species of indigo. Some species may actually be hepatotoxic.

Significant research is lacking overall.

Significant research is lacking.

The broad array of touted benefits is certainly a concern.

Almost any mineral, vitamin, amino acid, herb, or supplement can have side effects. Many of the specific side

**What They Told You**

**What They Did Not Tell You**

effects of indium are not known, but in excess it could be toxic. It has been reported to cause headaches.

### Indole-3-Carbinol—Cancer Prevention

Orally, indole-3-carbinol is touted for prevention of breast cancer, colon cancer, and other types of cancer. Indole-3-carbinol is also touted for fibromyalgia, laryngeal papillomatosis, cervical dysplasia, and systemic lupus erythematosus (SLE). It is also used to balance hormone levels, detoxify the intestines and liver, and to support the immune system.

There is some concern that certain patients might be at risk for tumor-promoting effects of indole-3-carbinol. Until more is known, it is not possible to determine if there is a real risk to humans or who might be susceptible to this risk.

### Inosine—Body Building

Inosine has been used by weight trainers in the belief that it builds muscle and endurance.

It also might help in stroke recovery.

Significant research is lacking in regard to muscle building.

There is interesting research in rats that demonstrated axon nerve growth from uninjured nerve cells to injured ones. This could have implications in human stroke victims, but research is needed.

### Inositol—OCD

**How it has been used:** Inositol has been used in OCD, depression, and anxiety in addition to insomnia and promoting hair growth.

**Some interesting data:** Breast milk is rich in inositol.

**The usual dose:** The usual dose is 4 to 18 grams per day; 500 to 1000 mg per day has also been recommended.

**Health concerns:** More studies are needed. "It may precipitate mania" (*Psychopharmacology Update,* 2000, Baylor College of Medicine, Houston).

High doses are needed.

It may worsen ADHD.

It causes gastrointestinal side effects such as gas and diarrhea.

One case of mania was reported when a dose of 3 grams per day was used.

**Clinical studies:** Inositol has been used in a number of psychiatric disorders but has been no better than placebo in some studies. It is possibly ineffective at times but may possibly help at times especially in OCD. More research is needed before recommendations can be made.

**The mechanism of action:** Inositol is an essential component of cell membrane activity. It is unclear whether taking exogenous inositol is useful in human physiology.

## What They Told You

### Inulin—Obesity
Orally, inulin is touted for hypercholesterolemia, hyper-triglyceridemia, hyperlipidemia, obesity and weight loss, and improving gastrointestinal function.

### Iodine—Diabetic Foot Ulcers
Iodine is a mineral used for treating goiter and hyperthyroidism.

It has been touted for fibrocystic disease.

It has been touted topically for treating diabetic foot ulcers.

### IP–6—Cancer
IP–6 is a compound consisting of the B vitamin inositol plus six phosphate groups. It is found in many foods—rice, wheat, and beans. It is also found in supplemental form. It has antioxidant effects.

IP–6 has also been touted for preventing heart attacks and enhancing the immune system.

### Ipecac—Expectorant
Ipecac comes from South America and has been used as an expectorant. It has been tried in bronchitis, hepatitis, amebic dysentery, and as an appetite stimulant.

### Ipriflavone—Osteoporosis
Ipriflavone has been used in osteoporosis. It is said to inhibit bone demineralization and to increase bone mineralization. It is touted to have no estrogenic activity.

Ipriflavone is often given in doses of 200 mg 3 times per day.

## What They Did Not Tell You

Side effects are usually limited to the gastrointestinal tract, becoming more bothersome at doses over 30 grams. Some people can experience severe allergic reactions to inulin-containing foods. There is one report of anaphylaxis following consumption of foods with a high concentration of inulin including salsify, artichoke leaves, and margarine with inulin as a food additive.

Iodine has been used effectively for treating goiter and hyperthyroidism. Topically, it might help some with diabetic foot ulcers.

Serious allergic reactions have occurred. Large amounts can cause many, many problems (acne, depression, thyroid adenoma, metallic taste, eye irritation, diarrhea, headache, pulmonary edema, and cough, to name just a few).

Topical iodine can cause irritation and burns in some cases.

Research is lacking. No studies in humans with cancer have been done apparently. This is certainly not up to treating cancer.

The safety of the supplements is not known. It might inhibit platelet aggregation and thus could potentially be dangerous with anticoagulant and antiplatelet agents.

Ipecac is an FDA-approved drug as an expectorant and as such is used in emergency rooms. It is not approved for any other use as the side effects can be difficult (nausea, vomiting, gastrointestinal irritation, dizziness, and rapid heartbeat). Chronic use has caused death.

Some research of ipriflavone indicates that it might be effective. It has been compared to calcitonin and with apparent good results, but studies on more advanced drugs such as Actonel are lacking.

It is a semisynthetic isoflavone manufactured in the laboratory from daidzein, a compound from soy.

Gastrointestinal distress and dizziness are possible side effects.

| What They Told You | What They Did Not Tell You |
|---|---|
| | Ipriflavone has been reported to increase the effects of estrogen in some studies, so those with breast cancer (especially) take note. |

### Iron—Anemia

Iron is used in iron-deficiency anemia. It has also been touted for ADHD, athletic enhancement, depression, Crohn's disease, infertility, and heavy menstrual periods.

It is found in several plants (anise seed, celery seed, basil leaves, flaxseed, parsley leaves, cumin seed, and dill leaves).

Iron is effective in iron-deficiency anemia.

Iron is important in several body functions (hemoglobin function, cytochromes activity, the Krebs cycle, and dopamine activity).

It can cause gastrointestinal irritation, constipation, diarrhea, and nausea. Overdose can result in death. It is the most common cause of pediatric poisoning deaths. The question of increased cancer risk has been raised with high level use.

It can interact with ciprofloxacin, methyldopa, penicillamine, tetracycline, and thyroid replacement therapy.

### Jaborandi—Glaucoma

Jaborandi has been touted to reduce intraoccular pressure.

Jaborandi contains pilocarpine, which has a muscarinic/acetylcholine effect, causing pupillary constriction and decreased intraoccular pressure.

It can interact with nonsteroidal anti-inflammatory drugs, beta-blockers, bethalcohol.

It can cause hypertension, dizziness, headaches, blurred vision, and allergic reactions, to name just a few possible side effects. It definitely should not be used by those with angle-closure glaucoma.

### Jamaican Dogwood—Insomnia

Jamaican dogwood has been touted for insomnia.

Jamaican dogwood can produce sedation, dizziness, vomiting, sweating, and tremors.

### Jambul—High Blood Sugar

Jambul has been touted to lower blood sugar.

Research is lacking. Effectiveness is highly in doubt.

### Jatoba—Infections

This is a rain forest herb touted for many uses (viral infections, bacterial infections, fungal infections, fatigue, etc.).

Research is lacking, and side effects are not known.

### Jiaogulan—Hypertension

Orally, jiaogulan is touted for hyperlipidemia, hypertension, strengthening immune function, and increasing stamina and endurance. It is also touted for appetite stimulation,

Orally, use of jiaogulan might cause severe nausea and increased bowel movements. Concomitant use of jiaogulan with herbs that inhibit platelet aggregation might increase the risk of bleeding in some people. Some of

**What They Told You**

chronic bronchitis, chronic gastritis, ulcers, constipation, gallstones, obesity, cancer, diabetes, insomnia, backache, and pain. Jiaogulan is also touted orally for improving memory, improving coronary and cardiovascular functions, stress, preventing hair loss, and as an antiaging agent. It is also touted as an anti-inflammatory agent, antioxidant, detoxifying agent, decongestant and cough suppressant, and as an "adaptogen" for increasing resistance to environmental stress.

### Jimsonweed—Parkinsonism
Jimsonweed has been touted for parkinsonism and IBS (irritable bowel syndrome).

### Jojoba—Chapped Lips
Jojoba has been touted topically to help in various skin disorders including chapped lips and hair loss.

### Jujube—Liver Disease
Orally, jujube is touted for improving muscular strength and to prophylax against liver diseases and stress ulcers. It is also touted as a sedative.

In Chinese medicine, it is touted for dry, itchy skin; neutralizing drug toxicities; lack of appetite; fatigue; diarrhea; hysteria; anemia; hypertension; purpura; and as a sedative.

In Arabic medicine, jujube is touted orally for fever wounds, ulcers, inflammation, asthma, and eye diseases.

### Juniper—Urinary Tract Infections
Juniper has been used for years for flavoring alcoholic beverages.

It has been touted to help in urinary tract infections (but dangerous in kidney disease and could even produce kidney damage with prolonged use). It is touted to have anti-inflammatory properties and thus has been used for various skin sores (but it can also inflame the skin). It has also been used to remove warts. Finally it has been used for herpes.

### Kan Jang—Common Cold
Kan jang has been touted for the common cold.

**What They Did Not Tell You**

these herbs include angelica, anise, arnica, asafoetida, bogbean, boldo, capsicum, celery, chamomile, clove, danshen, fenugreek, feverfew, garlic, ginger, gingko, Panax ginseng, horse chestnut, horseradish, licorice, meadowsweet, prickly ash, onion, papain, passionflower, poplar, quassia, red clover, turmeric, vitamin E, wild carrot, wild lettuce, willow, and others.

When one of the authors was growing up on a farm, his father always said, "Don't let the horses eat the jimsonweed. It will make them crazy."

Jimsonweed is highly toxic, capable of producing confusion, seizures, and death.

Allergic reactions are possible.

Reliable information is insufficient.

Research is needed.

Reliable information is insufficient.

## What They Told You

### Kaolin—Diarrhea
Kaolin is often used in combination with pectin for diarrhea. It is a naturally occurring clay.

### Karaya Gum—Constipation
Karaya gum has been used as a laxative.

### Kava—Anxiety
**How it has been used:** Kava is used to treat anxiety disorders, stress, insomnia, and restlessness. It is also used for epilepsy, psychosis, and depression. In folk medicine, kava is used orally as a sedative, to promote wound healing, to treat headaches including migraines, cold and respiratory tract infections, tuberculosis, and rheumatism. It is used to treat urogenital infections including chronic cystitis, venereal disease, uterine inflammation, menstrual problems, and vaginal prolapse, and at times is used as an aphrodisiac. In folk medicine, kava juice is used topically to treat skin diseases including leprosy. It has been used as a poultice for intestinal problems, otitis, and abscesses, and may be used as a ceremonial beverage.

**Interesting data:** Ships visiting the Polynesian islands in the 1700s describe kava-intoxicated British seamen left behind by Captain Cook. Some of these sailors' skin had turned yellow.

The distributors cannot claim that their product is a treatment for a specific condition, such as anxiety disorder, but they do use phrases such as "It helps you to relax." It is usually described as inducing pleasant, cheerful, and calm feelings.

**Historical data:** It was used by the Pacific Islanders and considered to be a "magical drink" because of its calming effects and promotion of sociability.

It is one of the best-selling herbal supplements in the nation with a reported sales growth of 437 percent in 1998.

**The usual dose:** The usual dose is 100 mg 3 times a day.

## What They Did Not Tell You

Kaolin can cause constipation. It can decrease absorption of some drugs.

Karaya gum might decrease blood sugar. It can cause gastrointestinal distress.

**Health concerns:** The double-blind, placebo-controlled studies of kava are limited. Three studies did suggest anxiolytic effects, but there are inadequate toxicity studies. There is a reported case of coma with alprazolam, there are reports of intoxication with kava alone, and it is synergistic with alcohol. Long-term users were reported to have poor health, facial swelling, scaly rash, and difficulty breathing. Serious liver toxicities have also been reported.

Other reported side effects include gastrointestinal disturbances and a yellowish tint to the skin. Effects on the fetus are unknown. It can be "intoxicating" (*Psychopharmacology Update,* 2000, Baylor College of Medicine, Houston). Recent cases of liver failure have been reported.

High doses of kava have been associated with severe adverse effects. Prolonged use of kava may lead to habituation and has also been associated with a kava dermopathy as well as loss of uterine tone. Use in pregnancy and breast-feeding is contraindicated.

The oral use of kava can cause gastrointestinal complaints, headache, dizziness, enlarged pupils, and disturbance of oculomotor equilibrium and accommodation, and rarely, allergic skin reactions. Use of normal doses of kava may affect the ability to drive or operate machinery, and driving under the influence (DUI) citations have been issued to individuals observed driving erratically after drinking large amounts of kava tea. Kava can cause drowsiness and may impair motor reflexes. Chewing kava can cause mouth numbness. Chronic use of high doses of kava has been associated with kava dermopathy, a pellagra-like syndrome unresponsive to niacinamide treatment. The long-term use of large amounts of kava is associated with poor health, including being significantly underweight, reduced protein levels, puffy faces, scaly rashes, hematuria, increased red blood cell volume, decreased platelets and lymphocytes, and possibly

**What They Told You**

**What They Did Not Tell You**

pulmonary hypertension. There have been reports of generalized abnormal movements of the body associated with high-dose, chronic kava use along with a case of recurrent, acute hepatitis.

There is one report of an individual who was hospitalized due to lethargy and disorientation when alprazolam and kava were used concomitantly. Concomitant use of alcohol, barbiturates, or benzodiazepines can increase drug effects and risk of adverse effects, and kava may interfere with levadopa.

**Clinical studies:** Most of the information regarding the mild calming effects of kava has been anecdotal. More reliable clinical studies are needed.

**The mechanism of action:** The active components, kava-lactones, act on the GABA receptors, thus the antianxiety effect. Other ingredients in the plant may have some local anesthetic and muscle-relaxing properties (*The Harvard Mental Health Letter*, November 2000, Vol. 17, No. 5, p. 8). Because kava acts on the GABA receptors as benzodiazepines (Xanax, Valium, Ativan, etc.) do, it too is probably potentially addicting.

### Kelp—Nutritional Support
Kelp is known as having exceptional nutritional power with many trace elements (chromium, zinc, iron, sulfur, silver, tin, silicon, magnesium, manganese); several vitamins (A, B-complex, C, D, E); several amino acids; iodine, calcium.

Kelp has also been used as a salt substitute (its sodium content is touted to be offset by potassium).

Whether this nutritional supplement proves valuable remains to be seen.

### Khat—Depression
Khat stem is chewed by people in Africa for its euphoric effect.

Khat can cause euphoric but also manic behavior, insomnia, increased blood pressure, heart palpitations, aggressiveness, occasional psychotic reactions, myocardial infarction, hepatic cirrhosis, and cerebral hemorrhage.

### Khella—Angina
Khella has been used for angina at 100 mg 3 times per day. It comes from Egypt and Pakistan.

Khella is a uterine stimulant and should not be used during pregnancy or by nursing mothers. It can cause insomnia, headaches, dizziness, skin cancer with topical use, stomach upset, and liver disease. It should not be used with blood thinners, antihypertensives, calcium channel blockers, or diuretics.

| What They Told You | What They Did Not Tell You |
|---|---|
| **Kira—Depression**<br>Kira contains extract LI 160, which is an extract of Saint-John's-wort. | Reliable information is insufficient. |
| **Kiwi—A Food**<br>Kiwi is used as a food and added to some drinks. | Kiwi is high in serotonin and vitamin C. |
| **Kombucha Tea**<br>Kombucha tea is usually a combination of substances (fermented yeast and bacteria, alcohol, vinegar, and sugar).<br><br>It has been touted for fatigue, poor memory, PMS, aging, high blood pressure, hair regrowth, and cancer. | Research is lacking in regard to effectiveness.<br><br>Possible contamination is a real concern.<br><br>Side effects have included gastrointestinal upset, yeast infections, jaundice, anthrax, and possibly death. |
| **Kudzu—Angina/Suppress Alcohol Intake**<br>Kudzu has *chemicals* (flavonid-like) that have been touted to improve blood flow and thus, has been used for angina. It also contains isoflavons that have been touted to decrease the urge to drink alcohol. It also has estrogen-like chemicals. | Kudzu should not be used with cardiac medicines such as those for arrhythmias.<br><br>As with most herbs or supplements, allergic reactions are possible with kudzu.<br><br>As with most herbs, it should not be used during pregnancy. |
| **Kwai—High Blood Pressure**<br>Kwai is an odor-free garlic and is touted for high blood pressure, cancer prevention, and high cholesterol. | Reliable information is insufficient. |
| **Kyolic—Heart Disease**<br>Kyolic, a form of garlic, is touted for cancer prevention, heart disease prevention, treatment of high blood pressure, and for enhancing the immune system. | Reliable information is insufficient. |
| **Lactoferrin—Infections**<br>Lactoferrin is a protein that has been touted to stimulate the immune system. | Significant research is lacking. |
| **Lady's Bedstraw—Wound Healing**<br>In folk medicine lady's bedstraw has been touted for oral use for treating swollen ankles, as a diuretic for bladder and kidney mucous discharge, for cancer, epilepsy, hysteria, spasms, tumors, and for relief of chest and lung ailments. It is also touted to induce sweating; as a tonic; to simulate appetite; as an aphrodisiac; and for astringent, cleansing, and purgative effects.<br><br>In folk medicine, lady's bedstraw is touted for topical use | Insufficient reliable information is available. No adverse effects have been reported. |

## What They Told You

for poorly healing wounds and to stop bleeding.

### Lady's Mantle—Bleeding

Lady's mantle can decrease bleeding.

### La Pacho—Yeast Infections

This herb has been touted to help in yeast infections and even in cancer.

### Laurelwood—HIV

Orally, the laurelwood constituent (+)-calanolide A is touted for HIV infection.

Topically, tamanu oil from the nut of the laurelwood is used for skin ailments including sunburn, rashes, burns, psoriasis, dermatitis, scratches, skin blemishes, acne, skin allergies, bedsores, rosacea, and hemorrhoids. It is also used topically for infant skin care.

In folk medicine, laurelwood was used for leprosy, piles, scabies, gonorrhea, vaginitis, and chicken pox.

### Lavender—Athlete's Foot and Insomnia

Lavender (topical application) has been used as an antifungus herb for athlete's foot. It has also been used for acne in topical form.

Just a little (one or two drops) of lavender oil in a bath mixture is touted to help induce sleep and calm emotions.

Lavender oil is still found in soap and perfume.

### L-Carnitine—Weight Loss

**How it has been used:** Weight loss and bodybuilding, increase weight gain in premature infants, and in treatment of chronic fatigue syndrome. It is FDA approved for intravenous use in people with end-stage renal disease who are undergoing hemodialysis and have L-carnitine deficiency.

**Historical data:** A number of individual amino acids have been available in health food stores for many years with a number of recommended uses.

**The usual dose:** The usual dose is 500 to 2000 micrograms 2 times a day.

## What They Did Not Tell You

Lady's mantle can also cause liver damage.

Good research is lacking as to the benefits of la pacho, but we do know it can be dangerous, with severe anemias occurring in chronic use. The general conclusion is: *not practical, too dangerous.*

The use of the laurelwood constituent, (+)-calanolide A, by healthy individuals can cause dizziness, oily aftertaste, headache, and nausea when taken orally.

Topically, there are no reported adverse reactions when tamanu oil from the nut of laurelwood is used.

This is interesting. Significant research is lacking.

**Health concerns:** The cost is high. They tend to be a waste of money if you eat an adequate diet. If you eat more protein than you need for growth, repair, and maintenance, the body will work harder to process the excess protein, putting more work on the liver and kidneys.

The racemic mixture is toxic.

**Clinical studies:** There is insufficient information available for effectiveness of L-carnitine with the exception of its use in inborn errors of metabolism and end-stage renal disease.

**The mechanism of action:** L-carnitine is an amino acid. Amino acids are building blocks of a more complex

**What They Told You**

**What They Did Not Tell You**

protein molecule in humans and animals. It plays an important role in transport of free fatty acids across mitochondrial membrane for energy production.

### Lecithin—Alzheimer's Disease

Lecithin contains phosphatidylcholine, which contains choline. Choline is related to the neurotransmitter acetylcholine. Lecithin has been touted for dementia, lowering cholesterol, myasthenia gravis, tardive dyskinesia, hepatic stenosis, gallbladder disease, liver disease, bipolar disorder, anxiety, and improving memory.

Lecithin can cause gastrointestinal complaints and hepatitis.

### Lemon Balm—Cold Sores

Lemon balm has a long folklore reputation for lifting mood. It has also been touted for several other disorders—cold sores (topical cream), colitis, herpes (topical cream), gastric conditions, migraines, hypertension, insomnia, and bronchitis. It is touted to be antiseptic, antibacterial, and antiviral.

Lemon is taken as an oil, tincture, or fresh fruit. Orally, lemon balm is used for promoting digestion, as an antispasmodic, for Grave's disease, and for functional gastrointestinal disorders with distention and gas. Topically, it is used for cold sores (herpes labialis). Traditionally, lemon balm has been used for promoting sweating, promoting menstrual flow, for female discomforts, nervous problems, insomnia, cramps, headache, toothache, sores, tumors, insect bites, nervous stomach, hysteria and melancholia, chronic bronchial mucous membrane inflammation, nervous palpitations, vomiting, and high blood pressure.

Research is lacking. Lemon balm is probably safe for most people but should not be given to pregnant women or children.

Lemon balm is contraindicated in hypothyroid conditions because lemon balm can exacerbate or interfere with treatment and thyroid replacement therapy. Some patients have been reported to be hypersensitive to lemon balm.

Theoretically, concomitant use with herbs that have sedative properties might enhance therapeutic and adverse effects. These include calamus, calendula, California poppy, catnip, capsicum, celery, couch grass, elecampane, ginseng, German chamomile, goldenseal, gotu kola, hops, Jamaican dogwood, kava, sage, Saint-John's-wort, sassafras, scullcap, shepherd's purse, stinging nettle, valerian, wild carrot, wild lettuce, withania root, and yerba mansa.

### Lemongrass—Upper Respiratory Infections

Lemongrass has been touted for pain, neuralgia, and upper respiratory infections (URI).

Effectiveness of lemongrass is not known.

### Lentinan—HIV Infections

Lentinan has been touted for cancer, HIV infections, bacterial infections, and viral infections.

It is possible that lentinan may cause some augmentation of natural killer cell activity and enhance T-helper cell functioning, but significant research is lacking.

### Licorice—Peptic Ulcers

Licorice comes from a small plant. Its use dates back thousands of years. It has been used for peptic ulcers, infections, and hepatitis.

Licorice has estrogen-like effects and aldosterone-like effects. Thus it may have benefits or side effects accordingly. A more prominent danger is present for those with high blood pressure, diabetes, and heart disease. It could especially be dangerous if used by those with renal failure or as digitalis preparations.

**What They Told You**

**What They Did Not Tell You**

It can be dangerous in large dosages (greater than 400 mg per day).

### Lily of the Valley—Heart Failure
Lily of the valley has been touted for heart failure.

The components of this herb might possibly increase the force of heart contraction but is no match for digitalis and other heart medications.

### Linden—Common Cold
Linden has been used for colds, coughs, and bronchitis.

It probably does have antispasmodic, sedative, and mild astringent effects.

It could damage the heart with frequent use, but this is rare. It usually does not interact with other drugs.

### Liver Extract
Liver extract has been touted for liver disease, body building, energy, and recovery from addictions.

Research is lacking in regard to effectiveness.

In regard to potential side effects, contamination is a concern since the extract can be made from liver in slaughterhouses. Mad cow disease (bovine spongiform encephalitis) is a concern.

### Lobelia ("Indian tobacco")—Smoking Deterrent
Native Americans used lobelia for its tobacco-like effects (Indian tobacco). It has been touted for use as an expectorant and as a smoking deterrent.

To use this herb for smoking deterrent is like burning down the barn to get rid of the rats. Deaths have been reported with its use.

### Lovage—Edema
Lovage has been touted as a diuretic.

Effectiveness of lovage is not known.

### L-Tryptophane
See Monoamine Precursors.

### L-Tyrosine (Catecholamine Precursor)
L-tyrosine is a precursor to dopamine, epinephrine, and norepinephrine. It has been tried in depression in dosages from 3200 to 8000 mg per day.

Controlled studies are lacking.

### Luffa—Cough
Orally, luffa is touted for treating and preventing colds, nasal inflammation, sinusitis, and suppuration of the sinuses.

Topically, luffa sponge is used to remove dead skin and stimulate the skin.

Luffa charcoal is used topically for shingles in the face and

| What They Told You | What They Did Not Tell You |
|---|---|
| eye region.<br>In Chinese medicine, luffa is used orally for arthritis and associated pain, muscle pain, chest pain, amenorrhea, and to promote lactation.<br><br>In cosmetics, powdered luffa is used in skin care products as an anti-inflammatory and detoxicant. | |

### Lungwort—URI
Lungwort has beet touted for upper respiratory infections (URIs).

Effectiveness of lungwort is not known.

It might increase bleeding time.

### Lutein—Cataracts
Orally, lutein is touted for preventing age-related macular degeneration, cataracts, and colon cancer.

Concomitant administration may reduce bioavailability of lutein and may reduce or increase bioavailability of beta-carotene.

### Lycopene—Cancer Prevention
Lycopene has been touted to have cancer, preventing effects. It is found in tomatoes.

Effectiveness of lycopene is not known.

### Lysine—Herpes
Lysine is an amino acid manufactured by the body, but it can also be found in dairy products, wheat germ, brewer's yeast, and meats.

It has been used to treat cold sores and even herpes. It has also been used in Bell's palsy and rheumatoid arthritis and to detoxify opiates.

Significant research is lacking.

Side effects are probably few. Gastrointestinal side effects are possible. Of course, it should not be used by pregnant women or children.

### Maca—Sexual Enhancement
Maca has been touted for sexual enhancement.

Significant research is lacking.

It might increase the risk of cancer in some individuals.

### Madder—Renal Stones
Madder has been touted for renal stones.

Madder can cause gastrointestinal symptoms and possibly liver cancer.

Effectiveness is not known.

### Magnesium—Fibromyalgia
Magnesium is one of the minerals of the human body. It has been touted to help in fibromyalgia. The reasoning is that it is important in ATP synthesis which is important in energy production which is usually low in fibromyalgia.

Magnesium is used for treating and preventing hypomag-

The reasoning is interesting but has some possible leaps in logic. Of course, magnesium is unlikely to have side effects at low dosages, but there is some concern at the doses often recommended.

It is conceivable that magnesium may have some minor antianxiety effects.

## What They Told You

nesemia as well as for a laxative for constipation and for preparation of the bowel for surgical or diagnostic procedures. It is used as an antacid for symptoms of gastric hyperacidity. Magnesium is used orally for treating symptoms of asthma and for cardiovascular diseases including angina, atrial fibrillation, cardiomyopathy, congestive heart failure, hypertension, intermittent claudication, low high-density lipoprotein (HDL) levels, mitral valve prolapse, myocardial infarction, and stroke.

It is also used for treating diabetes, eosinophilia myalgia syndrome, fatigue, fibromyalgia, glaucoma, hearing loss, hypoglycemia, kidney stones, migraine, osteoporosis, premenstrual syndrome, and preventing hearing loss. Magnesium has also been used by athletes to increase energy and endurance. In combination with malic acid, magnesium has been used orally for decreasing pain and tenderness associated with fibromyalgia. It is sometimes added to antidepressants to enhance the antidepressant effect of medications. Magnesium is also used for treating infected skin ulcers, boils, and carbuncles; and for speeding wound healing.

It is also used as a cold compress in the treatment of erysipelas, and as a hot compress for deep-seated skin infections. Intravenously, magnesium is used for acute hypomagnesemia occurring in conditions such as pancreatitis, malabsorption disorders, cirrhosis, and as an additive to total parenteral nutrition (TPN) for prevention of pomagnesemia. It is also used intravenously for controlling seizures in patients with epilepsy, merulonephritis and uremia, hypothyroidism, and eclampsia in patients with hypomagnesemia. It has also been used for the treatment of life-threatening arrhythmias such as torsade de pointes, cardiac arrest, and for preventing arrhythmias after myocardial infarction. Magnesium is also used intravenously for treating acute exacerbations of asthma, chronic obstructive pulmonary disease (COPD), as an osmotic agent for cerebral edema, and for tetanus.

For fibromyalgia some have recommended as high as 500 mg tablets—6 tablets, 2 times per day.

## What They Did Not Tell You

Orally, magnesium can cause gastrointestinal irritation, nausea, vomiting, and diarrhea, and rarely, large amounts may cause hypermagnesernia with symptoms including thirst, hypotension, drowsiness, confusion, loss of tendon reflexes, muscle weakness, respiratory depression, cardiac arrhythmias, coma, cardiac arrest, and death.

Urticaria has been reported with IV administration. Chronic use of magnesium-containing antacids, especially those which do not contain aluminum, can cause diarrhea leading to fluid and electrolyte imbalances. Topically, prolonged use of magnesium sulfate in the treatment of boils and carbuncles can cause skin damage. Boron can increase serum magnesium levels.

Concomitant administration decreases absorption of the fluoroquinolones (ciprofloxacin, levofloxacin, etc.). Profound hypotension or neuromuscular blockade can occur in individuals using oral nifedipine concomitantly with intravenous magnesium sulfate.

Parenteral magnesium could potentiate the effects of skeletal muscle relaxants, e.g., tubocurarine chloride.

Concomitant use of urinary excretion-enhancing can reduce the effects of supplemental magnesium, which include amphotericin B, cisplatin, aminoglycoside antibiotics, cyclosporine, thiazide and loop diuretics, mannitol, and intravenous glucose.

Concomitant use of excretion-reducing drugs can increase the effects of supplemental magnesium and magnesium serum levels. Urinary excretion-reducing drugs include calcitonin, glucagon, and potassium-sparing diuretics.

Digoxin can decrease renal tubule reabsorption and increase excretion of magnesium. Use of loop diuretics and thiazide diuretics can increase urinary magnesium loss and reduce serum levels. Use of estrogens and estrogen-containing oral contraceptives might shift magnesium from the serum to storage in other tissues, decreasing serum magnesium levels. Penicillamine can reduce serum magnesium levels.

## Magnolia Flower—Nasal Congestion

Magnolia flower, a Chinese herb, has been touted for nasal

Animal data suggest antibacterial, antifungal, antiviral, anti-inflammatory effects, but data in humans is lacking.

## What They Told You

## What They Did Not Tell You

congestion, the common cold, headaches, and facial dark spots. Topically, it has been used for toothaches and on the skin as a whitener.

Overall, serious reported adverse reactions have been few. In overdoses dizziness and red eyes have been reported.

Orally, people using large amounts may experience emesis.

### Maidenhair Fern—Bronchitis
Orally, maidenhair fern is touted for bronchitis, coughs, whooping cough, and painful and excessive menstruation. It is also used orally as an expectorant and demulcent.

Historically, it was used orally for various respiratory tract illnesses and severe coughs. It was also used topically for hair loss and to promote dark hair color.

### Maitake (grifola frondosa)—Herpes
Maitake is a mushroom that has been used to boost the immune system in several diseases (cancer, HIV). It has been used for hypertension, obesity, high cholesterol, and diabetes.

Good research is meager at best. We seriously doubt it will prove to be the "miracle herb" that the Orient thinks it is.

Standardized extracts of maitake apparently are not recommended.

Maitake has been used to treat herpes, warts, and other viral illness such as colds.

Two tablets of 350 mg made from grifola frondosa mushrooms are recommended.

### Malabar Tamarind—Weight Loss
Malabar tamarind has been touted for weight loss.

Effectiveness is not proven and is, in fact, in doubt. Reported adverse reactions have been few, and drug interactions also seem low.

### Male Fern—Tapeworm
Male fern has been used against tapeworm.

Male fern can have side effects: damage to the liver, gastrointestinal symptoms, heart failure, seizures, and death.

### Malic Acid—Fibromyalgia
Malic acid is a natural organic acid found in apples. It has been touted to help in fibromyalgia when combined with magnesium because of possible benefits in ATP formation and thus energy.

The theory is interesting. Research is needed. Side effects are unlikely in sensible amounts.

### Mallow—URIs
Mallow has been touted for upper respiratory infections (URIs).

Research is lacking. Effectiveness of mallow is not known.

### Maltsupex—Constipation
Maltsupex is touted for use in constipation.

Reliable information is insufficient.

| What They Told You | What They Did Not Tell You |
| --- | --- |
| **Manganese—PMS**<br>Manganese plus copper, zinc, and calcium has been touted to help in osteoporosis and PMS. | Significant research is lacking except for its use in manganese deficiencies.<br><br>Manganese-like minerals, herbs, and supplements become more toxic as the dose is increased. At high dosages it might cause parkinsonism. Some of those exposed to it in their occupation have developed depression and dementia. |
| **Marigold—Cancer**<br>Marigold has been touted for cancer. | Effectiveness of marigold is not known. Significant research is lacking.<br><br>It can cause gastrointestinal upset. |
| **Marijuana**<br>Marijuana is used for euphoria. The prescription-only, synthetic dronabinol (Marinol) product is used for the treatment of anorexia or appetite loss associated with AIDS and for cancer chemotherapy-induced nausea and vomiting unresponsive to traditional medications. As an inhalant, marijuana is used for treating nausea, reducing intraocular pressure, stimulation of appetite, altering senses (psychoactivity), euphoria, mucous membrane inflammation, leprosy, fever, dandruff, hemorrhoids, obesity, asthma, urinary tract infections, cough, and treating anorexia associated with weight loss in AIDS patients. Marijuana reduces intraocular pressure in some patients with glaucoma. | While short-term inhalation increases bronchodilation and reduces bronchospasm, long-term use impairs lung function, which can result in constrictive lung disease. Marijuana can cause tachycardia and transient hypertension. The cannabinoids in marijuana are allergenic in animal models.<br><br>When used orally or inhaled, marijuana passes through the placenta and can reduce fetal growth. Marijuana use during pregnancy is also associated with childhood leukemia and should not be used during breast-feeding because dronabinol is concentrated and excreted in breast milk.<br><br>The use of marijuana can cause nausea and vomiting. The chronic use of marijuana can cause laryngitis, bronchitis, apathy, psychic decline, sexual dysfunction, and has been associated with several cases of an unusual pattern of bullous emphysema. Signs of acute poisoning from marijuana include nausea, vomiting, lacrimation, hacking cough, disturbed cardiac function, and limb numbness. Marijuana has a high abuse potential. Regular use of marijuana in middle-aged persons has been associated with an increased risk of myocardial infarction, with a 4.8 fold increase in relative risk of myocardial infarction within the first hour following smoking marijuana. Marijuana can have additive or synergistic effects when used with herbs that possess CNS depressant or stimulant effects, and it can decrease barbiturate clearance rate.<br><br>Concomitant use of marijuana with fluoxetine and disulfiram can cause transient hypomanic episodes. |

**What They Told You**

**What They Did Not Tell You**

Concomitant use can increase theophylline metabolism. Use of dronabinol can have additive or synergistic effects with amphetamines, anticholinergics, antihistamines, cocaine, hypnotics, psychomimetics, sedatives, and sympathomimetics. Concomitant use of alcohol with dronabinol can have additive or synergistic CNS effects.

Marijuana has the potential to cause tachycardia and transient hypertension. Theoretically, inhalation of marijuana smoke containing aspergillus spores increases the risk of fungal infections and sensitization in individuals with compromised immune function. Long-term use of marijuana can exacerbate respiratory conditions. Marijuana could exacerbate seizure disorders in some individuals.

### Marjoram—Insomnia

This inhaled oil is touted to help in insomnia.

Research is lacking if existing at all.

Marjoram has also been touted topically for eczema.

Marjoram can cause gastrointestinal upset.

### Marsh Blazing Star—Kidney Disorders

Orally, marsh blazing star is touted for kidney disorders, dysmenorrhea, gonorrhea, and as a diuretic.

Orally, marsh blazing star, which contains coumarin, can be associated with nausea and vomiting, diarrhea, dizziness, insomnia, asymptomatic SGOT elevations, and liver toxicity.

Topically, handling the plant can cause contact dermatitis.

Marsh blazing star can cause an allergic reaction in individuals sensitive to the asteraceae/compositae family. Members of this family include ragweed, chrysanthemums, marigolds, daisies, and many other herbs.

### Marshmallow—Irritations of the Mouth, Throat, and Stomach

Wild marshmallows have been eaten in Europe for centuries. Marshmallows contain mucilage polysaccharides that soothe mucous membranes and skin inflammations. It has been used to soothe irritations in the mouth, throat, and stomach. It has been used to suppress cough. There have been some reports of hypoglycemic effects.

Marshmallows are usually safe and taste great. They do soothe mucous membranes.

### Mastic—Skin Cuts

Orally, mastic is used for gastric and duodenal ulcers, respiratory conditions, muscle aches, and to improve circulation.

Children using mastic may develop diarrhea.

## What They Told You

Topically, it is used for skin cuts and as an insect repellent.

### Maté—Fatigue

Maté has been used for fatigue. It has also been used as a diuretic and for weight loss.

It is a common South American beverage.

### Mayapple—Warts

Mayapple has been touted for topical use to remove warts.

### Meadowsweet—Fever

This North American herb has long been used for fever, infections, and pain.

### Melatonin—Insomnia

**How it has been used:** Melatonin has been used for insomnia and in cluster headaches.

**Some interesting data:** Melatonin is a hormone we all have that is secreted at night by the pineal gland. As people grow older, the pineal gland may calcify and secrete inadequate amounts of melatonin. Thus difficulty falling asleep may develop, and the addition of melatonin may help.

**Historical data:** It has been efficacious in jet lag. It may help in insomnia. It has been used in attempting better seizure control.

**The usual dose:** 0.1 to 0.3 mg at bedtime. Extreme doses as high as 3 to 10 mg have been used. Smaller doses of 0.3 to 1 mg often seem more appropriate if this hormone is to be used.

## What They Did Not Tell You

Maté contains caffeine with its central nervous-system stimulating effects. It also may have appetite suppressant, lipolytic, and glycogenolytic effects.

Long-term use is associated with cancer of the esophagus, mouth, larynx, kidney, bladder, and lung. The caffeine can cause anxiety and insomnia.

It can possibly interact with many drugs.

Significant research is lacking.

Mayapple can have many side effects when used orally (seizures, liver toxicity, low platelets, gastrointestinal upset, and apnea).

The chemicals of meadowsweet are similar to those in willow bark from which we obtain aspirin.

Research is needed to see if the gastrointestinal irritation is less than that of its cousin, aspirin.

**Health concern:** "The quality of products highly suspect" (*Psychopharmacology Update*, 1999, Baylor College of Medicine, Houston).

Reduced alertness, fatigue, headache, transient depression, and irritability have been reported. Driving or operating machinery for 4 to 5 hours after taking melatonin is not recommended.

Some health food stores sell melatonin preparations containing 2.5 to 3 mg—10 times the dose that promotes normal sleep. At this dose, blood melatonin levels may rise to 30 times the normal nighttime level. When too much of the hormone remains in the body too long, it can cause daytime drowsiness or dizziness. It may also interfere with physiological rhythm and the rise and fall of natural melatonin, possibly causing lower body temperature, nightmares, and nighttime headaches or disorientation. It possibly has induced depression (*The Harvard Mental Health Letter*, Vol. 17, No. 12, June 1996).

**Clinical studies:** It is a strong antioxidant and in some animal and human studies seemed to have anticarcino-

**What They Told You**

**What They Did Not Tell You**

genic effects especially for estrogen receptor-positive tumors such as those of the breast, prostate, melanoma, and glioma. We are lacking in long-term data use with melatonin, but we are also lacking in data on the long-term use of conventional sedative hypnotics. Unlike the sleep induced by many of the sedative-hypnotic drugs, melatonin-induced sleep often seems normal. Since aspirin and ibuprofen (Motrin) may inhibit normal melatonin synthesis, extra melatonin may help.

**The mechanism of action:** Melatonin is a naturally occurring hormone produced by the pineal gland. It is involved in the endogenous circadian rhythm (sleep-wake cycle). Levels of melatonin peak between the ages of 1 and 3.

Decreased melatonin has been found in individuals suffering from insomnia. Taking low doses of melatonin appears to have rapid mild sleep-inducing effects. It lowers alertness, body temperature, and performance for 3 to 4 hours after ingestion. It is thought to regulate circadian rhythm and sleep patterns by interacting with melatonin receptors in the brain. Other mechanisms reported are antioxidant properties, improved immune function, as well as inhibition of certain types of cancer cells.

*Menthol Cream—Poison Ivy*
Menthol cream has been used for the itch of poison ivy.

Significant research is lacking.

*Methionine—Aging*
Methionine is an amino acid with antioxidant effects and as such has been touted to have antiaging effects.

Significant research is lacking.

*Milk Thistle—Liver Disease*
**How it has been used:** Milk thistle has been used in hepatitis, other liver problems, digestive disorders, colic, gallbladder problems, poor appetite, breast milk deficiency, hemorrhoids, malaria, to aid in treatment of toxins from ingesting poison mushrooms, and for menstrual pain.

**Some interesting data:** It has been called the Virgin Mary's breast milk.

**Historical data:** For over 2000 years, this plant has been used for liver ailments. It grows in Europe and in North America.

**Health concerns:** Milk thistle may cause allergic reactions in people who are sensitive to plants such as ragweeds or marigolds; may cause diarrhea. Milk thistle seems fairly innocuous, and since there is often little in modern medicine (except interferon) that may help in the treatment of some liver disorders, it might be considered a possibility if interferon or other upcoming medicines cannot be used for some reason.

**Clinical studies:** Clinical studies involve research in animals showing improvement in liver cell regeneration.

**The mechanism of action:** Silymarin contained in the plant is responsible for the biochemical action which is

**What They Told You**

**The usual dose:** The usual dose is 420 to 840 mg daily.

**What They Did Not Tell You**

reportedly capable of altering liver cell membranes to prevent the uptake of toxins, promoting antioxidant activity, and increasing glutathione levels (*Pharmacist's Letter/Prescriber's Letter,* p. 25).

---

**Minerals**

"It's only a mineral. Take a lot of them."

Selenium has been used in weight-loss formulas, and zinc is famous for the common cold. Magnesium is known for its sedative effects. It may require concomitant $B_6$. It has been tried in bipolar studies.

Minerals too can be toxic in megadoses at times (*Current Medical Diagnosis and Treatment and the American Medical Associates Encyclopedia of Medicine,* N.Y.: Random House, 1989, p. 1058).

Megadose supplementation of selenium induces hair loss, dermatitis, and irritability.

Zinc may cause gastrointestinal irritation, vomiting.

Magnesium may depress deep tendon reflexes and respiration.

---

**Mistletoe**

Mistletoe grows on the bark of various trees.

Because of fatal poisonings that have occurred, mistletoe is an especially dangerous herb.

---

**Moleskin—Blisters**

Moleskin is an herbal oil that has been used for blisters on the feet. It is touted to be antiseptic and germicidal.

Significant research is lacking.

---

**Molybdenum**

Orally, chelated minerals are touted as mineral supplements (marketed to be more bioavailable than nonchelated minerals), for supporting normal growth, building strong muscles and bones, improving immune protection, healthy blood, and glowing skin.

Reliable information is insufficient.

---

**Monascus—High Cholesterol**

Monascus has been touted to lower cholesterol and possibly have an antidepressant effect.

Significant research is lacking.

In rare cases monascus can damage the liver. It can cause gastrointestinal upset.

---

**Monoamine Precursors (dopamine, epinephrine, norepinephrine, serotonin, and L-tryptophane)**

L-tryptophane was banned in the United States after deaths with eosinophelia-myalgia syndrome. All of these monoamine precursors have been tried for antidepressant hopes.

There is little controlled data.

---

**Morinda—Smallpox**

Reliable information is insufficient on the effectiveness of

## What They Told You

A fruit typically found in Polynesia and the Pacific Islands, morinda is also known as Indian mulberry, hog apple, and wild pine. It has been used for colic, convulsions, diabetes, constipation, malarial fever, nausea, bone and joint problems, depression, and digestive problems as well as numerous other disorders. Topically, the fruit has been used as a wrap to reduce signs of aging and to reduce the pain of arthritis. Historically, it was used to treat smallpox by applying the preparation directly on the lesions.

Usual dosage is 1 to 10 ounces of the fruit juice. Capsules of 200 mg of morinda are also marketed. Reportedly, 1200 mg from capsules is equal to one ounce of the juice.

### Mormon Tea—Kidney Disorders
Mormon tea has been used for syphilis, gonorrhea, colds, kidney disorders, and as a "spring tonic."

### Motherwort—Rapid Heart Rate
Motherwort has been used for heart disease, rapid heartbeat, and hyperthyroidism.

### MSM (Methylsufonylmethane)—Arthritis
MSM is a naturally occurring organic sulfur compound. It has been touted to help in the healing of injuries, pain relief, inflammation reduction, arthritis, and muscle pain.

It is often given at 1–2 mg per day.

### Mucilage—High Cholesterol
See Fiber.

### Mugwort—Insomnia
This inhaled oil has been used for insomnia and PMS.

### Muira Puama—Impotence
Muira puama (potency wood) comes from the Amazon jungle. It has long been used in the Amazon for impotence.

The usual touted dose is ½ to 1 teaspoon liquid before sexual activity. One milliliter should be about 500 milligrams. One milliliter is equal to 1 cc, and 5 cc's is one teaspoon.

## What They Did Not Tell You

morinda.

The fruit of morinda contains essential oils, hexoic acids, paraffin, and alcohol esters. Other ingredients are thought to work at the cellular level to repair damage such as xeronine, which is contained in the morinda fruit. Morinda contains a high level of potassium, which can be toxic to individuals suffering from renal insufficiency.

The fruit can discolor urine to a pink or rust tinge. The smell is unpleasant, and the cost is high.

Significant research is lacking.

Several different actions have been theorized: uterine stimulation (possibly through actions of lonurine and stachydrine); increase in force of myocardial contraction; anticoagulant effects, antianxiety effects, and effects that improve thyroid function.

More research is needed since it could cause uterine stimulation. It should not be used in pregnancy.

Significant research is needed.

Research is lacking if existing at all.

Effectiveness is not known or safety proven although few if any adverse reactions have been reported as to date. No drug interactions are reported.

## What They Told You

### Mullein—Upper Respiratory Infections

Mullein has been used to treat many forms of upper respiratory infections—colds, coughs, bronchitis, sore throat, and asthma. It has also been used to treat urinary tract infections and herpes simplex virus.

### Mussel—Arthritis

Mussel is touted to have anti-inflammatory effects and has been used for arthritis.

### Mustard—URIs

Mustard has been touted to help in upper respiratory infections (URIs), gas, arthritis, and cancer.

### Myrrh—Sore Throat

Myrrh has been used topically for mild inflammations of the mouth and throat. It has been touted for colds, ulcers, and cough. Topically, it has been used for bedsores, skin abrasions, bad breath, and hemorrhoids.

It is used as a fragrance in perfumes and cosmetics.

### Myrtle—Diabetes Mellitus

Myrtle has been touted to lower blood sugar.

### NAC (N-Acetylcysteine)—Aging

NAC is a sulfur-containing amino acid and as such has been touted to have antiaging effects. It has also been touted to decrease infections.

### NADH (niacinamide adenine dinucleotide—reduced form)—High Cholesterol

NADH has been touted for Alzheimer's dementia, fatigue, Parkinson's disease, and cognitive decline of aging.

Niacin has been used for treating pellagra. Niacin has also been used as a second live treatment for high cholesterol and high triglycerides.

It has been touted as a secondary prevention for myocar-

## What They Did Not Tell You

Mullein might help to a degree for some in congestion and sore throat. It contains mucilage, which alleviates local pain. The sporins in mullein might have an expectorant effect and some activity against herpes simplex virus, but this is unproven.

Mullein can cause drowsiness, nausea, and hypersensitivity reactions.

Significant research is lacking.

Mussel can cause gastrointestinal side effects.

Significant research is lacking.

Mustard can irritate the skin, accentuate asthma, and damage the thyroid gland.

Myrrh is probably antimicrobial, deodorizing, and anti-inflammatory. It might lower blood sugar.

Side effects are possible: fever, increased systemic inflammation, increased uterine bleeding, diarrhea, kidney irritation, and rapid heart rate.

Myrtle could possibly be dangerous with other drugs that lower blood sugar. It could possibly damage the liver.

Significant research is lacking.

NAC might interfere with insulin.

NADH is the activated form of vitamin $B_3$ (niacin).

Niacin has been effective for pellagra. It has helped some with mixed hyperlipidemia.

Niacin is high in possible adverse side effects (headaches, dizziness, nausea, vomiting, diarrhea, liver damage, high blood sugar, flushing, itching, and dental pain). The side effects increase as the dose is increased.

## What They Told You

dial infarction. It has even been touted for schizophrenia. Niacinamide has been touted for diabetes.

### Neem—Gingivitis
Neem has been used as an insecticide in commercial preparations. It has been used in humans for worm infections, malaria, and gingivitis. It is contained in some commercial preparations of toothpaste. It has also been used in diabetes to lower blood sugar.

### Neroli—Insomnia
Neroli is an oil and should not be consumed but rather breathed. It is touted to help insomnia, help sad mood, and decrease anxiety.

### Nerve Root—Insomnia
Nerve root has been touted for insomnia, anxiety, diarrhea, and heavy menstrual bleeding.

### Nettle—Hay Fever
Nettle is literally found all around the world. It is rich in iron. Iron is important in the production of red blood cells and hemoglobin. It also is touted to contain natural antihistamines (that would help in hay fever) and anti-inflammatories that would help in arthritis, prostatitis, and urinary tract infections. It is touted to help in benign prostate enlargement, bed wetting, and kidney stones.

### Niacin (Vitamin B₃)—High Cholesterol
See NADH.

### Niacinamide—Diabetes Mellitus
See NADH.

### Norepinephrine
See Monoamine Precursors.

### Notoginseng Root (panax pseudoginseng)—Bleeding
Notoginseng, from China, has been touted to stop bleeding such as nosebleeds and injuries. It has also been touted to improve stamina and Crohn's disease.

It is touted to stop bleeding without making a blood clot.

## What They Did Not Tell You

Concerns have been raised about potential insulin resistance in regard to its being tried for diabetes.

Effectiveness has not been established for any of the claims. It is certainly more safe when the oil is used orally in small amounts. The seeds especially can cause poisoning. It can cause confusion, convulsions, and even death in excessive amounts, even more so in children.

In animals it has reduced blood sugar substantially.

Research is lacking if existing at all.

Significant research is lacking.

Nerve root can cause hallucinations, anxiety, headache, and insomnia.

Nettle is safe for most people. Gastrointestinal side effects and an allergic skin reaction are possible.

Research is lacking. The use is apparently based on folklore. Side effects are largely unknown except it could cause a miscarriage in pregnancy.

The claim of stopping bleeding without clotting is hard to believe.

**What They Told You**

**What They Did Not Tell You**

### Nutmeg

Nutmeg is often used in custard pies. But it has also been used for bad breath, indigestion, anxiety, diarrhea, joint pain, and as an aphrodisiac. It is touted to have antiinflammatory, hypolipidemic, and chemoprotective actions.

A little nutmeg may taste good in custard pie, but when taken for medicinal purposes, dangerous reactions are possible: death, confusion, seizures, vomiting, constipation, and spontaneous abortion. Indeed nutmeg can be toxic, especially in large doses.

### Nux Vomica

Nux vomica is used for impotence, diseases of the gastrointestinal tract, circulatory problems, depression, migraine headaches, neuralgias, and menstrual discomfort. Historically, nux vomica has been used as an oral tonic for increasing appetite. It has also been used as a rodenticide.

Dosage safety has not been determined.

Nux vomica has been used in over-the-counter homeopathic products for headaches.

Nux vomica is unsafe due to its contents of strychnine. One to two grams of nux vomica contains 60–90 mg of strychnine and can cause severe adverse effects. Chronic ingestion over several weeks of lesser amounts can lead to death. Strychnine is a centrally acting neurotoxin and in sufficient amounts can lead to a full contraction of all voluntary muscles. Death results from impaired respirations or exhaustion.

Nux vomica is considered toxic and should be avoided.

### Oak—Kidney Stones

Oak has been touted for kidney stones.

Significant research is lacking.

### Oat Bran—High Cholesterol

See Bran.

### Oats (avera sativa)

Oatmeal has a reputation for being soothing, nourishing, tasty, and healthy.

It has been used to help lower cholesterol.

In this case especially, what they told you on the opposite side of the page is true.

### Octacosanol—Athletic Performance

Octacosanol has been touted to lower triglycerides and increase athletic performance.

Significant research is lacking.

It can cause movement disorders, anxiety, and can interact with sinemet that is used for parkinsonism.

### Olive—High Blood Pressure

Olive oil has been used as a mild laxative. It has also been touted to reduce the risk of asthrosclerotic heart disease, breast cancer, rheumatoid arthritis, and hypertension.

Olive leaf has been used for lowering blood pressure.

Some preliminary scientific data points to a degree of effectiveness for those issues touted on the left side of the page.

Other preliminary data on the leaf points toward some hypoglycemic, antispasmodic, hypotensive, antiarrhythmic, bronchodilator, or coronary dilator, and diuretic

## What They Told You

## What They Did Not Tell You

effects. More research is needed to see if the various seemingly beneficial effects bear out.

It is usually safe for most with the amounts in foods.

### Omega-3 Fatty Acids—Mood Stabilizer

**How it has been used:** It seems to have at times potential benefits in bipolar disorder, some data for unipolar depression, well-tolerated often, no known drug interactions, and other possible health benefits on the heart, GI tract, and joints. It has also been used for weight loss. It is relatively inexpensive. Crohn's disease symptoms have been reported to decrease with it at times. Also, cognitive enhancement has been reported. There have been suggestions that it might help in schizophrenia and ADHD. It has also been promoted for cardiovascular health and to lower blood pressure.

**Some interesting data:** Antioxidants (C, E, etc.) may prevent in vivo degradation of omega-3 fatty acid.

**Historical data:** Around 100 years ago the human diet contained about an equal amount of omega-6 and omega-3 fatty acids. The vegetable oil industry changed and began to hydrogenate oil which decreased omega-3 content, and the livestock industry began to use more grains to prepare the animal for slaughter. Grains are rich in omega-6 and low in omega-3. The American diet now consists of about a 25 to 1 ratio of omega-6 to omega-3, resulting in a diet that is perhaps too high in omega-6 and too low in omega-3. Omega-6 is helpful when a person is injured by causing the blood to clot and the blood vessels to constrict, preventing further blood loss. Omega-3 inhibits clotting and relaxes vascular smooth muscle. The ratio of omega-6 to omega-3 may be a factor in heart disease (Goldberg, p. 181).

**The usual dose:** The usual dose is 3–5 grams per day.

More clinical data is needed. GI distress may occur. One may smell like a fish and have a fishy aftertaste with some brands. There is at least a theoretical risk of increased bleeding, so it could be dangerous with aspirin, NSAIDs, and anticoagulants.

Are there any long-term risks? There are reports of either "mania, hypomania, or worsening of a mixed state" (*Information Drug Therapy Newsletter,* 21 September 2000).

**Clinical studies:** Early double-blind, placebo-controlled studies suggest that omega-3 fatty acids may improve the course of bipolar disorder. Also in one study in geriatric patients, omega-3 fatty acids significantly reduced apathy and withdrawal.

**The mechanism of action:** Omega-3 fatty acid is the best natural source of alpha-linolenic acid, which is required for the structural integrity of all cell membranes. It may reduce serum triglyceride levels in some people. Omega-3 fatty acid also relaxes vascular smooth muscle and is reported to have an antiarrhythmic effect.

### Onion—Common Cold

Onion is well-known as a food or for its seasoning ability. It has also been touted to help in colds, coughing, high cholesterol, diabetes, high blood pressure, asthma, and tumors.

It is often given as 1 teaspoon of onion juice 3 times per day or 1/2 of a cup of chopped onions per day.

Interesting! Wouldn't it be interesting if indeed this common food proves helpful for some people? Needless to say, volunteers are not lining up for double-blind studies (because of onion breath to what is otherwise usually an innocuous substance).

### Oregana—Upper Respiratory Infections

Significant research is lacking.

## What They Told You

Oregana has been touted for upper respiratory infections.

### Oregon Grape—Psoriasis
Oregon grape has been used for psoriasis and many other ailments.

### Oswego Tea—Flatulence
Orally, oswego tea is touted for digestive disorders including flatulence and premenstrual syndrome. It is also touted as an antispasmodic and diuretic.

### Pancreatin—Flatulence
Orally, pancreatin is touted to treat malabsorption syndromes associated with pancreatic insufficiency in cystic fibrosis, chronic pancreatitis, or pancreas removal. It is also touted orally for flatulence or as a digestive aid.

### Pantethine—High Cholesterol
Pantethine is touted for lowering cholesterol and triglyceride levels.

### Pantothenic Acid—Rheumatoid Arthritis
Orally, pantothenic acid is touted for treating dietary deficiencies, acne, alcoholism, allergies, alopecia, asthma, autism, carpal tunnel syndrome, respiratory disorders, colitis, convulsions, and cystitis. It is also touted for dandruff, depression, headache, hypoglycemia, insomnia, irritability, low blood pressure, multiple sclerosis, muscular dystrophy, osteoarthritis, rheumatoid arthritis, Parkinson's disease, PMS, reducing signs of aging, skin disorders, vertigo, and wound healing.

Topically, dexpanthenol, an analog of pantothenic acid, is used for itching, promoting healing of mild eczemas and dermatoses, insect stings, bites, poison ivy, diaper rash, acne, and preventing and treating acute radiotherapy skin reactions.

Intramuscularly or by intravenous infusion, dexpanthenol is used for stimulating intestinal peristalsis, to minimize the possibility of paralytic ileus after major abdominal surgery,

## What They Did Not Tell You

Oregana can cause gastrointestinal upset, edema, and inability to breathe.

Significant research is lacking.

Oregon grape can be dangerous. More than 500 mg have been associated with many side effects (fatigue, nosebleed, hemorrhagic nephritis, cardiac damage, diarrhea, respiratory arrest, and death).

Insufficient reliable information is available. No adverse effects have been reported.

Orally, excessive doses of pancreatin can cause nausea, vomiting, diarrhea or other transient intestinal upset, and perianal soreness. Extremely high doses have been associated with high uric acid level in blood and urine and colon strictures. Pancreatin powder is irritating to the skin, eyes, mucous membranes, and respiratory tract.

Reliable information is insufficient.

Orally, large amounts of pantothenic acid can cause diarrhea or eosinophilic pleuropericardial effusion.

Topically, dexpanthenol, an alcohol analog of pantothenic acid, can cause chronic dermatitis.

**What They Told You**

for intestinal atony causing abdominal distension, postoperative or postpartum flatus, and for postoperative delay in resumption of intestinal motility.

### Papain—Inflammation
Orally, papain is touted for inflammation and edema following trauma and surgery, as a digestive aid, for treating parasitic worms, inflammation of the throat and pharynx, herpes zoster symptoms, chronic diarrhea, hay fever, nasal drainage, and psoriasis. Papain is also touted as an adjuvant treatment for tumors.

Topically, it is touted to treat infected wounds, sores, and ulcers.

### Papaya—Intestinal Parasites
Papaya is an orange fruit from South America that has been added to some beer preparations, is eaten for breakfast, is in some commercial jellies, is touted to help heartburn, thin the blood, and work against intestinal parasites.

### Parsley—Bad Breath
Parsley was used by the ancient Greeks for bad breath.

It has long been used for flavoring in soups and sauces. Of course it is often used around meats in restaurants.

### Partridge Berry—Menstrual Cramps
Partridge berry was used by Native American females for menstrual cramps. They used it topically for nipple soreness from nursing.

### Pav D'arco—Yeast Infections
This is a Brazilian herb, which has been touted to have antitumor effects. It has also been used for fungal and yeast infections.

### PC Specs—Prostate Health
This is a dietary supplement touted for prostate health.

### Peanut Oil—Heart Disease Prevention

**What They Did Not Tell You**

Orally, large amounts of papain can cause esophageal perforation. Ingestion of papaya latex (raw papain) can cause severe gastritis.

Topically, papaya latex can cause severe irritation and blisters. Topical use of papain can cause itching. Severe allergic reactions have been reported in sensitive individuals.

Effectiveness is not proven. It seems unstable in digestive juices, which raises the question of whether it could be effective. It could possibly cause bradycardia in some and even potentially have paralytic effects in some. Large amounts could even cause esophageal perforation.

Parsley is usually safe but in high doses could conceivably cause or intensify a variety of problems—kidney problems, intensify MAOI antidepressants, liver damage, heart disease.

Effectiveness and safety of partridge berries are not known. We are not aware of reported adverse reactions.

This herb can be lethal. Other less serious side effects include nausea, diarrhea, and weight loss.

This supplement has estrogen-like effects. Some samples have been found to be contaminated with the anticoagulant warfarin (Coumadin), other samples have been touted to be contaminated with the benzodiazepine alprasolam (Xanax), other samples have contained indomethacin (Indocin), and yet others contained the estrogen diethylstilbestrol.

Research is lacking regarding its effectiveness. The high

## What They Told You

Peanut oil has been touted for lowering cholesterol, preventing heart disease and cancer, and for weight loss, joint pain, and skin care.

## What They Did Not Tell You

monounsaturated fat content is thought to lower cholesterol and prevent heart disease. However, animal studies suggest it may cause asthroscleretic heart disease.

A few severe allergic reactions and deaths have occurred after eating peanuts.

### Pectin—High Cholesterol

Pectin, a fiber found in fruits and vegetables, has been touted to lower cholesterol and even reduce the risk of radiation therapy.

It has been used for diarrhea and has also been touted in diabetes.

Pectin is possibly not effective in lowering cholesterol in some. It can help in diarrhea.

For those who inhale too much pectin in their occupation, it can cause asthma.

### Pennyroyal

Pennyroyal is a member in the mint family. It has been used to induce abortions.

Pennyroyal is highly toxic and has resulted in numerous deaths.

### Peppermint—IBS

Mints have been used for medicinal purposes for thousands of years. The most popular is peppermint. It has been used to treat indigestion, gas, irritable bowel syndrome, gallstones, and colds. Externally it has been used for analgesic purposes. It is often used for flavoring. In fact, it is found everywhere today—in toothpastes, mouthwashes, candy, laxatives, antacids, and cold preparations.

The dosage for internal use is often 1 to 2 capsules (0.2 milliliters per capsule) 3 times daily between meals. Externally, a cream containing 1 to 16 percent menthol is applied to the affected area 3 times daily.

Side effects of peppermint may include skin rash, heartburn, slow heart rate, and tremors. It could possibly be a danger in liver disease or gallbladder disease. Infants should not take it.

However, having said the above, doses in moderation in most people are usually safe.

### Perilla—Asthma

Perilla, a plant from Asia, has been touted to help in asthma.

Research is needed. It might help some in asthma, but research is inadequate.

Allergic reactions are possible with topical use.

### Periwinkle—Dementia

Periwinkle has been touted for improving brain productivity, decreasing hypertension, and for blood purification.

Periwinkle contains toxic alkaloids such as vincristine, which can damage the liver and kidneys. It can cause leukocytopenia and lymphocytopenia due to its immunosuppressant effects.

### Perna

Perna is obtained from the New Zealand green-lipped mussel. People use this for symptoms of rheumatoid

Reliable information is insufficient about the safety and effectiveness of perna mussel. It may cause diarrhea, nausea, and flatulence.

## What They Told You

arthritis and osteoarthritis.
Dosage used is from 300 to 350 mg 3 times per day.

### Peru Balsam—Pain

Topically, peru balsam has been touted for infected and poorly healing wounds, burns, bed sores, frost bite, bruises caused by prosthetics, hemorrhoids, diaper rash, and intertrigo.

In dentistry, peru balsam is a component of dental preparations for treating dry sockets and as an ingredient in some dental impression materials. It is also used in toothpaste and tooth powder.

In traditional medicine, peru balsam has been used for cancer, to stop bleeding, to promote wound healing, as a diuretic, and to expel worms.

### Phenylalanine—Parkinsonism and Depression

Phenylalanine has been touted for parkinsonism and depression.

Phenylalanine is an amino acid. It is a precursor of tyrosine, which is a precursor of dopamine. By increasing the neurotransmitter, dopamine, in depressed individuals, mood, energy, and motivation might be enhanced. Increasing dopamine might also help in parkinsonism.

The usual dose is 200 to 500 mg per day.

### Phosphate Salts—Kidney Stones

Orally, phosphate salts are touted for treating hypophosphatemia and hypercalcemia, hypophosphatemic rickets or osteomalacia, and for prevention of recurrent nephrolithiasis (kidney stones). Phosphate salts are also touted for enhancing exercise performance, as an antacid for gastroesophageal reflux disease (GERD), and as a laxative for presurgical bowel preparation.

Topically, phosphate salts are used with calcium in dentistry for sensitive teeth.

Rectally, phosphate salts are used as a laxative for presurgical bowel preparation.

## What They Did Not Tell You

One case of hepatitis was associated with the New Zealand green-lipped mussel.

The product is thought to contain a prostaglandin inhibitor that exerts an anti-inflammatory effect, possibly aiding in relief of arthritis symptoms.

Orally, peru balsam can cause kidney damage with consumption of large amounts.

Topically, peru balsam can cause allergic skin reactions and contact dermatitis, including urticaria, recurring aphthoid oral ulcers, Quincke's disease, and diffuse purpurea. It has the potential to cause photodermatitis and phototoxicity. Kidney damage can also occur with the external use of large amounts.

The logic is interesting and worthy of more research. However, there is quite a jump in logic from exogenous phenylalanine to endogenous dopamine.

Phenylalanine is contraindicated in alkaptonuria, hypertension, phenylketonuria, schizophrenia, stroke, and those on levodopa, antipsychotics, and MAOIs. It can exacerbate tardive dyskinesia, tremor, and rigidity. Birth defects have occurred with its use.

Orally, phosphate salts can cause gastrointestinal irritation, fluid and electrolyte disturbances including hyperphosphatemia and hypocalcemia, and extraskeletal calcification. Potassium phosphates can cause hyperkalemia. Sodium phosphates can cause hypernatremia and hypokalemia. Sodium and potassium phosphates can cause diarrhea. Aluminum phosphate can cause constipation.

Rectally, phosphate salts can cause fluid and electrolyte disturbances including hyperphosphatemia and hypocalcemia, gastrointestinal irritation, and perforation of the rectum.

**What They Told You**

**What They Did Not Tell You**

Intravenously, potassium phosphate is used for hypophosphatemia and hypokalemia, preventing hypophosphatemia in people receiving parenteral nutrition, and treating hypercalcemia.

### Phosphatidyl Choline (PC)—Memory Loss
PC has been touted to lower cholesterol, help in memory loss, and help in depression.

PC has been used orally in combination with interferon for hepatitis C. Otherwise, research is lacking. It can induce gastrointestinal upset.

### Phosphatidylserine (PS)
Phosphatidylserine (PS) has been advertised as a product that helps keep the brain functioning in the way it does in youth. It is touted to have a positive effect on brain aging. A number of claims have been made about PS including: keeps cell membranes more flexible and permeable, increases dopamine release, restores youthful synaptic plasticity, augments brain glucose metabolism, increases the number of neurotransmitter receptor sites, and spurs the release of the acetylcholine. Many of the proponents of phosphatidylserine suggest memory function is enhanced.

Phosphatidylserine (PS) has been known to cause gastrointestinal upset and insomnia. Most PS supplements used to come from bovine cortex, so there was concern about possible contamination with mad cow disease. Using supplements from diseased animals might present a health hazard. Most manufacturers now use soy or cabbage to obtain PS. Reliable information is not available concerning PS and interaction with herbs, drugs, foods, or other supplements.

PS has been reported to be more effective in patients with less severe symptoms and may lose some of its effectiveness with extended use.

PS reportedly enters the bloodstream within 30 minutes of ingestion and is soon found in the liver and shortly thereafter in the brain, where it readily crosses the blood-brain barrier. Its action in the brain is concentrated on the nerve cell membrane that controls the movement of nutrients, waste products, ions, neurotransmitters, and other molecules into and out of the cell. PS is the most dominant of the 5 types of phospholipid that comprise cell membranes. It has been described as a kind of "biologic detergent" to help keep fatty substances soluble and cell membranes fluid, enabling hormones, neurotransmitters, and other substances to be more effectively transported for use by the cell. PS may halt the destruction of neuronal dendrite spines, the loss of which is associated with aging.

At least two randomized, double-blind studies are reported on the use of PS for memory enhancement. Dr. T. Crock of the Memory Assessment Clinics in Bethesda, Maryland, reported significant improvement in learning names and faces, recalling names and faces and facial recognition in addition to recalling telephone numbers and improved concentration while reading in study subjects taking PS versus placebo. Some evidence suggests PS may reduce exercise-induced stress by lowering cortisol.

| What They Told You | What They Did Not Tell You |
|---|---|
| Phosphatidylserine is usually supplied in 100 mg capsules. The usual dose is 100 mg 3 to 4 times a day. | |

### Phyllanthus—Hepatitis and HIV

Phyllanthus has been touted to help in hepatitis and HIV.

It comes in a liquid extract.

Effectiveness and safety are not proven.

### Phytodolor—Arthritis

Phytodolor has been touted for both osteoarthritis and rheumatoid arthritis. It has also been touted to help in the treatment of trauma and athletic injury.

There is insufficient reliable information available.

### Picrorrhiza—Hepatitis

Picrorrhiza has been touted for hepatitis.

Picrorrhiza can cause gas, diarrhea, and a skin rash.

Effectiveness and safety are not proven.

### Pimpinella Root—Inflammation

Orally, pimpinella root is touted for upper respiratory tract mucous membrane inflammation.

Topically, pimpinella root is touted for inflammation of the oral and pharyngeal mucous membranes and as a bath additive for poorly healing wounds.

In folk medicine pimpinella root is used for urinary tract disorders and inflammation, bladder and kidney stones, edema, and "flushing out" therapy for urinary tract bacterial inflammation.

No adverse side effects have been reported. However, it may cause photosensitivity in fair-skinned individuals.

### Pineapple—Arthritis

See Bromelain.

### Pipsissewa—High Blood Sugar

Pipsissewa has been touted for many ailments (diabetes mellitus, anxiety, gastrointestinal upset, seizures, and kidney stones).

Significant research is lacking.

Pipsissewa can cause gastrointestinal upset. Other side effects are not fully known.

### Piracetam—Cognitive Enhancement

Piracetam has been described as an intelligence booster and central nervous system stimulant with no apparent toxicity or addictive potential. The word *nootropic* was prompted by the invention, in Belgium, of piracetam. Nootropic is a Greek term meaning "acting on the brain." Piracetam, which has been around for about 30 years, is

Piracetam may increase the effects of certain drugs such as amphetamines and medications used to treat anxiety, depression, and other psychiatric disorders. Adverse effects may include insomnia, psychomotor agitation, nausea, upset stomach, and headaches. More studies need to be done to evaluate its safety and effectiveness in humans.

**What They Told You**

similar in structure to amino acids. It is a derivative of GABA (gamma amino butyric acid, a neurotransmitter) but does not appear to work through the GABAnergic system. Piracetam is thought to enhance memory and learning and has been used outside the USA for disorders affecting cognition caused from lack of oxygen to the brain tissues, alcoholism, stroke, vertigo, senile dementia, and sickle cell anemia. Studies in mice indicate an increase in muscarinic cholinergic receptors in the frontal cortexes, and older mice had higher density of these receptors after treatment with piracetam.

A September 2001 article in the neurology journal *Stroke* indicated stoke victims' brain scans showed more activity in areas of the brain that control language skills after treatment with 4800 mg of piracetam daily. There are reports of its use in ADHD and dyslexia.

Piracetam is supplied in 400 mg to 800 mg capsules or tablets. The usual dose is 2400 to 4800 mg per day in 3 divided doses. Some individuals have reported taking up to 8000 mg daily.

**What They Did Not Tell You**

*Plantain—Constipation*

Psyllium, the well-known laxative (but also used for diarrhea), is from plantain. Plantain also has a long history of being used for skin irritations.

Plantain can have gastrointestinal side effects (nausea, diarrhea, obstruction).

It can decrease the effectiveness of Tegratol and lithium and increase the effects of some cardiac drugs such as beta-blockers, calcium channel blockers, and cardiac glycosides.

*Pleurisy Root—Pleurisy*

Pleurisy root has been touted for pleurisy.

Pleurisy root is probably unsafe for most because it contains digitalis-like cardenolide glycosides. Thus, it could cause digitalis-like poisoning especially at higher doses. Also, it can cause nausea, vomiting, and uterine stimulation.

Effectiveness is not proven.

It could interact with digoxin, antidepressants, and hormones.

*Poison Ivy—Pain*

In folk medicine poison ivy was used as a narcotic.

Reliable information is insufficient about the effectiveness of poison ivy.

Orally, the plant can cause severe mucous membrane irritation, nausea, vomiting, intestinal colic, diarrhea, dizzi-

| What They Told You | What They Did Not Tell You |
|---|---|
| | ness, stupor, nephritis, hematuria, fever, and unconsciousness. |
| | Topically, the plant can cause severe contact dermatitis, reddening, swelling, and herpes-like blisters. |
| | Eye contact can cause severe conjunctivitis, corneal inflammations, or loss of sight. |
| | Inhalation due to burning the plant can result in fever, major lung infection, and death from throat swelling. |

**Pokeweed—Laxative**
Pokeweed has been touted to be antiviral, antifungal, and anticancer. It has also been used as a laxative.

Significant research is lacking.

It can have side effects potentially (gastrointestinal upset, confusion, seizures, hypotension, and many others).

**Policosanol—Plaque**
Orally, policosanol is touted for hyperlipidemia, for intermittent claudication, for decreasing myocardial ischemia in patients with coronary heart disease, and as an antiplaque agent.

Orally, policosanol can cause erythema, migraines, insomnia, somnolence, irritability, dizziness, upset stomach, polyphagia, dysuria, weight loss, skin rash, and nose and gum bleeding.

**Polygonum (fo-gi)—Schizophrenia**
Polygonum is a Chinese herb touted for a wide variety of disorders including insomnia and even schizophrenia.

Polygonum has been associated with nausea, vomiting, and diarrhea. There are serious questions about its safety.

It is certainly not up to treating schizophrenia.

**Pomegranate—Tapeworm**
Pomegranate has been touted for various intestinal worms. It has also been touted for diabetes mellitus. Finally, it has been touted to have antiviral effects.

Pomegranate can cause gastrointestinal upset, liver damage, and possibly even cancer. In high doses it can even cause death.

**Poplar—Arthritis**
Poplar has been touted for upper respiratory infections and arthritis.

Poplar contains a salicylate similar to that in commercial aspirin.

It can increase bleeding time, damage the liver, and cause ear ringing.

**Poppy—Pain**
Poppy has been used for its analgesic effects.

Poppy has been used to make opiates, which is illegal.

**Potassium—Hypertension**
Oral potassium has been used to treat hypokalemia. It has

The list of touted treatments goes on almost endlessly. Of course, potassium does help in hypokalemia, and it

**What They Told You**

also been touted for hypertension, insulin resistance, heart attacks, stroke prevention, fatigue, allergies, and Alzheimer's disease.

### Potato—Weight Loss

Raw potato has been touted for gastrointestinal disorders. An extract has been tried in weight loss.

### Precatory Bean

In folk medicine, precatory bean is used orally to quicken labor, as an abortifacient, oral contraceptive, and as an analgesic in terminally ill patients. The whole plant is used for ophthalmic inflammations.

### Pregnenolone—Aging

Pregnenolone has been touted for aging, depression, PMS, poor memory, MS, psoriasis, seizures, injuries, and BPH.

### Prickly Ash—High Blood Pressure

Prickly ash has been touted for high blood pressure, fever, gas, and arthritis.

### Probiotics

Probiotics are bacteria that are helpful in normal digestion. They include acidophilus and bifidobacteria.

**What They Did Not Tell You**

might help lower blood pressure a little in some people. Research is largely lacking for the rest.

Potato is abundant in vitamin C, vitamin $B_2$, iron, and carbohydrates. Satietrol (a proteinase inhibitor) could theoretically decrease appetite, but in general significant intake of potatoes would lead to weight gain.

Orally, the seeds that are chewed or with cracked shells can cause stomach cramping, nausea, vomiting, severe diarrhea (possibly bloody), cold sweat, fever, weakness, tachycardia, coma, circulatory collapse, cerebral edema, and death. Signs of toxicity, including gastroenteritis usually occurs several hours after ingestion of the seeds, followed by the development of bloody diarrhea. Symptoms may last for up to 10 days. Fatalities have usually occurred 3–4 days after ingestion of the seeds.

Topically, the seeds when used as a necklace can cause dermatitis. Eye contact with the seed's contents can cause necrotizing conjunctivitis. There is no known antidote. There is no method for enhancing elimination. Patients seen within four hours of seed ingestion should be treated with usual decontamination methods including lavage, charcoal, and cathartics. In cases of diarrhea, the need for cathartics may be unnecessary.

Pregnenolone is a precursor of all of the steroid hormones (DHEA, progesterone, cortisol, testosterone, estrogen, aldosterone). Thus, it could potentially cause multiple steroid-like side effects.

Effectiveness of prickly ash is not proven.

It can be a uterine stimulant.

One study identified hepatic carcinogen enzymes present after this herb was used.

Toxicity can result in hypotension.

At times they probably do help return digestion to normal as when antibiotics have upset the digestive system.

## What They Told You

## What They Did Not Tell You

### Progesterone (Natural Progesterone)—Anxiety
Natural progesterone has been used for antianxiety, antianger, and mood-stabilizing effects.

The usual dose is 100–200 mg 2 to 3 times per day.

Natural progesterone may cause depression and weight gain. It is touted to have fewer side effects than synthetic properties.

### Propolis—Infections
Propolis has been touted to have antiviral, anticancer, anti-inflammatory, and antibacterial effects.

Propolis can cause contact dermatitis.

### Psyllium—Obesity
Please see Plantain.

In addition to its use as a laxative, it has been used for weight loss and might even result in lower blood sugar. It is what Metamucil, a famous over-the-counter laxative, is made of. It pulls fluid into the gut, creates a feeling of fullness, and then suppresses appetite. By pulling fluid into the gut, it softens its contents and thus, is a laxative.

One tablespoon in 8 ounces of water per day is often recommended, or 4 to 6 psyllium capsules daily is often recommended.

Psyllium could cause constipation. It should not be used simultaneously with other drugs since absorption of the other drug will be affected and decrease the other drug's effectiveness. It may lower blood sugar levels in diabetics. It should not be used with drugs such as Imodium, designed to slow intestinal motility.

### Pulsatilla—Otitis Media
Pulsatilla has been touted to help in otitis media, insomnia, anxiety, and cataracts.

Pulsatilla can cause gastrointestinal upset, proteinuria, and hematuria. In high doses it has caused seizures and kidney damage.

### Pumpkin—Benign Prostate Hypertrophy (BPH)
Pumpkin has been used for the pain associated with BPH. Pumpkin seed has been used because of its diuretic effect to relieve bladder discomfort and thus, help in BPH.

Pumpkin is probably effective in the manner described, at least to a mild degree in some men.

### Puncture Vine—Low Sex Drive
Puncture vine has been touted to improve sex drive.

Research is lacking and side effects are not known.

### Pycnogenol
See Grape Seed Extract.

### Pygeum—Benign Prostate Hypertrophy (BPH)
Pygeum has been used in benign prostate hypertrophy.

It is usually given at 75 to 150 mg per day.

Side effects of pygeum appear to be low.

Some research suggests that pygeum may partially work by antiproliferative effects on fibroblasts. Others feel the benefit comes from ferulic acid esters of fatty acids that reduce prostatic cholesterol levels. Others feel the phytosterols help by inhibiting prostaglandin biosynthesis. Others point to possible anti-inflammatory effects from triterpenes.

**What They Told You**

**What They Did Not Tell You**

In summary, by whatever mechanism it is likely effective, at least for some, for symptoms of benign prostate hypertrophy.

One huge problem is that some men think they have BPH when they really have prostatic cancer. We would highly encourage checking with your doctor. This is one mistake not to be made.

### Pyrethrum—Head Lice

Topically, pyrethrum is touted as an insecticide, particularly for head lice, crablice and their nits, and as an antiscabies agent.

Symptoms of overdose include headache, tinnitus, nausea, tingling of fingers and toes, respiratory disturbances, and other symptoms of neurotoxicity. The pyrethrum flower or derivatives of it might cause an allergic reaction in individuals sensitive to the Asteraceae/Compositae family.

### Pyridoxine (Vitamin B₆)—PMS

Vitamin B$_6$ has been touted for many disorders (PMS, autism, high cholesterol, diabetic neuropathy, protecting against cancer, leg cramps, asthma, stimulating appetite, menopause, infertility, dizziness, etc.).

Vitamin B$_6$ has obviously been overtouted. It is appropriate in vitamin B$_6$ deficiencies. Also, it may help at times with the nausea of pregnancy. It is not appropriate for autism, diabetic neuropathy, high cholesterol, and most of the many disorders often touted, and is probably not effective in PMS.

It can cause nausea, vomiting, headache, increased liver function, breast soreness, photosensitivity, and neuropathy to name a few.

### Queen Anne's Lace—Liver Damage

Queen Anne's lace has been touted to protect the liver and to relax most muscles.

Significant research is lacking.

This herb can lower blood pressure, be sedating, increase depression, and upset the stomach.

### Quercetin—Cancer

Orally, quercetin is touted for treating atherosclerosis, hypercholesterolemia, coronary heart disease, diabetes, cataracts, allergies, peptic ulcer, schizophrenia, inflammation, asthma, gout, viral infections, preventing cancer, and for treating chronic, bacterial prostatitis.

Intravenously and intraperitoneally, quercetin is used for treating cancer.

Orally, quercetin can cause headache and tingling of the extremities.

Intravenous administration of quercetin is associated with flushing, sweating, dyspnea, nausea, and vomiting. Injection pain can be minimized by premedicating patient with 10 mg of morphine and administering amounts greater than 945 mg/m2 over 5 minutes. Nephrotoxicity has been reported with use of amounts greater than 945 mg/m2.

| What They Told You | What They Did Not Tell You |
|---|---|
| **Quince—Gonorrhea**<br>Quince has been touted to help in gonorrhea. | Significant research is lacking.<br>The seeds can be toxic. |
| **Quinine—Malaria**<br>Quinine has been used to treat malaria. | Quinine has been used for malaria, but malaria is a disease that only an internist should tackle.<br><br>Potential side effects of quinine are varied and many (heart failure, seizures, severe gastrointestinal upset, kidney damage, bleeding, severe skin reactions, and confusion). |
| **Raspberry—PMS**<br>This fruit is tasty and has been touted for menstrual cramps. | Studies of the use of raspberry are conflicting and contradicting. Does it cause uterine relaxation or stimulation? Thus, it should not be used during pregnancy although at this time it often is. |
| **Rauwolfia—High Blood Pressure**<br>Rauwolfia has been used for high blood pressure. | Reserpine came from rauwolfia and was used many years for high blood pressure. However, it has been largely replaced by newer, more effective medication with fewer side effects overall.<br><br>The potential side effects are many (bleeding, gastrointestinal upset, depression, sedation, seizures, and parkinsonism).<br><br>The potential interactions with various medications (alcohol, opioids, digoxin, beta-blockers, amphetamines, MAOIs, etc.) are many. |
| **Red Bush Tea—Antiaging**<br>Red bush tea has been touted for antiaging. | Significant research is lacking. |
| **Red Clover—PMS**<br>Red clover comes from Europe but has done well in North America and is, in fact, the state flower of Vermont. It has estrogen-like compounds and has been used for PMS and menopause. | The debate is intense between those who warn that red clover may contribute to cancer (breast, prostate, etc.) and those who feel it is safe.<br><br>Certainly pregnant females should not take it. Neither should those with estrogen-related cancers. |
| **Red Maple—Eye Conditions**<br>In Native American folk medicine, red maple was used topically for eye conditions and as an astringent. | Reliable information is insufficient about the effectiveness of red maple. No adverse effects reported. |
| **Red Yeast—High Cholesterol** | Red yeast can be dangerous when used with several of |

**What They Told You**

Red yeast is fermented rice by monascus purpureus yeast. It has been used to lower cholesterol and triglycerides.

**What They Did Not Tell You**

the common cholesterol-lowering drugs because of drug interactions. It too contains statins (primarily levastatin) just as they do. The statins block cholesterol biosynthesis.

Side effects are certainly possible (elevated liver enzymes, gastritis, renal dysfunction, and skeletal muscle destruction).

High cholesterol is too dangerous to treat without a medical doctor, and side effects are too serious to treat oneself.

### Reishi—Aging

Reshi has been used for years in China for its touted anti-aging effects.

Significant research is lacking.

### Rhubarb—Constipation

Rhubarb pie sounds tempting to some. In addition, rhubarb has been touted for use in constipation, diarrhea, gastritis, and hemorrhoids.

Rhubarb can cause abdominal cramps and diarrhea. Chronic use can accelerate bone deterioration, cause hyperaldersteronism, lead to electrolyte loss, and cause hematuria, just to name a few possible adverse reactions.

### Riboflavin (Vitamin B₂)—Migraines

Riboflavin has been used for riboflavin deficiencies.

It has been touted for migraine headaches and cataract prevention.

More research is needed.

It can cause diarrhea and polyuria. It can cause an orange urine.

It can interact with aspirin, Retrovir, and other antiviral drugs.

It might be more effective for some in migraine prevention when combined with beta-blockers.

### RNA/DNA—Alzheimer's Dementia

RNA/DNA combinations are touted to improve memory. They have been used in depression, fatigue, low sex drive, and aging. The combination includes omega-3 fatty acids and arginine.

RNA might help in recovery time after surgery for some. It might help in serious illness for some. It probably does not do a lot for mental sharpness.

### Rose Hips—URIs

Rose hips has been touted for upper respiratory infections (URIs), urinary tract infections (UTIs), constipation, and arthritis.

It is high in vitamin C.

Rose hips can cause gastrointestinal upset.

| What They Told You | What They Did Not Tell You |
|---|---|
| **Rosemary—Alzheimer's Dementia** | Rosemary is usually safe for most people. However, it contains camphor, which can cause convulsions, so it should not be used in epilepsy or in excess. |
| Rosemary, a scented herb originally from Spain, has been used for arthritis, indigestion problems, circulatory problems, and liver problems. It, along with gingko biloba and sage, has also been used for Alzheimer's dementia. | |
| **Roseroot—Increasing Energy** | There is insufficient reliable information available. |
| Orally, roseroot is touted for increasing energy, stamina, strength, and mental capacity, and as a so-called "adaptogen" to help the body adapt to and resist physical, chemical, and environmental stress. It is also touted for improving athletic performance, improving sexual function, depression, and for cardiac disorders such as arrhythmias and hyperlipidemia. Roseroot is also touted for treating cancer, tuberculosis, and diabetes; preventing cold and flu, aging, and liver damage; improving hearing; strengthening the nervous system; enhancing immunity; and shortening recovery time after prolonged workouts. | |
| **Royal Jelly—High Cholesterol** | Significant research is lacking. |
| Royal jelly comes from bees. It contains the B vitamins, acetylcholine, minerals, enzymes, hormones, and amino acids. | It appears safe for many but certainly less safe in those with asthma who are more prone to allergic reactions. Topically, allergic reactions are possible also. |
| It has been touted to lower high cholesterol and to help in asthma, liver disease, insomnia, ulcers, kidney disease, and skin disorders. | |
| **Rue—Snakebites** | Significant research is lacking. |
| Rue has been touted for arthritis, anxiety, and snakebites. | Rue can cause spontaneous abortions, lower blood pressure, and interact with heart and blood pressure medications. |
| **Rutin—Osteoarthritis** | Orally, rutin may cause headaches, flushing, rashes, or mild gastrointestinal disturbance. |
| Orally, rutin is touted as a vascular protectant; for reducing capillary permeability, fragility, and bleeding; for treating varicose vein symptoms; and prophylaxis of mucositis associated with cancer treatments. In combination with trypsin and bromelain, rutin is touted orally for osteoarthritis. | |
| In Chinese medicine, rutin has been used orally to treat internal bleeding and bleeding hemorrhoids and to prevent strokes. | |
| **Safflower—High Blood Pressure** | Significant research is lacking. |
| Safflower has been touted for arthritis, URIs, yeast infections, high blood pressure, and constipation. | It appears safflower might lower blood pressure and is often low on side effects, but only time will tell. |

## What They Told You

### What They Did Not Tell You

*Sage—Menopausal Night Sweats*
This mintlike herb has been used for perspiration as in menopausal night sweats. Sage has also been touted to help in bad breath and indigestion. Some drink it in tea form for indigestion and Alzheimer's dementia. Others gargle it for sore throat or bad breath. It has been used for excessive perspiration.

Research of sage is lacking.

Sage is safe for most people. Often the danger of herbs comes from excess use. Even sage could conceivably cause convulsions, dizziness, and rapid heartbeat.

*Saint-John's-Wort (hypericum perferatum)—*
*Depression*
Saint-John's-wort has been called "nature's Prozac."

Saint-John's-wort is *no* Prozac!

**Health concerns:** For some it is probably more effective than placebo in the treatment of mild to moderate depression. Major depression can be a lethal disease and should not usually be treated lightly with Saint-John's-wort.

**How it has been used:** A number of unscientific articles indicate Saint-John's-wort is good for depression, anxiety, burns, indigestion, myalgia, seasonal affective disorder (SAD), alcoholism, arthritis, chickenpox, flu, hepatitis, herpes, HIV, vertigo, bed-wetting, gallbladder problems, hemorrhoids, kidney disease, and worms.

Some individuals taking this product have complained of dry mouth, dizziness, constipation, confusion, and other gastrointestinal discomfort.

Orally, Saint-John's-wort is used for depression and dysthymic disorder, and in Germany the herb outsells and is more prescribed than are many prescription antidepressants. It is also used to treat secondary symptoms associated with depression such as fatigue, loss of appetite, insomnia, anxiety, or nervous unrest; obsessive-compulsive mood disturbances associated with menopause (4); migraine headache; neuralgia; disorder (OCD), excitability; fibrositis; sciatica, lack of drive; palpitations; exhaustion; headache, and muscle pain. It is also used orally for treating cancer, vitiligo, and as a diuretic. Oily Saint-John's-wort preparations are used orally for gastric indigestion. Topically, oily Saint-John's-wort preparations are used for treating bruises and abrasions, muscle pain, first-degree burns, hemorrhoids, relieving inflammation, promoting healing, and neuralgia. Saint-John's-wort and its constituents, hypericin and pseudohypericin, have been shown to have activity against viruses and bacteria including influenza virus, herpes simplex virus types I and II, sindbis virus, poliovirus, retrovirus, murine cytomegalovirus, hepatitis C, and Gram negative and Gram positive bacteria. Hyperforin has been shown to inhibit growth of penicillin- and methicillin-resistant staphylococcus aureus and other Gram positive organisms, but not Gram negative organisms.

It could be potentially dangerous with antidepressants. It can cause sunburn. Recent evidence indicated interactions with digoxin, l-dopa, 5-hydroxtryptophan theophylline, protease inhibitors, and drugs used to combat transplant rejection. It may also cause Serotonin Syndrome if used with other antidepressants. Certain foods should also be avoided if taking Saint-John's-wort including cheeses, beer, wine, pickled herring, and yeast. Animals grazing on the plant suffered severe photosensitivity and skin problems (Murray, p. 300).

"It occasionally causes GI upset, agitation, and phototoxicity" (*Psychopharmacology Update*, 2000, Baylor College of Medicine, Houston).

It causes significant induction of an enzyme system in the liver (CYP4503A4) and, thus, could be dangerous when used with other medications.

Saint-John's-wort can seriously interfere with a variety of drugs, to include those used to treat the AIDS virus as well as antirejection medications used with transplant recipients.

**Some interesting data:** It is named after John the Baptist plus wort, an old English name for plant. "It was thought to be so obnoxious to evil spirits that a whiff of it

Saint-John's-wort extracts have also been shown to prolong narcotic-induced sleep time, decrease barbiturate-induced sleep time, and antagonize the effects of

## What They Told You

could cause them to depart" (Murray, p. 295).

**Historical data:** Saint-John's-wort is a common plant and is considered a weed in many locales. It has a long history of folk use. Many of the founding fathers in medicine (as Hippocrates) used it to treat many illnesses. It is often well tolerated and has no sexual side effects. It has been used for many ailments over the years. Initially it was thought that this botanical supplement rarely, if ever, led to any drug interactions. In Europe, it has a long history of use as a folk remedy especially in depression.

**The usual dose:** The usual dose is 300 mg 3 times per day.

## What They Did Not Tell You

reserpine. Hypericin is photodynamically active and is thought to be the constituent responsible for phototoxicity reactions, and its use in strong sunlight should be questioned. The polar fraction of a methanolic Saint-John's-wort extract, but not isolated hypericin, inhibits cytochrome P450 3A4 (CYP3A4) activity in human liver microsomes. These are major metabolic liver pathways, and Saint-John's-wort may as a result interfere with a large number of agents normally metabolized via these pathways. Clinical evidence suggests that Saint-John's-wort actually induces these enzymes. Evidence suggests that Saint-John's-wort may also affect the activity of P-glycoprotein, which mediates the absorption and elimination of digoxin and other drugs. Saint-John's-wort does not appear to affect CYPIA2 or Nacetyltransferase (NAT2).

Saint-John's-wort use has been associated with reports of intermenstrual bleeding and one report of changed menstrual bleeding. Most of the women in these reports were taking an oral contraceptive, and the changes in menstrual bleeding may be the result of a drug interaction.

Photosensitivity and photodermatitis have been reported. Light or fair-skinned people should employ protective measures against direct sunlight when using Saint-John's-wort due to its potential photosensitivity effects. Neuropathy after sun exposure has also been reported with the use of Saint-John's-wort. There is some indication that Saint-John's-wort may be associated with a higher incidence of cataracts. The hypericin constituent is photoactive and, in the presence of light, may damage lens proteins, leading to cataracts. Some evidence suggests that high doses of Saint-John's-wort may reduce male and female fertility, but this effect has not been demonstrated in humans. Saint-John's-wort could lead to withdrawal effects similar to those found with conventional antidepressants, including headache, nausea, dizziness, insomnia, paresthesias, confusion, and fatigue. Topically, Saint-John's-wort oil may irritate the skin.

Concomitant use of Saint-John's-wort with digitalis could reduce therapeutic effects. Saint-John's-wort extract decreases digoxin serum levels in healthy people, and Saint-John's-wort seems to lower digoxin serum concentrations.

**What They Told You**

**What They Did Not Tell You**

The concomitant use of Saint-John's-wort with selective serotonin agonists and reuptake inhibitors could increase the risk of serotonergic adverse effects and serotonin syndrome. Saint-John's-wort can also decrease barbiturate-induced sleep time.

Concomitant use may decrease plasma cyclosporine levels. There are multiple case reports of patients with heart, kidney, or liver transplants treated with cyclosporine, in whom use of Saint-John's-wort was associated with a drop in plasma cyclosporine to subtherapeutic levels and in some cases resulted in acute transplant rejection.

Concomitant use with nonnucleoside reverse transcriptase inhibitors (NNRTIs) may decrease serum levels of NNRTIs. Since NNRTIs and protease inhibitors are metabolized through similar routes, NNRTIs may also be affected. Subtherapeutic concentrations are associated with therapeutic failure, development of viral resistance, and development of drug class resistance. Saint-John's-wort is thought to induce cytochrome P450 enzymes. NNRTI-type antiretroviral drugs include nevirapine (Viramune), delavirdine (Rescriptor), and efavirenz (Sustiva).

Concomitant use with oral contraceptives may decrease steroid concentrations, resulting in breakthrough bleeding and irregular menstrual bleeding. There are multiple reports of breakthrough bleeding and irregular menstrual bleeding in women concomitantly taking oral contraceptives and Saint-John's-wort. Saint-John's-wort is thought to induce the cytochrome P450 3A4 enzymes, which are responsible for steroid metabolism. Women taking Saint-John's-wort and oral contraceptives concurrently should use an alternative form of birth control.

Concomitant use is thought to decrease the therapeutic effects of warfarin. Multiple cases of decreased International Normalized Ratio (INR) have been reported, although none have involved thromboembolic complications. Saint-John's-wort is thought to induce the cytochrome P450 2C9 enzyme, which is involved in warfarin's metabolism.

Saint-John's-wort can induce hypomania or mania when used in patients with bipolar disorder or depressed patients with occult bipolar disorder. Theoretically, like other antidepressants, Saint-John's-wort may also induce

**What They Told You**

**What They Did Not Tell You**

rapid cycling between depression and mania in patients with bipolar disorder. Some evidence suggests that Saint-John's-wort may inhibit oocyte fertilization and alter sperm DNA, but this effect has not yet been demonstrated in humans.

When used orally, Saint-John's-wort is thought to increase muscle tone of the uterus and should be avoided during pregnancy. Colic, drowsiness, and lethargy have been reported in infants whose mothers used St. John's wort while breast-feeding.

**Clinical studies:** Research has been done more in Europe than the United States. In Germany, over 37 randomized trials have been published. These studies concluded that Saint-John's-wort was superior to placebo and compared effectively with tricyclic antidepressants in the treatment of mild to moderate depression (*American Family Physician,* October 1998). However, Richard Shelton, a psychiatry professor at Vanderbilt University, has recently concluded from his studies that serious questions arise as to the effectiveness of Saint-John's-wort in moderate to severe depression. His conclusions came from 200 adult outpatients with major depression at 11 academic medical centers in the United States. The studies were double-blind and placebo controlled.

**The mechanism of action:** Extracts of this product appear to inhibit the breakdown of certain nerve impulse transmitters—specifically those that effect mood. In some respects it may act similar to an MAO inhibitor. It may also act as a weak neurotransmitter reuptake inhibitor of serotonin, norepinephrine, and dopamine. It binds to GABA receptors in vitro, but whether it crosses the blood-brain barrier is currently unknown.

Concentrations of the active ingredient—hypericum—reach peak levels in about 5 hours and a steady state in about 4 days. Half-life is about 4 days. Excretion and how it is metabolized is unknown (*The Medical Letter,* Vol. 39, 21 November, 1997, p. 107). It may have affinity for other receptors (Sigma) as well. Its possible effectiveness may be attributable to a combination of mechanisms (including MAO inhibition).

This herb has probably become the most commonly written-about herb in the medical literature in regard to

**What They Told You**

**What They Did Not Tell You**

possible drug interactions. Here are just a few: the trip-tans (Imitrex, Zomig, Amerge, Maxalt) for migraines, amitriptyline (Elaiul) for depression, the SSRIs (Paxil and Zoloft) for depression, nafazodone (Serzone) for depression, barbiturates, cyclosporine, digoxin, indinavir for AIDS, nortriptyline (Pamalar) for depression, oral contraceptives, tetracycline antibiotics, sulfa drugs, reser-pine for high blood pressure, theophyline for asthma, warfarin for blood thinning, some chemotherapeutic agents such as vincristine, antifungals such as beto-conazide, orneprazole (Prilosec) for GERD, and fexo-fonadine (Allegra) for sinusitis.

### SAMe—Depression

**How it has been used:** SAMe has been used for antide-pressant effects and arthritic pain. Some people have used it to improve liver health. It has also been helpful for ADHD and fibromyalgia and protection against coronary artery disease.

SAMe is likely to be effective when used orally for reliev-ing symptoms of osteoarthritis.

SAMe is possibly as effective as intravenous or oral tri-cyclic antidepressants, and SAMe is therefore often used for the treatment of depression.

Multiple clinical trials have also shown that short-term SAMe therapy is superior to placebo in decreasing pruri-tus, fatigue, alkaline phosphatase levels, and total and con-jugated bilirubin. One clinical trial using intravenous SAMe during the third trimester of pregnancy demonstrated sig-nificant benefit compared to placebo for normalizing liver function tests, decreasing associated symptoms, and pre-venting premature labor and low infant birth weight in pregnant women.

SAMe can normalize liver enzymes, decrease bilirubin, and decrease symptoms associated with various forms of chronic liver disease. SAMe supplementation may be ben-eficial in osteoarthritis due to analgesic and anti-inflamma-tory effects. Preliminary evidence suggests SAMe may also stimulate articular cartilage growth and repair. SAMe seems to protect against hepatic dysfunction caused by acetaminophen, alcohol, estrogens, monoamine oxidase inhibitors, phenobarbital, phenytoin, and steroids.

**Some interesting data:** S-adenosylmethionine, the

**Health concerns:** More safety and efficacy data is needed. Side effects of SAMe, if they occur, are usually mild and temporary; headaches, diarrhea, anxiety, and insomnia. There have been a few reports of cardiac pal-pitations.

When taken orally, SAMe can cause headache, flatulence, nausea, vomiting, and diarrhea. SAMe synthesis is closely linked to vitamin $B_{12}$ and folate metabolism. Deficiencies of these vitamins can result in decreased SAMe concen-trations in the central nervous system.

Anxiety has occurred in people with depression and hypomania in people with bipolar disorder. When used as an injection, SAMe has caused mania in people with bipolar disorder.

Possible interactions with antidepressants may be caused by the additive serotonergic effects and serotonin syn-drome-like effects, including agitation, tremors, anxiety, tachycardia, tachypnea, diarrhea, hyperreflexia, shivering, and diaphoresis. Concurrent use of SAMe with imipramirte (Toftanil) has resulted in a more rapid onset of antidepressant action. Use of SAMe can cause patients to convert from a depressed state to a hypomanic or manic state.

**Clinical studies:** In the few studies that did seem to show efficacy in depression, the dose was high (approxi-mately 1800 mg/day), and the cost was also very *high* (approximately $360 per month at 1800 mg/day).

There is also the possibility of inducing mania and hypo-mania in bipolar patients not receiving mood stabilizers. Some patients have become anxious. Some patients

## What They Told You

generic name for SAMe, was first discovered in 1952 and is available by prescription in Europe. It is a natural substance found in every cell of our bodies. It is one of the basic molecules of life.

**Historical data:** SAMe became available in Italy in the late 1970s and later in Spain, Germany, and other countries in Europe in the 1980s.

**The usual dose:** Doses are recommended at 200 mg 2 times per day to 800 mg 2 times per day.

## What They Did Not Tell You

show an increased level of homocysteine, a risk factor in heart attacks.

Finally, it encourages self-treatment of a potentially lethal medical condition—major depressive disorder.

**The mechanism of action:** It appears to heighten the activity of the mood-regulating neurotransmitters dopamine, norepinephrine, and serotonin. It is considered essential for three central pathways of metabolism that in turn stimulate other essential pathways. Transmethylation (donation of carbon), transulfuration (donation of sulfur), and transaminopropulation (generation of polyamines) are the 3 essential chemical pathways involved. Apparently, SAMe acts as an antidepressant, as an anti-inflammatory, and as a memory enhancer. It appears that it usually does not interact with other drugs and does not appear to have effects on cytochrome P450 metabolism in the liver. It does help in depression. It may be that its onset of action is half that of the old tricyclic antidepressants.

### Sangre de Grado—Infections

This is a rain-forest herb touted for various kinds of infections.

Research is lacking, and side effects are not known.

### Sarsaparilla—Hepatitis

Sarsaparilla was used in the past for syphilis. Today it is touted for psoriasis, liver protection, dieresis, and athletic enhancement.

Effectiveness is not proven.

It can interact with many drugs taken at the same time.

It definitely is not effective for syphilis.

### Sassafras—A Tonic and "Blood Purifier"

Sassafras has been touted for blood purification, syphilis, high blood pressure, arthritis, and cancer.

Sassafras probably does none or little of what it is touted to do.

It can cause hot flashes. Large doses can cause hallucinations, hypertension, liver cancer, and death.

### Saw Palmetto—BPH

**How it has been used:** Saw palmetto has been used mostly for BPH (benign-prostatic enlargement) with hope for improved sexual functioning. Other uses include gallbladder problems, hair loss, inflammation, prostatitis, urethral inflammation, cystitis, micromastia, URIs, gastrointestinal problems, and urinary disorders.

**Health concerns:** There are no long-term studies (greater than 90 days) on saw palmetto extract.

**Clinical studies:** Numerous double-blind, placebo-controlled clinical trials show saw palmetto as effective treatment for BPH. A number of studies suggest that saw palmetto is associated with a significant increase in urinary flow rate and perhaps a 50 percent decrease in

**What They Told You**

**Some interesting data:** Saw palmetto is a small palm tree that grows in the West Indies and the warm regions of the Atlantic Coast.

**Historical data:** American Indians used saw palmetto berries for GU problems and for inflammation of the breasts.

**The usual dose:** The usual dose is 160 mg 2 times a day. Some clients have reported improvement within a week or 2 at a dose of 320 mg per day.

**What They Did Not Tell You**

residual urine volume. At around age 45, free testosterone may drop in some men. Conversely, estrogen, prolactin, and sex hormone binding globulin may rise. The estrogen in turn may inhibit the clearance of DHT (dihydrotestosterone) and thereby increases DHT. The major components in saw palmetto are the sitosterols, which lower DHT and thereby may decrease inflammation in the prostate. Generally, saw palmetto is thought to take a number of months to work optimally. Some authors (*Review of Psychiatry*, Vol. 19) report better results when the combination of saw palmetto, pygeum, and stinging nettle are used. We feel more studies need to be done. In one study only 2 percent of men on saw palmetto stopped treatment because of side effects (transient headaches, nausea, etc.) compared to 11 percent on Proscar. Thus side effects appear to be low, but more studies are needed.

**The mechanism of action:** Saw palmetto inhibits the intraprostatic conversion of testosterone to dihydrotestosterone. DHT causes the cells of the prostate to multiply, enlarging the prostate.

### Saw Palmetto + Pygeum + Stinging Nettle—BPH

**How it has been used:** This combination has been used mainly for male menopause symptoms such as prostate enlargement.

**Some interesting data:** After age 45, there are hormonal changes in males that appear to be responsible for stimulating growth of the prostate. Modern medical treatment for prostate hypertrophy has tended to be costly, ineffective, and to pose significant side effects.

**Historical data:** This combination as well as separate use of each have been common in Europe for many years.

**The usual dose:** Saw palmetto has been used in the 320 mg per day range; pygeum generally is dosed at 75–150 mg per day; and stinging nettle often is recommended at the 300 mg per day dose.

**Health concerns:** Transient headaches and stomach upsets have been reported with saw palmetto. So far few side effects have been reported with pygeum. Overall, it seems that at least to date side effects are often negligible.

**Clinical studies:** Data from several studies suggest that saw palmetto use results in significant increase in urinary flow and a decrease in residual urine volume by apparently reducing the inflammation and size of the prostate. Saw palmetto may take a number of months to work optimally. Pygeum bark extract has been helpful in decreasing inflammation and inhibiting prostate cell growth. It seems to increase nocturnal erections and sexual activity in elderly men. Nettle blocks prostate cell growth receptors and acts as an anti-inflammatory. Studies have also indicated the use of these 3 in combination work better than 1 alone or 2 in combination.

**The mechanism of action:** Active compounds including sitosterols, anthranilic, caffeic, and chlorogeneic acids are apparently active in decreasing androgenic and inflammatory processes in the prostate. Inhibition of 5-alpha-reductase results in less dihydrotestosterone, which in turn decreases the growth of prostate cells.

| What They Told You | What They Did Not Tell You |
|---|---|
| | Pygeum reportedly decreases cell growth by inhibiting inflammation and reducing prolactin, increases prostate secretions, and lowers estrogen/testosterone levels. |
| | Pygeum inhibits prostate cell growth. Nettle blocks prostate cell growth receptors, blocks 5-alpha-reductase, inhibits aromatase and its binding capacity, and reduces inflammation of the prostate. |

### Scarlet Pimpernel—Depression

Orally, scarlet pimpernel is touted for depression, mucous membrane disorders, liver disorders, herpes, and as supportive therapy for carcinomas. It is also used orally for painful kidney disorders, particularly those with inflammation and an increase in urination.

Topically, scarlet pimpernel is used for poorly healing wounds and pruritus. It is used both orally and topically to treat painful joints.

Gastrointeritis and nephritis may occur with large oral doses or long-term administration.

### Schisandra—Hepatitis

This Chinese herb has been used in hepatitis to help improve liver functions. It has also been used in an attempt to improve concentration and endurance.

Schisandra is often given in 500 mg tabs—1 in the morning and 1 in the evening.

What is said appears to have some truth. However, schisandra can cause indigestion, allergic skin reactions, and severe depression in some but more so at higher dosages.

### Scotch Broom—Heart Disorders

Orally, scotch broom herb is touted for heart and circulatory disorders.

Historically, people used scotch broom herb for edema, cardiac arrhythmia, racing heartbeat, low blood pressure, heavy menstruation, hemorrhaging after birth, as a contraction stimulant, for bleeding gums, hemophilia, gout, rheumatism, sciatica, gallbladder and kidney stones, enlarged spleen, jaundice, bronchial conditions, and snake bites.

Orally, sparteine toxicity can occur with doses greater than 300 mg of sparteine, which is roughly equivalent to 30 grams of scotch broom. Symptoms of this toxicity include dizziness, headache, palpitations, prickling in the extremities, feeling of weakness in the legs, sweating, sleepiness, pupil dilation, and ocular palsy.

### Sea Buckthorn (topical)—Antiwrinkles

This herb from Asia, Europe, and Canada is touted to reduce age-induced wrinkles. It is often an ingredient in beauty lotions. It has also been used topically for pain or inflammation of the skin.

Significant research is lacking.

### Sea Cucumber—Arthritis

Sea cucumbers are marine animals touted for arthritis.

Significant research is lacking.

## What They Told You

## What They Did Not Tell You

### Sea Mussel—Arthritis
Sea mussel is a shellfish that contains amino acids, minerals, and enzymes. They have been touted for arthritis.

Significant research is lacking.

### Selenium—Cancer
Selenium is a mineral that has been touted to be helpful in cancer.

It has been touted for hair growth.

Significant research is lacking.

Toxicity can cause many symptoms including hair loss, fatigue, anger, nausea, vomiting, odor, and metallic taste.

### Senegra—Snakebites
Senegra has been used for URIs and snakebites.

Significant research is lacking.

Senegra can decrease the effectiveness of diabetic medications. It can increase bleeding time, can be sedating, and can cause anxiety and gastrointestinal upset.

### Senna—Laxative
Senna is used worldwide as a laxative. It causes stimulation of the bowel.

It has been sold under various names (black draught, Fletcher's Castoria, Gentlax, Dr. Caldwell's Dosalax).

As with most herbs and supplements, senna should not be used by pregnant females or by children. It can cause extreme cramping of the intestines. It especially should not be used by alcoholics.

### Shark Cartilage—Arthritis
Shark cartilage comes from the hammerhead and spiny dogfish sharks in the Pacific Ocean. It has been used primarily for arthritis in addition to cancer, psoriasis, diabetic retinopathy, macular degeneration, and to aid in wound healing. It has been tried rectally for advanced stage breast cancer, advanced stage colon cancer, and for spinal and intercranial tumors.

Dosages vary from 500 mg to 4500 mg in divided doses 2 to 6 times daily.

Shark cartilage is made up of about 40 percent protein, 5-20 percent glucosaminoglycans, and the rest is calcium salts. Enthusiasts tout its use to stimulate the immune system and its helpfulness in decreasing tumors by inhibiting the growth of new blood vessels. Reliable information is insufficient on its safety or usefulness. Studies professing the usefulness of shark cartilage in cancer treatment have not been repeated, thus its efficacy and safety for this purpose is unknown. The FDA is seeking an injunction against companies marketing shark cartilage for treatment of cancer.

Oral use can cause a bad taste in the mouth, stomach upsets, constipation, low blood pressure, dizziness, increased blood sugar, increased blood levels of calcium, altered mental status, and fatigue.

Adverse reactions and symptoms have been reported including elevated liver enzymes, acute hepatitis, jaundice, yellowing of the eyes, and right upper quadrant tenderness.

Those taking shark cartilage should have their liver function evaluated periodically in view of its possible toxic effect on the liver.

| What They Told You | What They Did Not Tell You |
|---|---|
| **Shepherd's Purse—Excessive Menstruation**<br>Shepherd's purse has been used for excessive menstruation, nosebleeds, and for bleeding wounds. | What is said is probably true.<br><br>It is probably safe for most people at small doses, but at high doses it has caused heart palpitations, changes in blood pressure, abnormal thyroid functions, sedation, paralysis, and death. |
| **Shitake—Arthritis**<br>Shitake is a mushroom from Japan that is high in vitamins. It has been used in Japan for help with joints. It has also been touted for heart disease and fatigue. | Significant research is lacking. |
| **Silymarin—Hepatitis**<br>Silymarin is an extract from milk thistle, which has been touted for liver disorders. | Silymarin is usually well tolerated. It can cause gastrointestinal upset. Allergic reactions are possible. |
| **Skullcap—Anxiety**<br>Skullcap has been used for high cholesterol, anxiety, in blood clots, and in strokes. | Skullcap, in overdose especially, can have toxic side effects—tremors, confusion, seizures, nausea, vomiting, and hypersensitivity reactions. It should not be taken in pregnancy or in childhood. |
| **Slippery Elm—Sore Throat**<br>Slippery elm was used by Native Americans for inflammations both inside and out. It has been used for gastrointestinal problems, sore throat, coughing, and infections of the bucial mucosa of the mouth. | Slippery elm is probably generally safe for most people. It may delay absorption of other medicines. Of course, allergic reactions are possible. |
| **Sneezewort—Nausea**<br>Orally, sneezewort is touted for rheumatic and painful disorders, toothache, diarrhea, nausea, vomiting, and flatulence.<br><br>Topically, sneezewort is touted for toothache.<br><br>In folk medicine, sneezewort was used for tiredness, urinary tract complaints, and as an appetite stimulant. | Orally, sneezewort may cause an allergic reaction. |
| **SOD (superoxide dismute)—Aging**<br>SOD is an enzyme with antioxidant effects and as such is touted to neutralize the aging effects of free radicals in the body. | Significant research is lacking. |
| **Solvents (sedative solvents)**<br>These agents have been used to heighten libido, in date rape, and to get high. | Most of these products have been recalled. They can lead to death. |

**What They Told You**

### Sorrel—Sinusitis

Orally, sorrel has been touted for acute and chronic inflammation of the nasal passages and respiratory tract and as an adjunct to antibacterial therapy. It is also used as a diuretic and to stimulate secretions. In combination with gentian root, European elder flower, verbena, and cowslip flower, sorrel is used orally for maintaining healthy sinuses and treating sinusitis.

### Soy—Menopause

**How it has been used:** Soy products are popular for menopausal symptoms and lowering cholesterol. Other uses include treatment for osteoporosis, skin disorders, and hepatitis. Soy has also been recommended for improving prostate health.

**Some interesting data:** Soy is a member of the bean family and has been considered a source of natural female hormones. It has been called tofu, imitation meat, miso, and high quality vegetable protein. Fewer than 20 percent of Japanese women with high soy diets have hot flashes compared with 65 percent of Canadian women.

**Historical data:** Chinese medicine has used soy compounds for more than 2000 years and has described soy as the "world's most versatile food."

**The usual dose:** The usual dose is from 300 mg up to 1 to 3 grams per day.

### Soybean Oil—High Cholesterol

Soybean oil has been touted as an excellent nutrient. It has also been touted to lower cholesterol.

### Spanish Broom—Laxative

Historically, Spanish broom has been used as a laxative and diuretic.

### Spearmint—Bad Breath

Spearmint, along with its cousins peppermint and watermint, belong to the popular mint family. It has been used for bad breath, colds, and gastrointestinal upset.

**What They Did Not Tell You**

Orally, excessive amounts of sorrel can cause diarrhea, nausea, polyuria, dermatitis, and gastrointestinal symptoms.

Oxalic acid (constituent) poisoning affects skin, eyes, respiratory system, and kidneys.

Oral symptoms of oxalate irritation include swelling of the mouth, tongue, and throat, with difficulty in speaking and suffocation. It has a corrosive effect on the digestive tract and can lead to oxalic acid crystals in the kidneys, blood vessels, heart, lungs, liver, and/or hypocalcemia.

**Health concerns:** Some individuals who take regular dosages of soy products have experienced gastric complaints including loose stools or diarrhea.

**Clinical studies:** Animal studies have shown soy to possibly have preventative benefits against breast cancer and other cancers with estrogen regulators.

**The mechanism of action:** Genistein, daidzein, and phytoestrogens found in soy are considered biological equivalents of the female hormones, estrogen and progesterone. Phytoestrogens are thought to reduce the more damaging effects of estrogen-like pollutants. Genistein is believed to inhibit angiogenesis, a process which occurs when malignant cells form blood vessels during tumor growth. Whole natural soy products may be better than isolated preparations (genistein).

It is true. Soybean oil is a good nutrient and possibly has some benefits in lowering total cholesterol.

Allergic reactions are possible just as with peanuts.

Reliable information is insufficient. No adverse effects have been reported.

Spearmint, along with peppermint, should not be used by those with liver disease. Also, those who have a gastrointestinal disorder known as achlorhydria should not

## What They Told You

## What They Did Not Tell You

use these mints. Those with gallbladder disease probably also should not use these mints.

### Spigelia—Migraines

Spigelia, also known as gelsemium or evening trumpet flower, is used as an analgesic for neuralgia and migraine headaches. It has also been used for asthma and respiratory problems.

Orally, people typically use 0.3 to 1 ml of the tincture.

Orally, this toxic alkaloid can be deadly. It can cause headache, dilated pupils, double vision, muscle weakness, seizures, shortness of breath, and failure of the respiratory muscles.

Spigelia may increase the effects of aspirin products.

There is a narrow margin of safety with this plant, and its affect can be unpredictable.

### Spinach—Stimulating Growth in Children

Spinach has been touted for stimulating growth in children, building energy, calming gastrointestinal complaints, lowering blood sugar, and decreasing the risk of stomach cancer.

Significant research is lacking.

Popeye made the myths popular, but spinach does not contain several vitamins and minerals. It is thought to have hypoglycemic effect in some, and consumption of fresh spinach does perhaps lower stomach cancer risk for some. Some research even suggests some antiaging effects. Perhaps Popeye was not totally wrong.

### Spirulina—Weight Loss

Spirulina is a blue-green algae product used as a dietary source of protein, B-vitamins, and iron. It has also been used for weight loss, ADHD, PMS, stress, fatigue, to improve memory, and to lower cholesterol.

Blue-green algae is found in tropical or subtropical alkaline waters that have a high salt content. There are thousands of species of blue-green algae also known as cyanophyta.

Spirulina contains high concentrations of protein, B-vitamins, phenylalanine, iron, and other minerals. The phenylalanine content is touted to be responsible for the suppression of appetite and subsequent weight loss. The iron in spirulina is highly bioavailable to humans. Some reports suggest blue-green algae may stimulate the immune system by increasing T-cells as well as having some antiviral activity. Others suggest it may help in lowering triglycerides and total cholesterol.

The usual dosage of spirulina blue-green algae is 3–5 grams daily before meals.

Spirulina has a high iodine content that may decrease the effectiveness of thyroid medications.

Some species of blue-green algae can be contaminated with microbes, heavy metals (mercury, cadmium, lead, or arsenic), and radioactive ions. Algae grown in uncontrolled settings such as lakes and ponds are more likely to be contaminated. Some types of blue-green algae are known to contain ingredients toxic to the liver. Commercial spirulina blue-green algae are usually grown under strict conditions and are unlikely to be contaminated. It is important to select blue-green algae products that have been tested to avoid preparations contaminated with heavy metals, microbes, and microcystins (poisonous materials).

The FDA has reviewed the claim of weight-loss potential of spirulina and has found no evidence to support that claim. Further research is needed to evaluate the usefulness and safety of blue-green algae in dietary supplementation.

### Spleen Extract—Inadequate Spleen Function

Orally, spleen extract is touted as replacement therapy

Spleen extract is derived from raw animal spleens gath-

**What They Told You**

after spleenectomy or in people with inadequate spleen function. It is also touted for treating people with low white blood cell counts, enhancing general immune function and immune function in people with cancer, and treating bacterial infections. Spleen extract is also touted for treating celiac disease, dermatitis herpetiformis, glomerulonephritis, HIV-related bacterial infections, rheumatoid arthritis, systemic lupus erythematosus, thrombocytopenia, ulcerative colitis, and vasculitis.

**What They Did Not Tell You**

ered from slaughterhouses, possibly from sick or diseased animals. Products made from contaminated or diseased organs might present a human health hazard. There is also concern that spleen extracts produced from cows in countries where bovine spongiform encephalitis (BSE) has been reported might be contaminated with diseased tissue.

### Spurge—Bronchitis

Spurge has been touted for bronchitis and other upper respiratory infections.

This herb can be toxic and can also interact with many prescription medications.

### Squawvine—PMS

Squawvine has been touted for menstrual cramps and anxiety. Topically, it has been used for treating sore nipples.

Effectiveness is not known.

Few side effects have been reported as of this date.

### Squill—Congestive Heart Failure

Squill has been used in congestive heart failure.

Squill can cause heart toxicity.

It can interact with heart medications, amphetamines, and steroids.

In regard to effectiveness, significant research is lacking.

### Star Anise—Bronchitis

Orally, star anise is touted for respiratory tract mucous membrane inflammation, peptic discomfort, flatulence, loss of appetite, cough, and bronchitis.

As an inhalant, it is touted for respiratory tract congestion.

In Chinese medicine, star anise is used for increasing milk secretion, promoting menstruation, facilitating childbirth, increasing libido, and treating symptoms of male climacteric.

Topically, use of the constituent anethole can cause dermatitis, including erythema, scaling, and vesiculation.

### Stevia—Sweetener

Stevia is an herb from Paraguay. Its ability to sweeten has been touted to be a few hundred times that of sugar. It is calorie free and can be used in baking and cooking without being destroyed. It is touted to be nontoxic.

Research of stevia is largely lacking.

In 1986 the FDA seized the inventories of stevia and in 1991 claimed it was not suitable as a food. It has been approved by the FDA as a dietary supplement only and not as a sweetening agent. It appears mutagenic in vitro and also caused reduced sperm production and testis size in rats.

## What They Told You

### Stone Root—Kidney Stones

Stone root has been used for stones—in the bladder, kidney, and urinary tract.

### Storax—Respiratory Congestion

Storax has been touted for use in vaporizers for respiratory congestion.

### Strawberry—Diuretic

Strawberry has been touted to have diuretic activity. It has also been touted for diarrhea, liver disease, gout, arthritis, anxiety, fever, weight loss, and slowing the aging of the nervous system.

### Suma—AIDS

Suma has been touted to boost the immune system.

### Sundew—Cough

Sundew is used as a cough suppressant.

### Sweet Annie—Malaria

Sweet Annie has been used for intestinal parasites and for malaria.

The semisynthetic derivatives of sweet Annie are used as prescription antimalarial drugs in Africa, Asia, and Europe.

### Sweet Gale—Digestive Disorders

Orally, sweet gale is touted for digestive disorders. Sweden, a strong brew of sweet gale dried bark, is used as an anthelmintic and to cure itching.

### Sweet Woodruff—Hemorrhoids

Orally, sweet woodruff is touted for preventing and treating respiratory tract, gastrointestinal tract, liver, gallbladder, and urinary tract disorders; for blood purification,

## What They Did Not Tell You

The effectiveness of stone root is not proven.

It might have some diuretic effects and antifungal effects.

It is usually safe but can cause intestinal tract irritation and pain. It can cause nausea and dizziness.

Significant research is lacking.

Strawberries taste good, but there is a lack of research to support all of the claims.

Allergic reactions are possible.

Effectiveness is not known.

Side effects reported so far are relatively few. It can precipitate asthma in some cases.

Sundew appears safe for most people. No drug interactions are known.

It is probably effective for some with antispasmodic, antimicrobial, and expectorant effects.

Effectiveness might help in some cases of malaria. Other uses lack proven effectiveness.

It is in the same family as ragweed, and allergic reactions could occur.

It is usually safe when used in appropriate amounts.

Orally, the volatile oil is considered toxic.

Orally, sweet woodruff above ground parts can be associated with headache, and in larger amounts, stupor. Long-term use can cause liver damage.

**What They Told You**

venous complaints, weak veins, hemorrhoids, vasodilation; spasms, abdominal discomforts; strengthening the nervous system, agitation, hysteria, nervous menstrual disorders, restlessness, insomnia, neuralgia; strengthening heart function, cardiac irregularity; stomachache, migraine, and bladder stones. Sweet woodruff is also touted orally for inducing sweating, as an antispasmodic, diuretic, or expectorant.

Topically, sweet woodruff is touted for use in skin diseases, treating wounds, venous conditions, hemorrhoids, and for reducing inflammation.

### Tamarind—Constipation

Orally, tamarind is touted for chronic or acute constipation, liver and gallbladder disorders, and to decrease fever.

Topically, a thick paste of the seeds is used as a cast for broken bones.

In China, tamarind is used to treat pregnancy-related nausea and as an anthelmintic in children.

In Arabia, it is used for stomach disorders, colds, and fevers.

### Tangerine Peel (mandarin orange)—Belching

Tangerine is touted for indigestion, gas, nausea, vomiting, belching, and diarrhea.

### Taumelloolch—Blood Poisoning

Orally, taumelloolch is touted for blood poisoning, cancer, cysts, dizziness, eczema, hemorrhage, idiocy, indurations, "knots," leprosy, migraine, nerve pain, nosebleeds, putrid flesh, sleeplessness, stomach cramps, involuntary dyskinetic movements, toothache, tumors, urinary incontinence, and colic.

Topically, taumelloolch is used as a poultice for skin diseases, to draw out splinters, and for broken bones.

In folk medicine taumelloolch is used orally for gangrene, headache, meningitis, neuralgia, rheumatism, and sciatica.

### Taurine—Congestive Heart Failure

Orally, taurine is touted for the treatment of congestive heart failure (CHF), high blood pressure, high cholesterol, seizure disorders (epilepsy), and as an antioxidant.

**What They Did Not Tell You**

No adverse reactions are reported; however, no sufficient reliable information is available.

Tangerine is usually benign but should not be eaten if one has a dry cough.

Symptoms of taumelloolch toxicity include colic, confusion, giddiness, weakness, dizziness, dilated pupils, headache, confusion, staggering, somnolence, trembling, vision and speech disorders, vomiting, delirium, and death from respiratory failure.

There is insufficient reliable information available.

## What They Told You

### Tea

Tea divides into black tea, so popular in America, and green tea, which is more popular in Asia. Both contain the stimulating effects of caffeine. Green tea has been touted for cavity prevention, cancer prevention, cognitive enhancement, and cholesterol lowering.

### Tea Tree Oil—Nail Infections

This herb comes from a small tree in Australia. It has been used topically for all kinds of infections of the skin, including acne, and fungal infections of the feet and toenails, including athlete's foot.

### Thiamine (Vitamin B₁)—Diabetic Neuropathy

Beriberi is treated with thiamine. It has also been touted for diabetic neuropathy and to help reduce the likelihood of cataracts.

### Thyme—Sinusitis

Thyme is from the Mediterranean and is a constituent of many soups, salads, sauces, and meats. It is touted to be helpful in sinusitis (bronchitis, coughing, whooping cough, respiratory infections). It is touted to facilitate breathing.

### Tobacco—Stimulant

Tobacco has been used for centuries for its stimulating and addicting effects. Next to coffee it has probably been used more than any other herb in history.

## What They Did Not Tell You

Green tea might have some of the benefits to a degree for some, under What They Told You, and it is safe for many when consumed in small and moderate amounts. However, it becomes unsafe when used in large amounts.

It can interact with many drugs (antiplatelet, some antipsychotics, some antianxiety drugs, some antidepressants, oral contraceptives, and some antiasthmatics, to name a few). It can interact with grapefruit juice. It can interfere with several lab tests (bleeding time, creatine, urine catacholamines, serum urate, and VMA).

It might aggravate ulcers, heart conditions, anxiety disorders, and kidney disease. It might lower blood sugar.

Topically, tea tree oil is usually safe (occasionally it can be irritating). It is toxic when ingested. Thus, if people are going to try this item, then use it topically. It also should be noted that it might exacerbate eczema. We would highly caution against vaginal use (in yeast infections).

Thiamine is effective for vitamin B₁ deficiency states. The other areas of potential benefit need research.

It can cause a hypersensitivity syndrome when given orally.

Thyme is usually safe in the amount in foods. It has constituents that are antibacterial, antispasmodic, antiflatulent, antitussive, and antihelmintic.

It can cause irritation of the gastrointestinal and urinary tract.

Tobacco is the most dangerous herb of all time, being responsible for more deaths than any other herb in history. It is responsible for perhaps one in every five deaths. It is a factor in many cancers. It causes wrinkles and premature aging. And yet, perhaps 1 in every 3 to 4 Americans continues to use this dangerous herb. The addicting attraction is strong, and the dangers are often delayed for a time; thus, it gives a misguided feeling of "It won't hurt me. I'm an exception."

**What They Told You**

**What They Did Not Tell You**

### Tomato

Almost everyone is familiar with the large red berry we call a tomato. It is high in antioxidants and touted to help in cancer, diabetes, high cholesterol, and prostate enlargement.

The antioxidants in tomatoes may help health in general, and it does taste good to many people.

### Tonka Bean—Nausea

Tonka bean has been touted to decrease nausea and vomiting.

Tonka bean contains coumarin compounds that increase bleeding.

### Touch-Me-Not (jewelweed)—Poison Ivy

Topical jewelweed has been used for itching in poison ivy.

Significant research is lacking.

### Tragacanth—Diarrhea

Orally, tragacanth is touted for both diarrhea and as a laxative.

Topically, it is an ingredient in toothpastes, hand lotions, and vaginal creams and jellies.

Orally, use of tragacanth requires ample fluid intake. Insufficient fluid intake can lead to obstruction ileus and esophageal closure. Tragacanth can cause asthma symptoms in people who are sensitive to quillaia bark.

### Trailing Arbutus—Urinary Tract Infections

Orally, trailing arbutus is touted for urinary tract conditions, as an astringent, and a diuretic.

Orally, chronic use of trailing arbutus may lead to hydroquinone toxicity. Symptoms of toxicity include tinnitus, vomiting, delirium, convulsions, and collapse. Liver damage, cachexia, hemolytic anemia, and hair depigmentation may also occur with long-term use. Overdosage could lead to inflammation of the mucous membranes of the bladder and urinary tract and may be accompanied by bloody urine, difficulty with urination, and painful urination.

### Tree of Heaven—Diarrhea

In Chinese medicine tree of heaven is used for pathological leukorrhea, chronic diarrhea, chronic dysentery, and dysmenorrhea.

In Africa, tree of heaven is used to treat asthma, cramps, epilepsy, fast heart rate, gonorrhea, malaria, and tapeworms.

Orally, large amounts of tree of heaven bark can cause queasiness, dizziness, headache, limb tingling, and diarrhea.

Topically, skin contact with the leaves can cause dermatitis.

### Trypsin—Osteoarthritis

Trypsin is a digestive enzyme found in the small intestines. It has been used in combination with bromelin and rutin for osteoarthritis.

In combination with rutin and bromelin, it may help some with osteoarthritis.

### Tung Seed—Constipation

Orally, tung seed is used for asthma, bloody diarrhea, dysentery, sprue, and as a bowel stimulant.

Orally, tung seed can cause severe stomach pain, violent vomiting, debility, diarrhea, slowed reflexes, slowed

## What They Told You

Topically, tung seed is used to stimulate hair growth and for constipation.

### Turmeric—Anti-inflammatory
Turmeric is an herb that is a cousin to the ginger family. It is a major ingredient in curry powder and mustard. It has been touted to have anticancer effects, anti-inflammatory effects, and cardiovascular benefits such as lowering cholesterol, hepatic benefits, and gastrointestinal benefits such as gas inhibition. It has also been used as a topical preparation for analgesia, as well as ringworm, bruising, and other inflammatory skin conditions.

Turmeric is rich in potassium and iron.

Typical doses are 0.5 to 1 gram of the powdered root several times daily between meals.

### Turtle Head
Orally, turtle head aboveground parts and roots are touted as a cathartic tonic.

### Usnea—Sore Throat
Usnea is used for mild inflammation of the mouth and throat.

It usually comes in lozenges and is taken 3 to 6 times per day.

It comes from a group of algae and fungi often found hanging from the trees of the Northern Hemisphere.

### Uva Ursi—Urinary Tract Infections and Heavy, Painful Menstrual Periods
See Bearberry.

### Valerian—Anxiety
Valerian is derived from the valerian root plant. It has been used for anxiety, muscle discomfort, and migraines. It is widely used in Europe.

Orally, valerian is used as a sedative-hypnotic and anxiolytic for restlessness and sleeping disorders associated with nervous conditions. It is also used for mood disorders such as depression, infantile convulsions, mild tremors, epilepsy, and attention deficit hyperactivity disorder (ADHD). It is used for rheumatic pain, conditions associated with psychological stress including anxiety, nervous asthma, nervous headaches, gastric spasms, colic,

## What They Did Not Tell You

breathing, and possibly death. Skin contact with tung seed can cause acute dermatitis.

Turmeric may in some respects work in a manner similar to Celebrex, a COX2 inhibitor. Use of turmeric with other herbs that have anitcoagulant or antiplatelet potential could increase the risk of bleeding.

With reasonable use it is safe for most people. Large doses could possibly be a factor at times in ulcers or even cancer.

Reliable information is insufficient about the effectiveness of turtle head. No adverse effects reported.

Usnea has at least some antimicrobial activity and is usually safe.

Valerian may work by inhibiting GABA degradation. It may have a bad smell ("dirty socks"). As with many GABA-augmenting agents, addiction should be considered as well as rebound insomnia.

The valepotriates possibly act as prodrugs in that they are thought to decompose rapidly to homobaldrinal in the intestine after ingestion. Valepotriates are highly unstable and rapidly decompose in acid or alkaline environments and at high temperatures. The presence of an epoxide group on the valepotriates has raised concern about possible cytotoxicity and carcinogenicity in

**What They Told You**

and menstrual cramps, as well as nervous complaints caused by menopause and hot flashes. Topically, valerian is used as a bath additive for restlessness and sleep disorders. Traditionally, valerian has been used for hysterical states, excitability, hypochondria, migraine, and rheumatic pains.

**What They Did Not Tell You**

animals. Valerenic acid also appears to inhibit the enzyme system responsible for the central catabolism of GABA, increasing GABA concentrations and decreasing CNS activity. There is some evidence that valerian might also contain other constituents such as ligands and GABA, which may also be responsible for the sedative effects of valerian.

Valerian taken orally can cause headache, excitability, uneasiness, cardiac disturbances, insomnia, and occasional morning drowsiness. Some reports suggest that impaired alertness and information processing may occur. Signs of valerian toxicity include difficulty in walking, hypothermia, and increased muscle relaxation.

Extended use can cause benzodiazepine-like withdrawal symptoms when treatment is discontinued. Patients should taper doses slowly after extended use. There have been several case reports of hepatotoxicity associated with use of multi-ingredient preparations containing valerian, but these preparations may have been adulterated with hepatotoxic agents. Four other cases of hepatotoxicity involving long-term use of single-ingredient valerian preparations have also been reported.

Possibly, concomitant use with herbs that have sedative properties could enhance therapeutic and adverse effects. These include calamus, calendula, California poppy, catnip, capsicum, celery, couch grass, elecampane, Siberian ginseng, German chamomile, goldenseal, gotu kola, hops, Jamaican dogwood, kava, lemon balm, sage, Saint-John's-wort, sassafras, scullcap, shepherd's purse, stinging nettle, wild carrot, wild lettuce, withania root, and yerba mansa.

Valerian can potentiate the sedative effects of alcohol, benzodiazepines, and barbiturates, causing additive therapeutic and adverse effects.

### Vanadium—Diabetes

Vanadium is a mineral that has been used for diabetes mellitus Types 1 and 2. It is also known by other names such as Vanadyl Sulfate.

Vanadium may be toxic in some cases.

### Vanilla—Aphrodisiac

Vanilla is usually used for its flavoring ability and as a perfume. It is touted to be an aphrodisiac. It has also been used for gas, itching, and as a stimulant.

Vanilla does have a great fragrance, but other scientific research of effectiveness is lacking.

**What They Told You**

*Verbena—Sore Throat*

Orally, verbena is touted for sore throats and other oral and pharyngeal inflammation, respiratory tract diseases, asthma, and angina.

Topically, verbena is used for poorly healing wounds, abscesses, gargle, contusions, itching, and minor burns.

*Viacreme*

Viacreme is described as a sexual response enhancer for women which works reportedly by increasing sensitivity and circulation. It is a compounded cream containing menthol and L-Arginine, an amino acid. Arginine supplements have been touted to treat impotence for some time. Women who have clinically tested Viacreme or similar products report improved response with continuing use including more interest in sexual activity and possibly more intense orgasms.

Arginine is a precursor to nitric oxide and works in a way similar to Viagra by causing dilation of blood vessels in the genital area. L-Arginine is a semi-essential amino acid synthesized by the body from ornithine. It is involved in protein synthesis and in the transport and storage of nitrogen.

Viacreme is applied topically to the external genitalia prior to or during sexual activity. Multiple applications are recommended if needed. Other products are currently being developed under different names with the basic formulation of menthol and L-Arginine plus additional ingredients including lubricants.

*Vinegar (Topical)—Bug Bites*

Vinegar has been used for help in athlete's foot (1/2 cup of white vinegar per gallon of water; soak for 15 minutes twice a day). White vinegar has also been used to rid oneself of ticks and chiggers.

*Vinpocetine—Poor Memory*

Vinpocetine has been touted for enhancing memory. It has also been touted for cerebrovascular disease.

*Vitamin A—Wrinkles*

Vitamin A has been touted for good vision, preventing glaucoma, preventing cataracts, improving wound healing,

**What They Did Not Tell You**

Excessive amounts of verbena can cause CNS paralysis, stupor, and convulsions.

There are numerous medical reasons that decrease female sexual responsiveness such as depression, anxiety, and hormonal imbalances. A number of medications are known to cause low libido. It is important to consult with licensed professionals about possible medical or psychological components contributing to female sexual dysfunction. Controlled studies on this compound and other similar products have not been done. There are no long-term toxicity studies. One source stated that Arginine taken by mouth has been reported to possibly predispose to herpes infection in short-term use, although little data is available at this time on the incidence or prevalence of herpes in individuals taking arginine.

It is important to note differences in various compounds containing L-Arginine. For example, L-Arginine 1000 is from free-base Arginine, which is 17 percent more potent that Arginine HCL. Arginine by mouth has been used for angina to dilate blood vessels to the myocardium. Headaches and visual disturbances may occur. Topical application in the amounts recommended for Viacreme is less likely to cause side effects or systemic changes than compounds taken by mouth.

Further scientific research is needed on products reported to enhance female sexuality.

This is interesting. Significant research is lacking.

Significant research is lacking.

Vitamin A is appropriate for vitamin A deficiency for various reasons.

## What They Told You

and skin conditions. Topically, it has been used for reducing wrinkles. It has also been touted for reducing the risk of breast cancer.

### Vitamin B Complex—Depression

(Please see individual vitamins by name.)

The B vitamins include $B_1$ (thiamine), $B_2$ (riboflavin), $B_3$ (niacin, nicotinic acid, niacinamide), $B_5$ (pantothenic acid), $B_6$ (pyridoxine), and $B_{12}$ (cyanocobalamin).

The B vitamins are often taken together since they can affect each other.

They have been touted for depression and other ailments.

### Vitamin C—Asthrosclerosis

Vitamin C has been used for treating scurvy and various nutritional problems.

It has been touted for many things (the common cold, wound healing, asthrosclerosis prevention, dementia, depression, arthritis, cancer, and drug withdrawal, to name a few). It has been used topically for wrinkled skin.

### Vitamin D—Rickets

Vitamin D has been used for rickets and other states in which vitamin D is deficient.

It has been touted to help in prevention of diabetes in children.

### Vitamin E

Orally, vitamin E is used for replacement therapy in vitamin E deficiency, treating and preventing cardiovascular disease, including slowing atherogenesis and preventing heart

## What They Did Not Tell You

Large amounts have been associated with many psychiatric symptoms including lethargy, anger, depression, and psychosis. It can cause gastrointestinal problems. Children on large doses may fail to gain weight and have various other symptoms.

Many other side effects of hypervitaminosis A can occur including gum disease, hair loss, brittle nails, skin pigmentation, and elevated liver function.

Vitamin C is effective for deficiency states.

It is possible that some people who consume fruits and vegetables high in vitamin C might help lessen the risk of cancer, but the question of causing cancer has also been raised with vitamin C supplements. It might lower cardiovascular risk for some. It is probably ineffective in preventing the common cold.

It can cause nausea, vomiting, diarrhea, heartburn, abdominal cramps, fatigue, headache, insomnia, and stones in the urinary tract.

Vitamin D is appropriate for deficiency states such as preventing hypocalcemia with chronic renal failure.

Vitamin D toxicity symptoms include weakness, fatigue, insomnia, decreased libido, kidney problems, osteoporosis in adults, decreased growth in children, pancreatitis, hyperpigmentation, and arrhythmias, to name a few.

Recent studies have indicated that loading up on vitamin E and other antioxidants may be worthless for many heart patients and may even interfere with widely used

## What They Told You

attacks. It is used for angina, thrombophlebitis, intermittent claudication, and preventing ischernia-reperfusion injury after coronary artery bypass surgery. Vitamin E is used for preventing cancer, particularly lung and oral cancer in smokers, colorectal cancer and polyps, and gastric, prostate, and pancreatic cancer. Vitamin E is used for Alzheimer's disease and other dementias, night cramps, and Parkinson's disease. Vitamin E is also used orally for preventing pre-eclampsia in high-risk women, for improving physical endurance, increasing energy, preventing allergies, for asthma and infections, for protecting against negative effects of air pollution, preventing aging, preventing cataracts, inflammatory skin disorders, burns, cystic fibrosis, oral leukoplakia, premenstrual syndrome, habitual abortion, menopausal syndrome, infertility, impotence, chronic cystic mastitis, mammary dysplasia, peptic ulcers, porphyria, tardive dyskinesia, neuromuscular disorders, Huntington's corea, chronic progressive hereditary chorea, and myotonic dystrophy. Additionally, vitamin E is used orally for preventing vitamin E deficiency in people with malabsorption syndromes or abetalipoproteinemia, treating hemolytic anemia caused by vitamin E deficiency in premature neonates, preventing retinopathy of prematurity, preventing bronchopulmonary dysplasia secondary to oxygen therapy in neonates, and preventing intraventricular hemorrhage in premature neonates.

Vitamin E is used for correcting erythrocyte membrane abnormalities in people with beta-thalassemia, for hereditary spherocytosis, glucose-6-phosphate dehydrogenase deficiency, or sickle-cell anemia.

### Vitamin K

Vitamin K is used for treating hypoprothrombinemia caused by vitamin K deficiency.

It has been touted to play a role in prevention of asthrosclerosis in some.

## What They Did Not Tell You

cholesterol-lowering drugs (the "statins"). Antioxidant nutrients, especially vitamin E, have been widely recommended over the past few years as a promising way of keeping the heart healthy. However, several recent large studies that tested this idea have failed to show a significant benefit to vitamin E, and now a new study raises the possibly that vitamin E might even be harmful for some patients. The latest study is relatively small and leaves some questions unanswered but nevertheless is discouraging news for what once seemed a cheap, simple way of warding off heart trouble. The study was funded by the National Institutes of Health and appeared in the *New England Journal of Medicine* and suggests that antioxidants such as vitamin E may actually blunt the benefits of statins and niacin, which are widely used to lower LDL, the "bad" cholesterol, and raise HDL levels, the "good" cholesterol. In addition, use of vitamin E in amounts greater than 10 units/kg per day can delay the response to iron therapy in children with iron-deficiency anemias. Omega-6 fatty acids are also known to inhibit antioxidant metabolism, resulting in an increase in vitamin E requirements, and mineral oil can decrease absorption. Vitamin E, on the other hand, increases the absorption of vitamin A and may protect against hypervitaminosis A.

Concomitant use of vitamin E with anticoagulants and antiplatelet agents may increase risk of bleeding, may reduce the effectiveness of anticancer agents, and prevents tolerance to nitrates. Agents known to affect vitamin E levels include cholestryramine, colestipol, gemfibrozil, mineral oil, and alcohol.

Finally, in all fairness vitamin E acts as a weak scavenger of free radicals in the brain and thus could possibly have some weak neuroprotective effects on the brain in Alzheimer's disease. It has also been tested in Parkinson's disease because of the weak scavenger effects on free radicals. And finally it might help some to have a more healthy heart, but this is not known, and more research is needed.

It is effective in treating hypoprothrombinemia caused by vitamin K deficiency. Research is needed otherwise.

**What They Told You**

Meadion (K3) has been touted to play a role in treating prostate and breast cancer when it is combined with vitamin C.

**What They Did Not Tell You**

## Vitamin O—Fatigue

Vitamin O (also called liquid oxygen) has been touted for increasing oxygen. It has also been touted for many other ailments.

Liquid oxygen only exists in a liquid form at temperatures below –183 degrees C. Thus, this is not liquid oxygen.

Great caution is warranted.

## Vitamins and Minerals

"It's only a vitamin. There is nothing wrong with megavitamins. They are good for your health."

$B_6$ has been given for depression and PMS under the theory that tryptophane is converted to serotonin with $B_6$.

$B_3$ (niacin) deficiency is touted to be related indirectly at times to low serotonin, and thus $B_3$ is touted to help some when depressed.

$B_1$ (thiamine) has been touted to play a role in fatigue at times since it is required to burn carbohydrates efficiently.

$B_{12}$ is important in acetylcholine production, which is a neurotransmitter important in brain functioning. Low $B_{12}$ is found in a severe form of anemia (pernicious anemia) that can manifest with severe depression.

Folic acid is important in the production of catacholamins, which give energy. Folic acid deficiencies have been found in some depressions.

Calcium deficiency has been touted to be important in some depressions and insomnia.

Magnesium is touted to have an antianxiety effect.

Vitamin C has been touted to extend life, help in stress, and help in resistance to the common cold.

Vitamin E has been used to promote health of the heart at 200–800 IU per day. It has also been used in tardive dyskinesia at 800–1600 IU per day.

Vitamin D has been used in winter depression at doses of 400–800 IU per day for 5 days. It has been used in prevention trials of diabetes Type I.

Anything that is used in essence as a medicine in a sense becomes a medicine. Vitamins can be toxic (*Current Medical Diagnosis and Treatment and The American Medical Associates Encyclopedia of Medicine*, N.Y.: Random House, 1989, p. 1058).

Vitamin A: This vitamin can cause headache, dizziness, nausea, skin sloughing, bone pain.

Vitamin K: Toxicity can be induced by water—dispersible analogues—hemolytic anemia, liver damage.

Vitamin $B_6$ (pyridoxine): Excessive intake has been reported to cause neuritis. Toxicity has occurred at doses from 50 to 4000 mg per day.

Vitamin $B_{12}$: No data exists to back its panacea use in the past for depression.

Vitamin E: Prolonged, excessive intake of Vitamin E may cause abdominal pain, nausea, vomiting, and diarrhea. It may also reduce intestinal absorption of Vitamins A, D, and K, which in severe cases produces symptoms of deficiency of these vitamins (complications with the eyes, softening of the bones, and affect blood-clotting ability). Headaches are another potential complication of excessive Vitamin E intake.

The evidence that Vitamin E improves memory in dementia is scant at best.

Vitamin C: The question of cancer promoting in high doses has been raised by recent studies. Some people, in the belief it prevents colds, take large doses. However, there is no convincing evidence to support this. Excessive intake has caused nausea, stomach cramps, diarrhea, and occasionally kidney stones.

**What They Told You**

Amino acids are found in protein. Two amino acids (tyrosine and aryptophane) have been used much in emotional issues—tryptophane for depression and insomnia and tyrosine for mental altertness.

Vitamins have been used for wound healing, youthful skin, and memory enhancement.

Copper, iron, selenium, and zinc have all been used for maintenance of healthy hair.

Zinc has been used in upper respiratory infections (mixed results) and to improve taste and smell.

Selenium has been used in depression at doses of 100–400 mcg per day.

Chromium has been used in depression, obesity, and diabetes.

Magnesium has long been used because of its sedative and anticonvulsant effects.

**What They Did Not Tell You**

Vitamin D: Excessive intake may cause weakness, abnormal thirst, increased urination, gastrointestinal disturbance, and depression. Over a long period, too much Vitamin D disrupts the balance of calcium and phosphate in the body, which may lead to abnormal calcium deposits in the soft tissues, kidneys, and blood vessel walls and sometimes retarded growth in children.

Selenium has caused neuropathy, fatigue, and irritability.

Toxic effects of chromium include iron deficiency and a question of malignancy.

Magnesium could be dangerous in renal insufficiency.

### Wahoo—Indigestion

Orally, wahoo root bark is touted for indigestion, to stimulate bile production, and as a laxative, diuretic, or tonic.

Wahoo is considered poisonous. Several hours after ingesting wahoo seeds, people experience severe upset stomach, sometimes with bloody diarrhea, fever, shortness of breath, circulatory problems, signs of collapse, stupor increasing to unconsciousness, alternating with motor restlessness, severe tonic-clonic spasms with locked-jaw muscles and coma.

### Watercress—Arthritis

Orally, watercress is touted for respiratory tract mucous membrane inflammation.

Topically, watercress is touted for arthritis, rheumatoid arthritis, earache, eczema, scabies, and warts.

In folk medicine, watercress is used orally for coughs, bronchitis, as a spring tonic, an appetite stimulant, improving digestion and stimulating appetite, alopecia, cancer, flu, goiter, polyps, scurvy, tuberculosis, gland tumors, as an abortifacient, aphrodisiac, bactericide, laxative, restorative, stimulant, and anthelmintic.

Orally, large amounts of watercress can cause gastrointestinal irritation. Theoretically, excessive or prolonged use might cause kidney damage.

### Wheat Bran—Diabetes

Wheat bran is high in vitamins and minerals. It has been touted for lowering lipids, helping in diabetes, and reduc-

Wheat bran, if used with a low-fat diet, would probably lower cholesterol in some. It might help in blood sugar

| What They Told You | What They Did Not Tell You |
|---|---|
| ing the risk of colon cancer. | control in some. It probably does not decrease the risk of colon cancer. |

### Wheatgrass—Cancer

| What They Told You | What They Did Not Tell You |
|---|---|
| Wheatgrass is high in vitamins and minerals. | Significant research is lacking. |
| It has been touted for nutrition, diabetes, anemia, and even cancer. | It is safe for most people. |

### White Cohosh—Menstrual Disorders

| What They Told You | What They Did Not Tell You |
|---|---|
| White cohosh has been touted for various menstrual disorders. | Significant research is lacking as to effectiveness. |
|  | This herb is toxic. It is not the same as black cohosh. |

### White Lily—Gynecological Disorders

| What They Told You | What They Did Not Tell You |
|---|---|
| Orally, white lily is touted for gynecological disorders. | Reliable information is insufficient. No adverse effects have been reported. |
| Topically, it has been touted for ulcers, inflammation, furuncles, finger ulcers, reddened skin, burns, and injuries. |  |
| Historically, it has been used as an astringent, anti-inflammatory, softener, pain reliever, diuretic, antihemorrhagic, and expectorant. |  |

### Wild Lettuce—Asthma

| What They Told You | What They Did Not Tell You |
|---|---|
| Orally, wild lettuce has been touted for whooping cough, mucous inflammations of the bronchial tract, asthma, urinary tract diseases, and irritable cough. | Orally, large amounts can cause sweating, increased respiration, tachycardia, pupil dilation, dizziness, ringing in the ear, vision disorders, pressure in the head, somnolence, excitatory states, respiratory depression, coma, and death. |
| The seed oil is touted orally for arteriosclerosis and as a substitute for wheat germ oil. |  |
| Topically, wild lettuce latex is used as an antiseptic. | Topically, wild lettuce can cause contact dermatitis. It can cause an allergic reaction in individuals sensitive to the asteraceae/compositae family, which includes ragweed, chrysanthemums, marigolds, daisies, and many other herbs. |
| Traditionally, wild lettuce has been used for insomnia, restlessness, and excitability in children, priapism, painful menses, nymphomania, muscular or joint pains, for aiding circulation, swollen genitals, and opium substitute in cough preparations. |  |
| By inhalation, wild lettuce is used for a recreational "high" or hallucinogenic effect. |  |

### Wild Yam—Menstrual Disorders

| What They Told You | What They Did Not Tell You |
|---|---|
| Wild yam has been used for various menstrual disorders. It has been touted as an alternative for estrogen replacement therapy to increase energy, sex drive, and breast enlargement. It has also been touted to enhance athletic performance and to slow aging. | Wild yam is a precursor of DHEA. It is related to both estrogen and testosterone. |
|  | Significant research is lacking. |

## What They Told You

### Willow Bark

Orally, willow bark is used for mild fevers, colds and mild infections, headaches, pain caused by inflammation, muscle and joint aches, influenza, respiratory tract and mucous membrane inflammation, gouty arthritis, ankylosing spondylitis, rheumatoid arthritis, other systemic connective tissue disorders characterized by inflammatory changes, diseases accompanied by fever, and rheumatic ailments. Willow bark has long been used as a folk remedy, the active ingredient of salicylate being the ingredient in prepared aspirin.

## What They Did Not Tell You

It may prove safer overall as a precursor than DHEA, but only time will tell for sure.

Based on a willow bark content of 7 percent salicin (superior quality willow bark), 1.5 gallons of willow bark tea per day would have to be consumed to obtain the pain relief of 4.5 grams of aspirin, the average daily dose used to treat arthritic-rheumatic disorders. Willow bark contains salicylates. which are excreted in breast milk and have been linked to macular rashes in breast-fed infants.

Willow constituents include flavonoids, tannins, and salicylates. Most of the information about willow is based on documented pharmacology for salicylates. These actions include anti-inflammatory, antipyretic, dose-dependent hyperglycemic/hypoglycemic, uricosuric/antiuricosuric activities, increase in blood clotting time and plasmaalbumin binding. Plants with at least 10 percent tannins can cause gastrointestinal disturbances, kidney damage, and necrotic conditions of the liver. Some evidence suggests that tannins may cause cancer, while other evidence shows they may prevent it. Regular consumption of herbs with high tannin concentrations correlates with increased incidence of esophageal or nasal cancer.

Possibly, gastrointestinal disturbances, kidney damage, and necrotic conditions of the liver may occur due to tannin content. Theoretically, adverse reactions associated with salicylates are possible including gastric and renal irritation, hypersensitivity, blood in stool, tinnitus, nausea, and vomiting. Salicin has been associated with skin rashes. Possibly, concomitant use may potentiate salicylate effects and adverse effects. Salicylate-containing herbs include aspen bark, black cohosh, poplar, sweet birch, and wintergreen. Concomitant use of herbs that affect platelet aggregation could theoretically increase the risk of bleeding.

Willow bark is possibly unsafe when used orally for viral infections. Although Reye's syndrome has not been reported, the similarity of constituents of willow bark to aspirin prompt concern. Willow bark should be avoided or used cautiously in individuals with aspirin hypersensitivity, asthma, active peptic ulcer disease, diabetes, gout, hemophilia, hypoprothrombinemia, and kidney or liver disease. Theoretically, oral use of willow bark is contraindicated in people with kidney or liver dysfunction

**What They Told You**

**What They Did Not Tell You**

because it might exacerbate these conditions. Plants with at least 10 percent tannins are reported to have the potential to cause kidney damage and liver necrosis.

### Wintergreen—Sore Throat

Wintergreen has been touted to soothe a sore throat and also help in urinary tract infections, digestion, and musculoskeletal pain. It is often used as a flavoring agent in food, candies, and teas.

Significant research is lacking.

It may be safe for most in the small amounts commonly found in foods but is probably not safe when used in higher amounts.

### Witch Hazel—Hemorrhoids

Witch hazel has been touted topically for hemorrhoids.

Witch hazel may be somewhat effective and safe for many when used topically in small amounts.

### Wobenzym N—Inflammation

Wobenzym N is promoted for reducing inflammation and edema and speeding recovery from certain injuries. Often it is used by individuals with arthritis and by athletes, including some professional and Olympic athletes. Enzymes in this product are thought to activate macrophages that attack inflammation-causing circulating immune complexes. Rutoside, an additional ingredient, acts as an antioxidant.

Adverse reactions reported after oral administration include loose stools, increased gas, and skin reactions. Wobenzym N contains enzymes with fibrinolytic activity and might affect coagulation. It should be used cautiously by people on anticoagulant medications. There is some concern about the safety of this product because it contains glandular or organ material derived from animals and therefore may harbor bovine spongiform encephalopathy (BSE, mad cow disease).

### Wood Sage—Liver Disorders

Orally, wood sage is touted for gastrointestinal tract disorders, tuberculosis, mucous membrane inflammation of the bronchi and nose, throat spasms, hypertension, healing wounds, and liver disorders.

Reliable information is insufficient. No adverse effects have been reported.

### Wormwood—Indigestion

Wormwood is used as a flavoring in some alcoholic beverages. It has been used for loss of appetite, biliary dyskinesia, indigestion, and other gastrointestinal complaints. Topically, it has been used for insect bites.

In small amounts, wormwood acts as an aromatic bitter. As the amount increases, it leads to increased salivation. Excessive amounts can lead to confusion, hallucinations, seizures, and even death. It is composed of up to 70 percent thujone, which has an active principal similar to marijuana. It contains a volatile oil that is poisonous.

### Yarrow—Wounds

Yarrow has been used topically to treat wounds since ancient times. It has also been used to treat menstrual bloating, high blood pressure, fever, digestive disorders, insomnia, and anxiety.

It is related to ragweed.

Yarrow contains many helpful substances: salicylic acid, folic acid, ascorbic acid, amino acids, flavonoids, and tannins just to name a few. It has antipyretic, hypotensive, diuretic, urinary antiseptic, spasmolytic, antiflatulant, and antibacterial effects.

It could theoretically interact with other herbs with

| What They Told You | What They Did Not Tell You |
|---|---|
| | sedative effects such as chamomile, valerian, kava, skull-cap, and hops. |
| | It contains thujone and could interact with other herbs that contain thujone such as sage, oak moss, tansy, cedar, wormwood, and tree moss. |
| | Yarrow can affect the menstrual cycle. It should not be used by pregnant females. |

### Yellow Dock—Constipation

Yellow dock has been used as a laxative, for anemia, for sore throat, and for nourishment for the liver.

It has been used topically.

Yellow dock can cause spontaneous abortion in the pregnant, severe electrolyte imbalance, gastrointestinal cramps, diarrhea, and dermatitis. Excessive amounts could cause intestinal atrophy and even death. However, it is usually safe when not used excessively.

### Yellow Toadflax—Digestive Disorders

Orally, yellow toadflax is touted for digestive and urinary tract disorders. It is also touted as an anti-inflammatory, diuretic, and to stimulate sweating.

Topically, yellow toadflax is touted for hemorrhoids, festering wounds, skin rashes, and ulcus cruris.

Insufficient reliable information is available. No adverse effects have been reported.

### Yerba Mansa—TB (Tuberculosis)

Yerba mansa has been touted for cancer, upper respiratory infections, TB, venereal diseases, and even anxiety.

Significant research is lacking.

### Yerba Mate—Kidney Stones

Yerba mate has been touted for depression, diabetes, UTIs, kidney stones, obesity, and aging.

Significant research is lacking.

Yerba mate can cause anxiety, liver damage, and gastrointestinal upset.

It can interact with antianxiety medications and caffeine.

### Yerba Santa—Bruises

Yerba santa has been touted for URIs, TB, and cancer. Topically, it has been touted for bruises, insect bites, and arthritic pain.

Effective research is lacking.

Yerba santa seems benign for many in small amounts.

### Yew—Ovarian Cancer

Yew has been used for ovarian cancer.

Yew bark is the source of paclitaxel (Taxol), the FDA-approved drug for breast and ovarian cancer.

This herb is poisonous and can cause death. Taxol under an MD's care is the way to go if this herbal derivative is to be used.

| **What They Told You** | **What They Did Not Tell You** |
|---|---|

### Yin Chen—Hepatitis

In Chinese and Japanese medicine, yin chen is used orally to treat hepatitis, infectious cholecystitis, and hyperlipidemia. Yin chen is used to stimulate the bile flow, liver, and gallbladder.

Orally, use of yin chen is associated with nausea, abdominal distention, and dizziness.

One study using yin chen and da zao orally to treat infectious hepatitis reported Adams-Stokes syndrome usually associated with heart block.

Yin chen can cause an allergic reaction in individuals sensitive to ragweed, chrysanthemums, marigolds, daisies, and many other herbs in the same family.

### Ylang Ylang—Aphrodisiac

Ylang ylang is touted to increase sex drive, decrease anxiety, and improve sleep. It is touted to have a unique scent. It is scented in the form of an oil and should not be taken internally.

Research is lacking if existing at all.

### Yohimbe—Impotence

The bark of this African tree has been used for many years for impotence in men.

Orally, yohimbe is used for impotence, as an aphrodisiac, for exhaustion, angina, hypertension, diabetic neuropathy, and postural hypotension. Yohimbine, the active constituent of yohimbe, has been used for sexual dysfunction caused by selective serotonin reuptake inhibitors. Yohimbe bark is also smoked or snuffed for its hallucinogenic effects.

Viagra is the new prescription drug that is now so popular for impotence. It has largely replaced yohimbe.

Yohimbe is an alpha-adrenergic blocker. It increases blood flow to the genitals.

Possible side effects are many including: elevated blood pressure, hallucinations, mania, dizziness, insomnia, and possible dangerous drug interactions with antidepressants.

The FDA considers the primary active ingredient, yohimbine, to be unsafe and ineffective for nonprescription use. Large doses can cause toxicity that includes severe hypotension, heart conduction disorders, and death. Children are more sensitive to the effects of yohimbe on the nervous system than adults. When yohimbe bark is used orally, it is contraindicated due to its potential as a uterine relaxant and fetal toxin, and it should not be used while breast-feeding.

Yohimbe can cause excitation, tremor, insomnia, anxiety, hypertension, tachycardia, nausea, and vomiting. The constituent, yohimbine, is associated with salivation, irritability, and fluid retention. Respiration is stimulated by relatively low amounts of yohimbe and depressed by larger amounts. There is one case report of fever, chills, malaise, itchy, scaly skin, progressive renal failure, and lupus-like syndrome associated with yohimbe. Yohimbe is reported to trigger psychosis in people predisposed to

**What They Told You**

**What They Did Not Tell You**

it; symptoms of toxicity include paralysis, severe hypotension, cardiac conduction disorders, cardiac failure, and death.

Theoretically, concomitant use of yohimbe with large amounts of caffeine-containing herbs or products can increase the risk of hypertensive crisis. Caffeine-containing herbs include coffee, cola, guarana, mate, and tea. Theoretically, concomitant use of large amounts of ephedra can increase the risk of hypertensive crisis due to ephedrine content. Theoretically, concomitant use of herbs with monoamine oxidase inhibiting (MAOI) activity with yohimbe can have additive therapeutic and adverse effects. Herbs with MAOI activity include California poppy, gingko, mate, and Saint-John's-wort.

Yohimbe is contraindicated with alpha 2-adrenergic-b locking drugs due to the risk of increased alpha-adrenergic blockade. Theoretically, concomitant use of yohimbe can interfere with antidiabetes drugs due to MAOL. Concomitant use of yohimbe can interfere with blood pressure control and should be used with caution with antihypertensive drugs.

Concomitant use of clonidine (Catapres), guanabenz (Wytensin) should be avoided because yohimbine antagonizes their effects.

Yohimbe is contraindicated with phenothiazines due to the risk of increased alpha 2-adrenergic antagonism and is contraindicated with tricyclic antidepressants due to its potential to increase or decrease blood pressure.

Consumption of large amounts of tyramine-containing foods should be avoided, due to the risk of hypertensive crisis. Tyramine-containing foods include aged cheeses, fermented meats, red wines, and others, as should consumption of large amounts of vasopressor-containing foods due to the risk of hypertensive crisis, such as over-ripe fava beans, coffee, tea, colas, and chocolate.

Due to the cardiovascular effects of the yohimbe constituent, yohimbine, its use is contraindicated in angina, heart disease, and anxiety and depression.

Theoretically, yohimbe might exacerbate symptoms of benign prostatic hyperplasia (BPH) due to the presynaptic alpha-2 blocking activity of the constituent yohimbine. Use should be avoided in diabetes due to the

**What They Told You**

**What They Did Not Tell You**

monoamine oxidase inhibiting (MAOI) activity of yohimbe. Use of MAO inhibitors in patients receiving insulin or oral antidiabetes drugs has been associated with hypoglycemic episodes.

### Yucca—High Blood Pressure

Yucca was a common food of Native Americans. Today it is often used as a flavoring agent in carbonated beverages.

It has been used for high blood pressure and lowering cholesterol. It has also been touted for PMS, menstrual pain, menopause, inflammations, and migraine headaches.

In experimental animals yucca seems to have some anti-inflammatory, antiviral, and anticancer effects.

It can cause gastrointestinal irritation. It is usually safe for most people.

Few, if any, drug interactions have been reported.

### Zedoary—Alzheimer's Disease

Zedoary is an herb originally from the Himalayas. It has been touted for improving digestion, stimulating bile flow, and as an anti-inflammatory. It has even been touted for Alzheimer's dementia.

Effectiveness is not proven.

It does have interesting constituents: zedoary that stimulates gallbladder emptying, sesquiterpene that evidences some anti-inflammatory effects and hepatoprotective effects, and finally some constituents that show antifungal and cytotoxic effects.

It appears to usually be safe in sensible amounts and with little drug interactions.

### Zinc—Common Cold

Orally, zinc is touted for the treatment and prevention of zinc deficiency. It is also used orally for treating the common cold, recurrent ear infections, macular degeneration, night blindness, cataracts, diabetes, hypertension, AIDS, psoriasis, eczema, acne, and many other diseases and ailments.

Zinc is unsafe taken in large amounts. Orally, zinc can cause nausea and vomiting.

There is concern that high daily doses above the tolerable upper intake level (UL) of 40 mg per day might increase the risk of copper deficiency. To prevent copper deficiency some clinicians give a small dose of copper when zinc is used in high doses, long-term.

*Appendix B*

# How Natural Products Work

Natural products work like any other medication. The mechanisms of action are the same. They are often less well known, but with research their mechanisms of action are elucidated. For example, the mechanism of action of the mold from which penicillin was originally derived was initially not understood, but it certainly is today. The mechanisms of action are not mysterious but operate on the same principles as drugs in allopathic medicine.

The following gives an overview of the mechanism of action of some well-known natural products:

## 1. Saint-John's-Wort in Depression

It "inhibits the uptake of serotonin, norepinephrine, and dopamine" (*The Medical Letter*, Vol. 39, 31 November 1997). It also binds to GABA receptors. Some of its constituents inhibit monoamine oxidase, but these concentrations appear to be low. Saint-John's-wort has many metabolites; its exact mechanism of action is not known, but it appears, in many regards, to act similar to the more traditional antidepressants.

## 2. SAMe in Depression

It is one of the basic molecules of life and is in all cells of the body. "It heightens the activity of the mood regulating neurotransmitters dopamine and serotonin" (*The Harvard Medical Health Letter*, Vol. 17, No. 7, January 2001).

## 3. Gingko Biloba in Cognitive Enhancement

The active ingredients are not completely known, and thus, its mechanism of action is not known either. Some of its constituents "scavenge free radicals which have been implicated in the pathogenesis of Alzheimer's Disease" (*The Medical Letter*, Vol. 40, 19 June 1998). "They may be antioxidants or simply mild antidepressants and stimulants" (*The Harvard Medical Letter*, Vol. 15, No. 3, September 1998), rather than a more complex mechanism of action.

## 4. Folic Acid in Depression

"Supplementation with folic acid resulted in improved response to fluoxetine (Prozac) in women, while male patients were not helped by the addition of folic acid" (*Psychiatric Drug Alert*, Vol. XIV). "Inadequate intake of the vitamins folate and $B_{12}$ is linked to both depression and low levels of SAMe in the brain" (*The Harvard Mental Health Letter*, Vol. 17, No 7, January 2001).

## 5. Valerian in Anxiety and Insomnia

"It presumably works through enhancing the activity of GABA" (*Directions in Psychiatry,* Vol. 19, lesson 4). "Valerian is thought to act by potentially binding *GABA A receptors*" (*Review of Psychiatry,* 2000, Vol. 19). Thus, its mechanism of action may be similar to minor tranquilizers. It should also be pointed out that the benzodiazepine minor tranquilizers actually bind to allosteric sites near GABA receptors and, thereby, enhance the activity of GABA.

## 6. Melatonin in Insomnia

Melatonin is a hormone secreted by the pineal gland. It is secreted more at night and is known to promote sleep. "In many older people, the pineal gland is highly calcified and secretes inadequate amounts of melatonin at night" (*The Harvard Medical Health Letter,* Vol. 12, No. 12, June 1996). Thus, it may help older people with insomnia. It has also been used in shift workers since it may work at any time and does not seem to alter normal sleep patterns. One danger could be the large doses that are in some of the preparations today. Just as we do not give large doses of other hormones (estrogen, thyroid) because we fear long-term side effects, the same may be true here. Long-term side effects are not known.

## 7. Kava in Anxiety

"The active components, which are known as Kava-lactones, interact with the same neuronal receptors (GABA receptors) that are affected by benzodiazepines. Other components of the plant may have local anesthetic and muscle-relaxing properties" (*The Harvard Mental Health Letter,* Vol. 17, No. 5, November 2000). Thus, it seems logical it could be abused. High doses have been known to produce intoxication, dizziness, and muscle weakness.

## 8. L-tryptophane in Depression, Insomnia, and Aggression

This most likely acts as a precursor in the synthesis of serotonin and thereby might have some of the effects listed above.

## 9. Echinacea in the Common Cold

Echinacea's mechanism of action is not known, but it may have interferon-like, antiviral effects. It increases lymphocyte activity and seems to stimulate an immune response. "Continued use beyond 8 weeks is not recommended" (*Directions in Psychiatry,* 1999, Vol. 19, Lesson 4).

## 10. Bilberry (Huckleberry by American Indians) in Diabetic Retinopathy

Bilberry contains anthrocyadin, which is thought to decrease vascular permeability, decrease basement membrane thickness, and aid in microvascular blood flow. It is reported to strengthen capillary walls, thus improving circulation and preventing leakage. It has been used "with varicose veins, easy bruising, hemorrhoids, and visual problems including retinopathy" (*Directions in Psychiatry,* 1999, Vol. 19, Lesson 4).

## 11. Milk Thistle (Silybrum Marianum) in Hepatitis

Milk thistle is an ancient remedy now recognized as hepato-protective due to its: (a) antioxidant activity, (b) protection of the hepaticellular membrane, and (c) stimulation of hepatocytes (*Directions in Psychiatry,* 1999, Vol. 19, Lesson 4).

## 12. GABA in Anxiety

GABA is the primary inhibitory neurotransmitter in the brain. Thus, it could theoretically have a calming effect. However, there are several potential problems with simply taking it by mouth: stomach acids, blood brain barrier, and being calm is more than just GABA.

## 13. Coenzyme Q10 in Congestive Heart Failure

Coenzyme Q10 is a vitamin-like compound that is a cofactor in many metabolic pathways such as the production of ATP (adrenosine triphosphate). It acts as an antioxidant and possibly helps in CHF by causing a decrease in oxidative damage.

## 14. Grape Seed Extract in Venous Insufficiency

Oligomeric proanthocyanidins in grape seed extract may have antioxidant and proteolytic enzyme inhibitory effects, which are important in preventing the destruction of the membranes of the vessels.

## 15. Folic Acid in Cardiovascular Disease

These studies are conflicted. Folic acid might decrease the risk of cardiovascular disease in those who have increased plasma homocystein levels since high levels of these seem to be linked to cardiovascular disease in some people. More research is needed.

Many of the herbs used for psychiatric purposes have mechanisms of action similar to standard psychiatric medication. Thus, the belief that somehow they work differently from psychiatric medication is nullified.

It is good to remember that while the mechanism of action may be similar at times, the benefits are not as good in general. Unknown dangers may lurk. There are at times significant limitations to the research; thus caution is essential. Research is not lacking with modern psychiatric medication. While research is certainly gaining in regard to the herbs and supplements, it is no match in general for the psychiatric medications today.

## Appendix C

# Drug-Herb Interactions—The P450 Enzyme System

We would be remiss if we did not provide our readers with a thorough discussion of a potential category of drawback in the use of alternative therapies. All drugs, active plant substances as well, have to be disposed of via a process called metabolism. This is not a simple, straightforward process in our bodies. The liver is the main organ for disposition of the vast majority of active herb substances (phytochemicals) found in alternative medical therapies, or in medications prescribed in the allopathic model for treating various illnesses and disease states. In the last two decades, our sophistication in understanding how our bodies process and get rid of (metabolize) medications by our liver enzyme systems has greatly expanded, and we would like to introduce you, our readers, to some of the concepts that are involved in this process. Before you scream, "They're trying to ram complicated biochemistry down my throat!" let us please assure you that we will assume no prior knowledge of any biologic processes or biochemistry on your part for the purposes of this chapter. We merely want you to be as informed as possible when you go out and evaluate the herbal preparations you might consider using on a daily basis. If you take any prescribed medications, this kind of discussion about possible negative interactions with prescribed medications with your regular physician may get her or him to think about herb-drug interactions more seriously. It may help your practitioner make safer or more effective choices for you.

Let's take a look at what the liver does in getting rid of medications or active principles from herbal preparations. The first principle of detoxification of any foreign substance is to make a substance that can be gotten rid of quickly and with less toxicity. For example, a compound that is less soluble (i.e., doesn't dissolve well in water) cannot be eliminated as readily as one that is more soluble. That is because our kidneys excrete substances that are in a water-based medium (i.e., urine), and our livers and the lining of our intestines are the principal factories for these changes. Therefore, a good deal of the metabolism of drugs has to do with making compounds more easily excretable. Another important function of the liver enzyme system is to change an active drug or substance into one that has little or no activity, compared with the original active substance. These are some of the main functions of liver enzyme systems. The major player in this is called the cytochrome P450 (CYP450) system. This represents a whole family of enzyme systems for metabolizing different classes of chemical compounds. The CYP450 system is found in cells of the liver, the intestinal wall, and the brain. It has a naming system that consists of a number, a letter of the alphabet, and another number. Although there are many subtypes, the most common is called 3A4. About 50 percent of all drugs are metabolized through this large system; 1A2,

2D6, and 3C19 are also commonly used enzyme systems by the liver. They each metabolize many drug substances. What we do not know at this point is which active principles from herbal preparations may interact with the P450 system and its components.

Medications or active principles, from plants and herbs, can be metabolized and therefore be eliminated from the body by the cytochrome P450 system. If it is processed or acted upon by the P450 system, it would be known as a substrate for the P450 subtype. So, in the case of the 3A4 subtype, drugs like those in Figure 1 are substrates and are going to be processed for elimination by the body.

Some drugs also increase the activity of the very system that is trying to get rid of them! These drugs are known as inducers of the P450 system. If the medication (or herbal product) has been taken for a while, the system is "revved up" for getting rid of it. If the substance is suddenly stopped and other drugs that are also metabolized by the same system are being given, then their metabolism will be slowed down and their elimination will take longer.

Other medications can do the reverse by interfering with a particular P450 enzyme system. For example, common antidepressant medications like the SSRI inhibitors (fluoxetine, flovoxamine, and sertraline), nefazodone, and common antibiotics like erythromycin act as inhibitors of the cytochrome P450 system. Even grapefruit juice can powerfully inhibit this system! That means an inhibitor prevents the P450 enzyme system from doing its job efficiently. In addition, if a particular system is inhibited by a drug or active plant principle, then any other drug that would normally be metabolized by that system will also have its elimination slowed down. That means that an ordinary dose of the drug (called substrate) might take longer to be gotten rid of by the body. Or, to look at it another way, a correct amount of a good thing can become just too much. Funny, though, that grapefruit juice can inhibit 3A4 enzyme systems in the gut while simultaneously inducing other metabolic systems in the liver.

This gets to be a complicated business with pharmaceuticals that are commonly prescribed for various ailments. In particular, certain antibiotics and antifungal agents can act as inhibitors of P450 subtypes, and physicians have to double-check on any potential drug-drug negative interactions. As you can imagine, it will get more complicated as we understand the molecular basis for the activities of substances found in herbs and plants. When you consider the staggeringly large number of chemical groups that the body has to eliminate after herbal products are taken (anthraquinones, glycosides, saponins, terpenes, essential oils, anthocyanins, coumarins, tannins, flavonoids, and many others), it is a sure bet that there will be positive and negative herb-drug and even herb-herb interactions. Many of these active principles will, no doubt, have inhibitory or inducing activity on P450 isoenzyme groups. There is a fair amount of test tube (in vitro) data that shows inhibitory effects of various plant constituents (saponins, coumarins, and flavonoids) that inhibit P450 enzyme subtypes. Data is lacking in the human test tube (in vivo). Consider that we are using, as a nation, herbal products that have sources all around the world. What is the likelihood that an herb that originates in South America might have a constituent that interacts badly with an herbal product from halfway around the world? The simple truth is that we just do not know. For example, common grapefruit juice is a powerful inhibitor of the P4503A4 system (while it can simultaneously induce metabolic enzymes). How about that?

That means that any drug or herbal constituent under the sun that has most of its metabolism accomplished by the 3A4 P450 subtype will probably have a blood drug level that is higher than it normally would be. This is because it cannot be gotten rid of (metabolized) as efficiently as normally would happen. Check with your doctor if you are on any medications that have their metabolism performed through the 3A4 system! This does include some common antidepressants, many of whom have their own inhibitory effects on 3A4. It may be a good idea to avoid grapefruit juice if you are taking certain medications.

Medications like fluoexetine (Prozac™), sertraline (Zoloft™), fluvoxamine (Luvox™), citalopram (Celexa™), and paroxetine (Paxil™), all of whom are SSRI-type antidepressants, as well as other substances that also antidepress, namely, venlafaxine (Effexor™), bupropion (Wellbutrin™), and also the old tricyclic antidepressants (like amitriptyline and its cousins), all inhibit 3A4. And this is only a partial list of psychiatric medications. There are many more that use this common P450 system for their metabolism.

How active principles from herbal preparations interact with the liver enzyme systems is largely unknown at this point. The truth is that research simply has not been done to look at the vast majority of herbal products and what they do in our bodies and with other pharmaceuticals; they are not subjected to any rigorous, scientific scrutiny to see if they have any adverse effects or if they interact poorly or negatively with other substances. We have almost no useful information on drug-herb interactions, be they positive or negative!

The business of getting rid of active herb principles or traditional medications is not as straightforward as we had thought in prior times. We have to watch out for potential drug-drug and drug-herb interactions, especially when it comes to the business of metabolism of active substances from the body. Undoubtedly, this area of medicine will get even more complicated in the future. But more complicated can also mean less dangerous.

When we consider drug-herb interactions, there are few scientifically documented and published reports of these kinds of problems. This is good, but it should not let everyone exhale. As our knowledge becomes more focused and detailed, we are certain that drug-herb interactions will become more defined and that we will be more aware of them. But for now there are few known problem areas, at least in the metabolism arena. It is not that many, if not most, physicians and health care providers do not accept the concept of so-called alternative or complementary therapies. It is that the vast majority of such therapies have not been subjected to the same kind of analysis as we perform for any common pharmaceutical product. While many other areas of the world have had positive, or at least no negative, experiences with many herbal substances, we are also aware that if we recommend them, we are doing so with little actual knowledge. This contradicts the usual scientific method that is at the heart of Western medicine. We hate to go on about this topic, but it will become more important as time goes on.

## Drug-Herb Interactions of Saint-John's-Wort

One of the best-documented and well-researched popular products, Saint-John's-wort (SJW) or hypericum perforatum, is an example of interaction with metabolic P450 systems and other biochemical mechanisms in the body. Flavonoids in SJW can inhibit 3A4 in the gut wall. They may also be additive in inhibiting the same enzyme system if grapefruit juice is taken with SJW. One problem is that often crude plant extracts are tested in vitro (in the test tube) as a screening method to see if there are any inhibitory properties against P450 enzymes. The concentrations of active substances are thousands of times higher than would be achieved after ordinary doses are ingested in the body. Also, there are hundreds of different plant constituents present at the same time, so there is no idea which item may be the culprit. A major active substance in SJW, hyperforin, has been shown in vitro to induce 3A4 in liver cells. This has also been shown in human volunteers using clinical doses of SJW.

One cell component, P-glycoprotein (PGP), is a factor in controlling the entry and exit of molecules into cells in many organs including the brain. SJW has recently been shown to induce the amount of this protein in cells. Grapefruit juice also has effects on the expression of this protein. Antioxidant substances from the rosemary plant act in the opposite manner and impede the ability of PGP to transport items to and from cells where they will be metabolized.

Another new scare has made the headlines. It is called the Call-Fleming syndrome and is drug induced; it is most commonly seen in women twenty to fifty years of age. The symptoms include sudden onset of headaches, seizures, and neurologic problems associated with constriction of blood vessels in the brain. Fortunately, this is reversible on stopping the offending drug, but strokes have been known to occur. A number of drugs that enhance the neurotransmitter serotonin, including prescription medications and Saint-John's-wort, have been implicated in this disorder. The evidence for Saint-John's-wort is weak (cf. *Neurology* 2002, Vol. 58, p. 130).

# Kava

Concomitant use of kava with herbs and supplements that have sedative properties might increase the risk of excessive drowsiness. Some of these include 5-HTP, calamus, calendula, California poppy, catnip, capsicum, celery, couch grass, elecampane, German chamomile, goldenseal, gotu kola, hops, Jamaican dogwood, lemon balm, melatonin, sage, Saint-John's-wort, sassafras, skullcap, shepherd's purse, Siberian ginseng, stinging nettle, valerian, wild carrot, wild lettuce, ashwaganda root, and yerba mansa.

There has been one report of an individual who was hospitalized due to lethargy and disorientation that occurred when alprazolam and kava were used concomitantly. The oral use of kava can cause gastrointestinal complaints, headache, dizziness, enlarged pupils, and disturbance of oculomotor equilibrium and accommodation, and rarely, allergic skin reactions. Use of normal doses of kava may affect the ability to drive or operate machinery, and driving under the influence (DUI) citations have been issued to individuals observed driving erratically after drinking large amounts of kava tea. Kava can cause drowsiness and may impair motor reflexes. Numbness in the mouth after chewing the root is another common side effect.

# Ephedra

Use of ephedra and other stimulant herbs such as those containing caffeine can increase the risk of common side effects such as insomnia, jitteriness, tremulousness, dizziness, etc. Using ephedra with other stimulants might also increase the risk of more serious adverse effects such as hypertension, myocardial infarction, stroke, and death. There are several reports of serious life-threatening or debilitating adverse events in patients taking ephedra in combination with caffeine and other stimulants, and over 150 deaths have been attributed to ephedra. Some herbs and supplements with significant caffeine content include black tea, coffee, cola nut, green tea, guarana, mate, and others. Theoretically, use of ephedra with digitalis might cause cardiac arrhythmias. Theoretically, concomitant use with amitriptyline might reduce the hypertensive effects of the ephedrine contained in ephedra. Amitriptyline blocks the hypertensive effects of ephedrine. Use of ephedra with caffeine can increase the risk of stimulatory adverse effects of ephedra and caffeine. There is also some evidence that using ephedra with caffeine might increase the risk of serious life-threatening or debilitating adverse effects such as hypertension, myocardial infarction, stroke, and death. Theoretically, concomitant use might reduce the effectiveness of dexamethasone, due to the ephedrine contained in ephedra. Ephedrine increases the clearance rate of dexamethasone.

Ephedra can raise blood glucose levels and interfere with diabetes drug therapy. Theoretically, concomitant use with Lanoxin might cause cardiac arrhythmias. Theoretically, concomitant use of ephedra and ergot alkaloids might cause hypertension, due to the ephedrine contained in ephedra. Concomitant use of ephedra with MAOIs might increase the risk of hypertension. A hypertensive crisis and subarachnoid hemorrhage were reported after a patient took a 50 mg dose of ephedrine and an MAOI drug. Ephedra might cause false-positive urine amphetamine or methamphetamine test results. One unpublished case involved a false-positive urine methamphetamine assay in a woman who experienced life-threatening adverse effects associated with the use of an ephedra/guarana product. Ephedra might increase blood glucose levels and test results. Current efforts are underway with the FDA to ban ephedra-containing products.

# SAMe

Concurrent use with antidepressants may cause additive serotonergic effects and serotonin syndrome-like effects, including agitation, tremors, anxiety, tachycardia, tachypnea, diarrhea, hyperreflexia, shivering, and diaphoresis. Theoretically, serotonen syndrome may also occur when SAMe is used with other tricyclic antidepressants and with non-tricyclic antidepressants. Concurrent use of SAMe with imipramine (Tofranil) has resulted in a more rapid onset of antidepressant action. Theoretically, this effect may also occur with other antidepressants. Theoretically, because SAMe affects serotonin and other neurotransmitters in a way similar to conventional antidepressants, concomitant use with MAOIs might have additive adverse effects, including hypertension, hyperthermia, agitation, confusion, coma, etc. SAMe should be avoided in patients taking MAOIs or within two weeks of discontinuation of an MAOI. Use of SAMe can cause patients to convert from a depressed state to a hypomanic or manic state.

The Japanese herbs Swertica japonica, kamikihi-to, and Cuban datura candida have anticholinergic properties that may interact with tricyclic antidepressants (TCAs), low potency neuroleptics, and clozapine. The elderly are especially sensitive to this interaction which can lead to blurred vision, constipation, urinary retention, confusion, psychosis, and delirium.

## Valerian

Extended use of Valerian can cause benzodiazepine-like withdrawal symptoms when treatment is discontinued. Patients should taper doses slowly after extended use. There have been several case reports of hepatotoxicity associated with use of multi-ingredient preparations containing valerian, but these preparations may have been adulterated with hepatotoxic agents. Four other cases of hepatotoxicity involving long-term use of single-ingredient valerian preparations have also been reported. Valerian taken orally can cause headache, excitability, uneasiness, cardiac disturbances, insomnia, and occasional morning drowsiness. Some reports suggest that impaired alertness and information processing may occur. Signs of valerian toxicity include trouble walking, hypothermia, and increased muscle relaxation.

## Willow Bark

Concomitant use of willow bark may potentiate salicylate effects and adverse effects. Salicylate-containing herbs include aspen bark, black cohosh, poplar, sweet birch, and wintergreen. Aspirin and Saint-John's-wort also decrease platelet aggregation. Concomitant use of herbs that affect platelet aggregation therefore may increase the risk of bleeding.

## Caffeine and Stimulants

Consumption of more than 300 milligrams of caffeine, which is equivalent to approximately five cups of green tea per day has been associated with significant adverse effects. Caffeine found in green tea crosses the placenta, producing fetal blood concentrations similar to maternal levels. Although controversial, some evidence suggests that high doses of caffeine might be associated with premature delivery, low birth weight, and loss of the fetus. Some sources suggest keeping caffeine consumption below 200 milligrams per day, and excessive use of green tea in pregnancy should be avoided. Concomitant use interacts with the caffeine in green tea and can increase the effects and risk of adverse effects. Natural products that contain caffeine include coffee, black tea, guarana, mate, and cola. Concomitant use of ephedra (ma huang) interacts with the caffeine in green tea and can potentiate the stimulant effects and risk of adverse effects. The concomitant use of iron and green tea can impair iron metabolism in infants and children, resulting in a high incidence of microcytic anemia.

## Others

The South American holly ilex guayusa has a high caffeine content which can worsen anxiety, akathesis caused by neuroleptics, and anxiety or agitation caused by selective serotonin reuptake inhibitors (SSRIs). The Nigerian root extract

Schumanniophyton problematicum is used to treat psychosis and is a sedative that may interact with benzodiazepines and neuroleptics.

Numerous other herbs are potent stimulators of cytochrome P450 enzymes: fructose Schizandrae, Corydalis bungeane diesl, Kopsina officinalis, Clauseana lansium, muscone, ginseng, and glycyrhhiza. These may increase the rate of metabolism of many psychotropics including antidepressants, anticonvulsants, and neuroleptics. Oleanolic acid inhibits the cytochrome P450 enzymes, which could lead to higher blood levels, increase in side effects, and toxicity (Henderson, 1995).

## Summary

Thus, in summary, many foods, herbs, and drugs induce or inhibit the CYP enzyme system. Grapefruit juice inhibits the metabolism of nifedipine (a calcium channel inhibitor and high blood pressure medication). It can also alter the metabolism of cyclosporine and diazepam (Valium), to name just a few. Also, Saint-John's-wort inhibits CYP3A4 and could theoretically interact with many medications. Since individuals with HIV, for example, are often on many medications, including Saint-John's-wort, great caution is in order. Saint-John's-wort could also theoretically interact with oral contraceptives, theophylline, and Tegretol. Gingko could be especially dangerous when combined with other drugs with anticoagulant effects. There have been several reports of spontaneous bleeding with gingko, a case of subdural hematomes, and a case of subarachnoid hemorrhage. Kava, especially when combined with alcohol, could be addictive. A case of coma resulted when kava was given to an individual on Xanax. Figure 2 lists natural products that are either inducers or inhibitors of the various families of the P450 enzyme system.

# Figure 1: Typical Medication Categories with Possible Herbal/Natural Agent Adverse Effects

| Medication Category | Herbal/Natural Agent |
|---|---|
| Benzodiazepines | Kava |
| | Valerian |
| Tricyclic antidepressants | Saint-John's-wort |
| MAOIs | Ephedra |
| | SAMe |
| | Grapefruit juice |
| | Tobacco |
| | Smoked foods |
| | Fructose schizandrae |
| | Corydalis bungeane diesl |
| | Kopsina officinalis |
| | Clauseana lansium |
| | Muscone |
| | Ginseng |
| | Glycyrhhiza |
| SSRI antidepressants | Saint-John's-wort |
| (citalopram least involved) | Ephedra |
| | SAMe |
| | Grapefruit juice |
| | Tobacco |
| | Smoked foods |
| | Fructose schizandrae |
| | Corydalis bungeane diesl |
| | Kopsina officinalis |
| | Clauseana lansium |
| | Muscone |

|  |  |
|---|---|
|  | Ginseng |
|  | Glycyrhhiza |
| Typical antipsychotics | Fructose schizandrae |
|  | Corydalis bungeane diesl |
|  | Kopsina officinalis |
|  | Clauseana lansium |
|  | Muscone |
|  | Ginseng |
|  | Glycyrhhiza |
| Novel antipsychotics | Saint-John's-wort |
|  | Ephedra |
|  | Grapefruit juice |
|  | Tobacco |
|  | Smoked foods |
| Beta-blockers | Kava |
|  | Valerian |
| Calcium channel blockers | Saint-John's-wort |
|  | Ephedra |
|  | Grapefruit juice |
|  | Tobacco |
|  | Smoked foods |
| Acetylcholinesterase inhibitors (used with Alzheimer's and dementias) | Saint-John's-wort |
|  | Ephedra |
|  | Grapefruit juice |
|  | Tobacco |
|  | Smoked foods |
| Birth control agents | Saint-John's-wort |
| Anticoagulants/aspirin | Saint-John's-wort |
|  | Aspen bark |
|  | Black cohosh |
|  | Poplar |
|  | Sweet birch |
|  | Wintergreen |
| Stimulants | Ephedra |

# Figure 2: P450 Enzyme System

| Medication | 1A2 | 2C | 2D6 | 3A4 | Other |
|---|---|---|---|---|---|
| 2∞ amine TCA (Pamelor, Norpramin) | | | S | | |
| 3∞ amine TCA (Anafranil, Elavil) | S | S | S | S | |
| Ace Inhibitors (Zestril, Accupril) | | S | | | |
| Acetominophen (Tylenol) | S | | | S | |
| Alfuzosin (Uroxatral) | | | | S | |
| Alprazolam (Xanax) | | | | S | |
| Aminophylline | S | | | | |
| Amiodarone (C-III antiarrythmic) | | Inh | Inh | S, Inh | |
| Amphetamine | | | S | | |
| Androgens | | | | S | |
| Angiotensin II receptor blocker (Atacand, Benicar) | | | | | |
| Antimalarials | | | Inh | | |

| | | | | | |
|---|---|---|---|---|---|
| Aripiprazole (Abilify) | | | S | S | |
| Astemizole | | | | S | |
| Atomoxetine (Strattera) | | | S | | |
| Atorvastatin (Lipitor) | | | | S | |
| Almotriptan (Axert) | | | | | Excreted by kidney |
| Barbiturates | | | | Ind | |
| Beta-blockers (Inderal, Toprol XL) | | | S | | |
| Bupropion (Wellbutrin) | | | Inh | | 2B6 |
| Buspirone (Buspar) | | | | S | |
| Caffeine | S | | | | |
| Calcium channel blockers (Verapamil, Norvasc) | | | | S, Inh | |
| Carbamazepine (Tegretol) | | | | S, Ind | |
| Celecoxib (Celebrex) | | S | | | |
| Cerivastatin (Baycol) | | | | S | |
| Cimetidine (Tagamet) | In | Inh | Inh | Inh | |
| Cisapride (Propulsid) | | | | S | |
| Citalopram (Celexa) | | S (partly) | | S (partly) | |
| Clarithromycin (Biaxin) | | | | Inh | |
| Clonazepam (Klonopin) | | | | S | |
| Clonidine | | | | | Excreted by kidney |
| Clozapine (Clozaril) | S | | S | S | |
| Codeine | | | S | S | |

| Drug | | | | | |
|---|---|---|---|---|---|
| Cyclophosphamide (chemotherapy) | | | S | | |
| Cyclosporin (immunosuppressant) | | | | S | |
| Debrisoquine | | | S | | |
| Desmopressin (DDAVP) | | | | | Excreted by kidney |
| Dexamethasone (Decadron) | | | | S, Inh, Ind | |
| Dextromethorphan (Dimetapp) | | | S | | |
| D-fenfluramine | | | S | | |
| Diazepam (Valium) | | S | | S | |
| Diltiazem (Tiazac) | | | | S, Inh | |
| Diphenhydramine (Benedryl) | | | | | Limited data-liver and kidney |
| Disulfiram (Antabuse) | | Inh | | | |
| Donezepil (Aricept) | | | S | S | |
| D-propoxyphene (Darvocet-N) | | Inh | | | |
| Duloxetine (Cymbalta) | S | | S | | |
| Eletriptan (Relpax) | | | | S | |
| Erythromycin | | | | S, Inh | |
| Escitalopram (Lexapro) | | | | S | |
| Estrogens | | | | | S |
| Ethosuximide (anticonvulsant) | | | | S | |
| Ezetimibe (Zetia) | | | | | Sm. Intestine; glucuronic conj. |
| Felbamate (Felbatol) | | Inh | | | |
| Felodipine (Plendil) | | | | S | |

| Drug | | | | | |
|---|---|---|---|---|---|
| Fentanyl (Duragesic) | | | | S | |
| Flecainide (C-I antiarrhythmic) | | | S | | |
| Fluconazole (Diflucan) | | Inh | | Inh | |
| Fluoroquinolines (Cipro) | Inh | | | | |
| Fluoxetine (Prozac) | | Inh | S, Inh | Inh | |
| Fluphenazine (Prolixin) | | | S, Inh | | |
| Fluvastatin (Lescol XL) | | S, Inh | | | |
| Fluvoxamine (Luvox) | Inh | Inh | Inh | Inh | |
| Frovatriptan (Frova) | S | | | | |
| Gabapentin (Neurontin) | | | | | Excreted by kidney |
| Galantamine (Reminyl) | | | S | S | |
| Glipizide (Glucatrol XL-oral hypoglycemic) | | S | | | |
| Haloperidol (Haldol) | | | S, Inh | | |
| Hydrocodone | | | S | | |
| Hydroxybupropion (Wellbutrin) | | | Inh | | |
| Ifosfamide (chemotherapy) | | | | S | |
| Imipramine (Tofranil) | | Inh | | | |
| Indinavir (Crixivan) | | | | Inh | |
| Indomethacin (Indocin) | | S | | | |
| Irbesartan (Avapro) | | S | | | |
| Itraconazole (Sporanox) | | | | Inh | |
| Ketoconazole (Nizoral) | | Inh | | Inh | |
| Lamotrigine (Lamictal) | | | | | Glucuronic acid |

| | | | | | conjugation |
|---|---|---|---|---|---|
| Lansoprazole (Prevacid) | | S | | | |
| Levetiracetam (Keppra) | | | | | Excreted by kidney |
| Lidocaine | | | | S | |
| Lithium carbonate | | | | | Excreted by kidney |
| Loratadine (Clariten) | | | | S | |
| Lovastatin (Altocor) | | | | S | |
| Memantine (Namenda) | | | | | Minimal P450 involvement |
| Mephobarbital | | S | | | |
| Methadone | | S | | Inh | S |
| Mexiletine (C-IB antiarrhythmic) | | | S | | |
| Mibefradil | Inh | | | Inh | |
| Miconazole (Monistat-azole antifungal) | | Inh | | | |
| Midazolam | | | | S | |
| Mirtazepine (Remeron) | | | S | S | |
| Moclobemide | Inh | S, Inh | Inh | | |
| Naringenin (grapefruit) | Inh | | | Inh | |
| Nefazodone (Serzone) | | | | S, Inh | |
| Nelfinavir (Viracept) | | S | | Inh | |
| Nifedipine (Procardia) | | | | S | |
| NSAIDS (Bextra, Celebrex) | | S | Inh | | |
| Olanzapine (Zyprexa) | S | | | | |

| | | | | |
|---|---|---|---|---|
| Omeprazole (Prilosec) | Ind | S, Inh | | S |
| Ondansetron (Zofran) | S | | S | S |
| Oxcarbazepine (Trileptal) | | Inh | | Ind |
| Oxybutynin (Ditropan XL) | | | | S |
| Oxycodone | | | S | |
| Paroxetine (Paxil) | | | S, Inh | |
| Perphenazine (Trilafon) | | | S, Inh | |
| Phenacetin | S | | | |
| Phenothiazines (Mellaril, Stelazine) | | | S, Inh | |
| Phenylbutazone | | Inh | | |
| Phenobarbitol | | | | Ind |
| Phenytoin (Dilantin) | | S, Inh, Ind | | Ind |
| Pioglitazone (Actos) | | | | Ind |
| Progesterone | | | | S |
| Propafenone (Rythmol) | | | S | S |
| Propanolol (Inderal) | S | S | | |
| Protease inhibitors | | | | S |
| Quetiapine (Seroquel) | | | | S |
| Quinidine (C-I antiarrhythmic) | | | Inh | S |
| Rifampin (Rifadin) | | Ind | | Ind |
| Risperidone (Risperdal) | | | S | |
| Ritonavir (Norvir) | | | Inh | Inh |
| Rivastigmine (Exelon) | | | | Minimal P450 involvement |

| | | | | | |
|---|---|---|---|---|---|
| Rofecoxib (Vioxx) | | | | | Reduction of cytosolic enz. |
| Rosiglitazone (Avandia) | | S | | | |
| R-warfarin (Coumadin) | | S | | | |
| Saquinavir (Invirase) | | | | Inh | |
| Secobarbital | | Ind | | | |
| Sertraline (Zoloft) | | Inh | Inh S, | Inh | |
| Sildenafil (Viagra) | | | | S * | |
| Simvastatin (Zocor) | | | | S | |
| S-mephenytoin | | S | | | |
| SSRs | | | S | | |
| Saint-John's-wort | | | Ind | | |
| Sumatriptan (Imitrex) | | | | | Excreted by kidney |
| S-warfarin (Coumadin) | | S | | | |
| Tacrine (Cognex) | S | | | | |
| Tacrolimus (Protopic- atopic dermatitis) | | | | S | |
| Tadalafil (Cialis) | | | | S * | |
| Tamoxifen (Nolvadex) | | | S | S | |
| Tegaserod (Zelnorm) | | | | | Minimal P450 involvement |
| Terbinafine (Lamisil) | | | | | Excreted by kidney |
| Testosterone | | | | S | |
| THC (marijuana) | | S | | | |

| | | | | | |
|---|---|---|---|---|---|
| Theophylline | S | | | | |
| Tiagabine (Gabitril) | | | | S | |
| Ticlopidine (Ticlid) | Inh | | | | |
| Timolol | | | S | | |
| Tobacco | Ind | | | | |
| Tolbutamide (Orinase) | | S | | | |
| Tolterodone (Detrol LA) | | | S | | |
| Topiramate (Topamax) | | | | | Carbonic anhydrase |
| Tranylcypromine (Parnate) | | Inh | | | |
| Trazadone (Desyryl) | | | S | | |
| Triazolam (Halcion) | | | | S | |
| Troleandomycin (TAO) | | | | Inh | |
| Valdecoxib (Bextra) | | S | | S | |
| Valproic acid (Depakote) | | | | | Liver |
| Vardenafil (Levitra) | | | | S * | |
| Venlafaxine (Effexor) | | | S | | |
| Vinblastine (Velban) | | | | S | |
| Vincristine (Oncovin) | | | | S | |
| Warfarin (Coumadin) | | | | S | |
| Yohimbine | | | Inh | | |
| Zafirlukast (Accolate-antiasthmatic) | | Inh | | | |
| Zaleplon (Sonata) | | | | S | Aldehyde oxidase |
| Ziprasidone (Geodon) | | | | S | Carbonic anhydrase |

| Zolpidem (Ambien) | S |
| Zonisamide (Zonegran) | Excreted by kidney |

S = Substrate
Inh = Inhibitor
Ind = Inducer
* = contraindicated with alpha blockers

# A List of Psychiatric Medications by Categories of Use

*Frank Minirth, M.D.*

The following is a list by category of usage of psychiatric medications. Some are used on-label; others are used off-label such as some of the anticonvulsants that are used for pain relief and mood stabilization. Most are available now; a few await future approval.

## Categories of Psychiatric Medications

I.   Antidepressants
    A.   Serotonin-Specific Reuptake Inhibitors (SSRIs)
        Citalopram (Celexa)
        Escitalopram (Lexapro)
        Fluoxetine (Prozac, Sarafem)
        Fluvoxamine (LuVox)
        Paraxetine (Paxil)
        Sertraline (Zoloft)
    B.   Tertiary Amine Tricyclic Antidepressants (TCAs)
        Amitriptyline (Elavil, Endep)
        Clomipramine (Anafranil)
        Dexepin (Adapin, Sinequan)
        Imipramine (Tofranil)
        Trimipramine (Surmontil)
    C.   Secondary Amine Tricyclic Antidepressants (TCAs)
        Desipramine (Norpramin)
        Nortriptyline (Pamelor, Aventyl)
        Portriptyline (Vivactil)

       D.   Tetracyclic Antidepressants
           Amoxapine (Asendin)
           Maprotiline (Ludiomil)
           Mirtazapine (Remeron)
       E.   Monoamine Oxidase Inhibitors (MAOIs)
           Phenelzine (Nardil)
           Tranylcypromine (Parnate)
           Moclobemide (Aurorix)—in Canada
       F.   Atypical Antidepressants
           Bupropion (Wellbutrin and Wellbutrin SR)
           Duloxetine (Cymbalta)
           Nefazodone (Serzone)
           Trazadone (Desyrel)
           Venlafaxine (Effexor and Effexor XR)

II.    Obsessive-Compulsive Disorder (OCD)
          SSRIs
          Clomipramine (Anafranil)
          Benzodiazepines
          Buspirone (BuSpar)
          Atypical Neuroleptics

III.   Generalized Anxiety Disorder
          SSRIs
          Benzodiazepines
          Buspirone (BuSpar)
          TCAs
          Neurontin
          Beta-Blockers
          Venlafaxine (Effexor XR)
          Nefazodone (Serzone)

IV.   Posttraumatic Stress Disorder
          SSRIs
          TCAs
          Beta-Blockers
          Buspirone (BuSpar)
          Mood Stabilizers
          Clonidine
          Neuroleptics

V.    Social Phobia
          SSRIs
          MAOIs
          B Blockers
          Benzodiazepines
          Neurontin

VI.   Specific Phobia
          Benzodiazepines
          Venlafaxine (Effexor XR)
          Nefazodone (Serzone)

VII.  Panic Disorder
          SSRIs

TCAs
MAOIs
Benzodiazepines
Venlafaxine (Effexor XR)
VIII.   Antipsychotics (Neuroleptics)
    A.   High-Potency Antipsychotics
        Fluphenazine (Prolixin)
        Haloperidol (Haldol)
        Pimozide (Orap)
        Thiothixene (Navane)
        Trifluoperazine (Stelazine)
    B.   Mid-Potency Antipsychotics
        Loxapine (Loxitane)
        Molindone (Moban)
        Perphenazine (Trilafon)
    C.   Low-Potency Antipsychotics
        Chlorpromazine (Thorazine)
        Mesoridazine (Serentil)
        Thioridazine (Mellaril)
    D.   Atypical Antipsychotics
        Arlplprazole (Abilify)
        Clozapine (Clozaril)
        Risperidone (Risperdal)
        Olanzapine (Zyprexa, Zydis)
        Quetiapine (Seroquel)
        Ziprasidone (Geodon)
IX.   Anxiolytics (Antianxiety Agents) and Sedative Hypnotics
    A.   Anxiolytic Benzodiazepines
        Alprazolam (Xanax)
        Chlordiazepoxide (Librium, Libritabs)
        Clonazepam (Klonopin)
        Clorazepate (Tranxene)
        Diazepam (Valium)
        Halazepam (Paxipam)
        Lorazepam (Ativan)
        Oxazepam (Serax)
    B.   Non-Benzodiazepine Anxiolytics
        Buspirone (BuSpar)
        Hydroxyzine (Atarax, Vistaril)
    C.   Benzodiazepine Hypnotics (Medications for Insomnia)
        Flurazepam (Dalmane)
        Estazolam (ProSom)
        Quazepam (Doral)
        Temazepam (Restoril)
        Triazolam (Halcion)
    D.   Non-Benzodiazepine Hypnotics (Medications for Insomnia)
        Eszopicolone (Estorra)
        Zolpidem (Ambien)
        Zaleplon (Sonata)

Diphenhydramine (Benadryl)
Chloral Hydrate (Somnote)
Doxylamine (Unisom)
Acetaminophen-diphenhydramine (Tylenol PM)
   E.   Barbiturates
Amobarbital (Amytal)
Phentobarbital (Nembutal)
   F.   Neuromodulators
Gabapentin (Neurontin)
Gabitril (Tiagabine)
X.   Mood Stabilizers (Neuromodulators)
   A.   Lithium Carbonate (Eskalith, Lithonate, Eskalith CR)
   B.   Anticonvulsants
Lamotrigine (Lamictal)
Levetiracetam (Keppra)
Carbamazepine (Tegretol)
Gabapentin (Neurontin)
Oxycabazepine (Trileptal)
Topiramate (Topamax)
Zonisamide (Zonegran)
Pregabalin
   C.   Olanzapine-fluoxetine (Symbyax)
   D.   Benzodiazepines
Clonazepam (Klonopin)
Alprazolam (Xanax)
Lorazepam (Ativan)
   E.   Calcium Channel Inhibitors
Verapamil (Calan)
Nifedipine (Procardia)
Nimodipine (Nimotop)
Isradipine (DynaCirc)
Amlodipine (Norvasc)
Nicardipine (Cardene)
Nisoldipine (Sular)
XI.   Attention-Deficit/Hyperactivity Disorder (ADHD)
   A.   Psychostimulants
Dextroamphetamine + Amphetamine (Adderall)
Dextroamphetamine (Dexadrine)
Methyphenidate (Concerta, Metadate, Methylin, Ritalin, Focalin)
Pemoline (Cylert)
   B.   Atomoxetine (Strattera)
   C.   Alpha Agonists
Clonidine (Catapress)
Guanfacine (Tenex)
   D.   Antidepressants
Bupropin (Wellbutrin)
Venlafaxine (Effexor)
   E.   Narcolepsy Medication
Modafinil (Provigil)

XII.    Substance Use Disorders
    A.    Management of Substance Dependence
        Clonidine (Catapres, Catapres-TTS)
        Disulfiram (Antabuse)
        Methadone (Dolophine)
        Naltrexone (ReVia)
        Bupropion (Zyban)
        Topiramate (Topamax)
    B.    Other Drugs That Have Been Used in Various Aspects of Substance Use Disorders
        Methadone (Dolophine)
        L-acetylmethadol (LAAM)
        Buprenorphine (Subutex)
        Buprenorphine plus Naloxone (Suboxone)
        Acamprosate
        Clonazepam (Klonopin)
        Carbamazepine (Tegretol)
        Chlordiazepoxide (Librium)
        Diazepam (Valium)
        Lorazepam (Ativan)
XIII.   Dementia (Alzheimer's Type)
    A.    Cholinesterase Inhibitors
        Donepezil (Aricept)
        Galantamine (Reminyl)
        Rivastigmine (Exelon)
        Tacrine (Cognex)
    B.    Glutamate Receptor (NMDA) Antagonists
        Mematine
        Alzhemed
    C.    Beta Amalyoid Inhibitors
    D.    Anti-inflammatory Ibuprofen (Motrin) Cox-2 Inhibitors
    E.    Estrogen Replacement Therapy
    F.    Free Radical Inhibitors
        Vitamin E
XIV.    Medications for Pain
    A.    Medications for Acute Migraine Headache Pain
        Isomethopetene (Midrin)
        Naratriptan (Amerge)
        Almotriptan (Axert)
        Ergotamine (Wygesic)
        Frovatriptan (Frova)
        Sumatriptan (Imitrex)
        Sumatriptan Nasal Spray (Imitrex)
        Zolmitriptan (Zomig)
        Dihydruergotamine Mesylate Nasal Spray (Migranal)
        Butalbital, Acetaminophen, Caffeine Combination (Esgic)
        Rizatriptan (Maxalt)
        Butorphanol Nasal Spray (Stadol)
    B.    Medications for the Prophylactic Treatment of Migraine
        Aspirin

Propranolol (Inderal)
Amitriptyline (Elavil)
Imipramine (Tofranil)
Sertraline (Zoloft)
Fluoxetine (Prozac)
Ergonovine (Maleate)
Cyproheptadine (Periactin)
Clonidine (Catapres)
Methysergide (Sansert)
Verapamil (Calan)

C.  Nonsterioidal Anti-Inflammatory Pain Medications
Acetaminophen (Tylenol, Datril)
Aspirin
Celecoxib (Celebrex)
Valdecoxib (Bextra)
Rofecoxib (Vioxx)
Choline Magnesium Salicylate (Trilasate)
Choline Salicylate (Arthropan)
Diclofenac (Voltaren, Cataflam)
Diclofenac Sustained Release (Voltaren-XR)
Diflunisal (Dolobid)
Etodolac (Lodine)
Fenoprofen Calcium (Nalfon)
Flurbiprofen (Ansaid)
Ibuprofen (Motrin, Advil, Rufen)
Indomethacin (Indocin, Indometh)
Ketoprofen (Orudis, Oruvail)
Ketorolac Tromethamine (Toradol)
Magnesium Salicylate
Meclofenamate Sodium (Meclomen)
Mefenamic Acid (Ponstel)
Nabumetone (Relafen)
Naproxen (Naprosyn, Anaprox, Aleve [OTC])
Oxaprozin (Daypro)
Piroxicam (Feldene)
Sodium Salicylate
Sulindac (Clinoril)
Tolmetin (Tolectin)

D.  Opioid Pain Medications
Morphine
Morphine Controlled Release (MS Contin, Roxanol, Oramorph)
Hydromorphone (Dilaudid)
Levorphanol (Levo-Dromoran)
Meperidine (Demerol)
Methadone (Dolophine)
Oxymorphone (Numorphan)
Codeine
Hydrocodone (in Lorcet, Lortab, Vicodin)
Oxycodone (Roxicodone, Percocet, Percodan, Tylox)

        Tramadol (Ultram)
- E. Neuropatic Pain Medications
  Tricyclic Antidepressants
  - Amitriptyline (Elavil)
  - Nortriptyline (Pamelor)
  - Desipramine (Norpramin)
  - SNRI Antidepressants (Serotonin-Norepinephrine Reuptake Inhibitors)
    - Venlafaxine (Effexor)
    - Duloxetine (Cymbalta)
  - Anticonvulsants
    - Carbamazepine (Tegretol)
    - Clonazepam (Klonopin)
    - Gabapentin (Neurontin)
    - Oxycabazepine (Trileptal)
    - Topiramate (Topamax)
    - Levetiracetam (Keppra)
    - Zonisamide (Zonegran)

XV. Antiparkinsonian Drugs
- A. Dopamine Precursors
  - Levadopa (Larodopa)
  - Carbidopa (Lodosyn)
  - Carbidopa-levadopa (Sinemet)
- B. Dopamine Agonists
  - Bromocriptine (Parlodel)
  - Ropinirole (Requip)
  - Pergolide (Permax)
  - Pramipexole (Mirapex)
  - Apomorphine
- C. COMT inhibitors (Catecholamine-o-Methyltransferase Inhibitors)
  - Entacapone (Comtan)
  - Tolcapone (Tasmar)
- D. Anticholinergic Medications
  - Benzotropine (Cogentin)
  - Trihexyphenidyl (Artane)
  - Biperiden (Akineton)
  - Ethopropazine (Parsidol)
  - Orphenadrine (Norflex)
  - Procyclidine (Kemadrin)
- E. Amantadine (Symmetrel)
- F. MAO-B Inhibitor
  - Selegiline (Eldepry)
- G. Antihistamine Medication
  - Diphenhydramine (Benadryl)
- H. Carbidopa-levadopa-entacapone (Stalevo)

XVI. Anorexiants (Weight-Loss Medication)
- A. Fat Blocker
  - Orlistat (Xenical)
- B. Serotonin, Norepinephrine Reuptake Inhibitor: Sibutramine (Meridia)
- C. Sympathomimetics

Amphetamine (Biphetamine)
Methanyshetamine (Desoxyn)
Mazindol (Mazanar, Sanorex)
Phentermine (Adipex, Fastin, Ionamin)
Diethylpropion (Tenuate)
Benzephetamine (Didrex)
Phenmetvazine (Preludin)
Phendimetrazine (Adipost, Bontril)

XVII.    Sexual Dysfunction
    A.   Erectile Dysfunction
        Tadalafil (Cialis)
        Sildendfil (Viagra)
        Vardenafil (Levitra)
        Bethanechol (Urecholine)
        Amantadine (Symmetrel)
        Yohimbine (Yocon)
        Alprostadil (Caverject)
    B.   Impaired Ejaculation
        Neostigmine (Prostigmin)
    C.   Inhibited Male Orgasm Secondary to Serotonergic Agents
        Cyprogeptadine (Periactin)
        Bupropion (Wellbutrin)
    D.   Inhibited Female Orgasm
        Cyproheptadine (Periactin)
    E.   Various Other Agents That Have Been Used in Sexual Dysfunction
        Buspirone (Buspar)
        Dextroamphetamine (Dexedrine)
        Gingko Biloba
        Mirtazapine
        Nefazodone
        Testosterone Cream
        Trazodone (Desyrel)
    F.   Hormones
        Estrogen
        Projesterone
        Testosterone
    G.   Premature Ejaculation
        SSRIs

XVIII.    Eating Disorders
    A.   Bulimia Nervosa
        Ondansetron (Zofran)
    B.   Anorexia Nervosa
        Fluoxetine (Prozac)

XIX.    Natural Products
        Omega-3 Fatty Acids
        Saint-John's-wort
        Kava
        Valerian
        Gingko

        S—Adenosymethionine (SAMe)
        Inositol
        Dehydroepianodrosterone (DHEA)
        Phenylalanine
        Tryptophane
        5HTP
        Glycine
        D—Cycloserine
        Serine
        Chromium
        Conjugated Linoleic Acid (CLA)
XX.     Narcolepsy
        A.    Sympathomimetics
              Methylphenidate (Ritalin, Concerta, Metadate)
              Dextroamphetamine (Dexedrine)
              Adderall (Amphetaine plus Dextroamphetamine)
        B.    Modafinil (Provigil)
        C.    Xyrem
XXI.    Movement Disorders
        A.    Tics
              Guanfacine (Tenex)
        B.    TD (Tardine Dyskinesia)
              Vitamin E
              Melatonin
              Gabapentin (Neurontin)
              Benzodiazepines
XXII.   Bed-wetting
              DDAVP
              Imipramine (Tofranil)
XXIII.  Premenstrual Mastalgia
              Lisuride
XXIV.   Smoking Cessation
              Bupropion (Zyban)
              Seleqiline (Eldepryl)
              Nicotine Gum and Nicotine Patch
XXV.    Fibromyalgia
              Milnacipran
XXVI.   Irritable Bowel Syndrome
              Tegaserod Maleate (Zelnorm)
              Alosetron (Lotronex)
              Dicyclomine (Bentyl)
              Diphenoxylate (Lomotil)
              Phenobarbital, Hyoscyamine, Atropine, Scopolamine (Donnatal)
              Loperamide (Imodium)
              Hyoscyamine (Nulev)
              Psyllium
              Metamucil
              Citrucel
              Senokot

# Endnotes

*Preface*

    1. Jonathan R. T. Davidson, and Kathryn M. Conner, "Evaluating Medicinal Herbs," *CNS Spectrums* 6, no. 10 (October 2001): 826.

*Chapter 2*

    1. Vincent Morelli and Roger J. Zoorob, "Alternative Therapies: Part I. Depression, Diabetes, Obesity," *American Family Physician* 62, no. 5 (1 September 2000): 1051.

*Chapter 3*

    1. George Andrew Ulett, "A Rational Approach to Alternative Medicine," *Directions in Psychiatry* 19, part 1, lesson 4 (1999): 59.

    2. *American Society of Clinical Psychopharmacology,* Progress Notes 10, no. left.

    3. Therese Zink and Jodi Chaffin, "Herbal 'Health' Products: What Family Physicians Need to Know," *American Family Physician* 58, no. 5 (1 October 1998): 1137.

    4. "Alternative Therapies," 1051.

*Chapter 4*

    1. Frank Minirth, *In Pursuit of Happiness* (Grand Rapids: Fleming H. Revel, 2004), 189–96.

# Bibliography

Abramowicz, Mark, ed. "Dehydroepiandrosterone (DHEA)." *The Medical Letter* 38, no. 985 (11 October 1996): 91–92.

_____. "Gingko Biloba for Dementia." *The Medical Letter* 40, no. 1029 (19 June 1998): 63–64.

_____. "PC Specs." *The Medical Letter* 43, no. 1098 (19 February 2001): 15–16.

_____. "Phenylpropanolamine and Other OTC Alpha-Adrenergic Agonists." *The Medical Letter* 42, no. 1094 (11 December 2000): 113.

_____. "Problems with Dietary Supplements." *The Medical Letter* 44, no. 1140 (30 September 2002): 84–85.

_____. "St. John's Wort." *The Medical Letter* 39, no. 1014 (21 November 1997): 107–8.

_____. "Vitamin Supplements." *The Medical Letter* 40, no. 1032 (31 July 1998): 75–77.

_____. "Zinc for the Common Cold." *The Medical Letter* 39, no. 993 (31 January 1997): 9–10.

Albers, Lawrence J., Rhoda K. Hahn, and Christopher Reist. *Current Clinical Strategies: Handbook of Psychiatric Drugs.* Laguna Hills, Calif.: Current Clinical Strategies Publishing, 2001.

Allen, James R. and Barbara Ann Allen. *Guide to Psychiatry.* New York: Medical Examination Publishing Co., 1978.

*American Psychiatric Association 2001 Annual Meeting New Research Abstracts.* Washington, D.C.: American Psychiatric Association, 2001.

Anderson, Lynn G. "University Researchers Confirm Three Most Important Factors in Weight Loss." *Journal of Longevity* 6 (2000).

Andreasen, Nancy C., and Donald W. Black. *Introductory Textbook of Psychiatry,* 2nd ed. Washington, D.C.: American Psychiatric Press, 1995.

"Androstenidione Supplements—Not Helpful, Maybe Harmful." *Journal Watch* 21 (January 2001): 2–3.

Arky, Ronald, medical consultant. *2001 Physician's Desk Reference.* Montvale, N.J.: Medical Economics Company, 1997.

Ayd, Frank J., Jr. "Expanding Clinical Indications and Treatment Strategies for Psychopharmacology in the New Millennium." *International Drug Therapy Newsletter* 35, no. 10 (October 2000): 73.

_____. "Omega3 Fatty Acids-Induced Hypomania/Mania." *International Drug Therapy Newsletter* 35, no. 10 (October 2000): 73–74.

Balch, James F., and Phyllis A. Balch. *Prescription for Nutritional Healing,* 2nd ed. Garden City Park, N.Y.: Avery Publishing Group, 1997.

Balch, Phyllis A., and James F. Balch. *Prescription for Nutritional Healing,* 3rd ed. New York: Avery Publishing Group, 2000.

Bannister, Roger. *Brain's Clinical Neurology,* 5th ed. Oxford: Oxford University Press, 1978.

Bartholomew, Anita. "Herbs That Turn Back the Clock." *Reader's Digest,* December 1999, 32.

Beers, Mark H., and Robert Berkow, eds. *The Merck Manual of Diagnosis and Therapy,* 17th ed. Whitehouse Station, N.J.: Merck Research Laboratories, 1999.

Benjamin, Ludy T., Jr., J. Roy Hopkins, and Jack R. Nation. *Psychology,* 3rd ed. New York: Macmillan Publishing Company, 1994.

Bergin, James D. *Medicine Recall.* Baltimore: Lippincott Williams & Wilkins, 1997.

Berkhof, Louis. *Systematic Theology.* Carlisle, Pa.: Banner of Truth Trust, 1958.

Bernstein, Carol A., Brian J. Ladds, Ann S. Maloney, and Elyse D. Weiner. *On Call Psychiatry.* Philadelphia: W. B. Saunders Company, 1997.

Birkmayer, Georg. *NADH: The Energizing Coenzyme.* Los Angeles: Keats Publishing, 1998.

Block, Mary Ann. *No More Antibiotics.* New York: Kensington Books, 1998.

_____. *No More Ritalin.* New York: Kensington Publishing Corp., 1996.

Bloomfield, Harold H., Mikael Nordfors, and Peter McWilliams. *Hypericum & Depression.* Los Angeles: Prelude Press, 1996.

Bognar, David. *Cancer: Increasing Your Odds for Survival.* Almeda, Calif.: Hunter House Inc., 1998.

Braunwald, Eugene, Kurt J. Isselbacher, Jean D. Wilson, Joseph B. Martin, Anthony S. Fauci, and Dennis Kasper, eds. *Harrison's Principles of Internal Medicine,* 13th ed. New York: McGraw-Hill Book Company, 1994.

_____. *Harrison's Principles of Internal Medicine—Companion Handbook,* 14th ed. New York: McGraw-Hill Book Company, 1998.

Brennan, Philip St. Vincent. *Bible Guide to Healthy Living.* Lontana, Fla.: Micro Mags, 1998.

Brett, A. S. "A Simple Treatment for Migraine Headaches . . . and Simple Prophylaxis for Migraine." *Journal Watch for Psychiatry* 4, no. 4 (April 1998): 34.

_____. "Do Vitamin Supplements Reduce the Risk for Cataracts?" *Journal Watch* 21, no. 1 (1 January 2001): 3.

_____. "Is Ginger Extract Effective for Osteoarthritis?" *Journal Watch* 21, no. 24 (15 December 2001): 196.

_____. "More on Estrogen and Cognitive Function." *Journal Watch* 21, no. 5 (1 March 2001): 37–38.

_____. "Testosterone and Aging." *Journal Watch* 21, no. 7 (1 April 2001): 55.

_____. "Yohimbine for Erectile Dysfunction." *Journal Watch* 18, no. 5 (1998): 39.

Brett, Allan S. "Vitamin and Mineral Supplements Don't Prevent Respiratory Infections." *Journal Watch* 22, no. 18 (15 September 2002): 140.

_____. "Magnesium Sulfate for Acute Severe Asthma." *Journal Watch* 22, no. 19 (1 October 2002): 151–52.

_____. "Vitamin D Deficiency: An Explanation for Nonspecific Aches and Pains?" *Journal Watch* 24, no. 2 (15 January 2004): 17.

Brown, Donald J. *Herbal Prescriptions for Better Health: Your Everyday Guide to Prevention, Treatment, and Care.* Rocklin, Calif.: Prima Publishing, 1996.

Brown, Thomas E., ed. *Attention-Deficit Disorders and Comorbidities in Children, Adolescents, and Adults.* Washington, D.C.: American Psychiatric Press, 2000.

Carey, Charles F., Hans H. Lee, and Keith F. Woeltje, eds. *The Washington Manual of Medical Therapeutics,* 29th ed. Philadelphia: Lippincott-Raven Publishers, 1998.

Carson, Robert C., James N. Butcher, and James C. Coleman. *Abnormal Psychology and Modern Life,* 8th ed. Upper Saddle River, N.J.: Scott Foresman, 1988.

Cassidy, Catherine M. *Home Remedies.* Emmaus, Pa.: Rodale Inc., 2000.

Cassidy, Catherine M., ed. "Women's Health Special: Healing Herbs." *Prevention.* Emmaus, Pa.: Rodale Inc., 2000.

Castleman, Michael. *The New Healing Herbs: The Classic Guide to Nature's Best Medicines Featuring the Top 100 Time-Tested Herbs.* Emmaus, Pa.: Rodale Inc., 2001.

Charney, Dennis S., Eric J. Nestler, and Benjamin S. Bunney, eds. *Neurobiology of Mental Illness.* Oxford: Oxford University Press, 1999.

"Chromium for Atypical Depression." *Psychiatry Drug Alerts* XVII, no. 4. Edited by John Roche (April 2003): 25–26.

Clark, Ronald G. *Manter and Gatz's Essentials of Clinical Neuroanatomy and Neurophysiology*, 5th ed. Philadelphia: F. A. Davis Company, 1975.

Cohen, Louise G. "Drug-Drug Interactions." *The Brown University Child and Adolescent Psychopharmacology Update* 3, no. 6 (June 2001): 1, 5.

Conner, Kathryn M., Rosario Hidalgo, and Jonathan R. T. Davidson. "What's in an Herb: Results of an Herbal Brand Survey." *International Drug Therapy Newsletter* 36, no. 3 (March 2001): 17–20.

Conners, C. Keith, and Juliet L. Jett. *Attention Deficit Hyperactivity Disorder (In Adults and Children)—The Latest Assessment and Treatment Strategies.* Kansas City: Compact Clinicals, 1999.

Cooper, Remi. *DHA: The Essential Omega-3 Fatty Acid.* Pleasant Grove, Utah: Woodland Publishing, 1998.

Coppen, A. "Folic Acid Enhances Antidepressant Response." *Psychiatric Drug Alerts* 14:1–8.

Coyle, J. "Seeing a Placebo Work in the Brain." *Journal Watch Psychiatry* 7, no. 11 (November 2001): 85–86.

Cupp, Melanie Johns. "Herbal Remedies: Adverse Effects and Drug Interactions." *American Family Physician* 59, no. 5 (1 March 1999): 1239–44.

Davis, Lisa. "Custom-Fit Vitamins." *Reader's Digest,* November 2001, 89.

Dershewitz, R. A. "Dementia and Statins." *Journal Watch* 21, no. 1 (1 January 2001): 3–4.

Dewey, Laurel. *Amazing Herbal Remedies.* Lontana, Fla.: Micro Mags, 1997.

_____. *Nature's Miracle Tonics.* Boca Raton, Fla.: American Media Mini Mags Inc., 2001.

DiCyan, Erwin. *A Beginner's Introduction to Trace Minerals.* New Canaan, Conn.: Keats Publishing, Inc., 1984.

DiGregorio, G. John, and Edward J. Barbieri. *Handbook of Commonly Prescribed Drugs,* 16th ed. Willow Grove, Pa.: Medical Surveillance Inc., 2001.

"'Dirty Dozen' of Dietary Supplements Named." Web MD with AOL Health. Online: http://aolsve.health.aol.com/content/Article/84/98372.htm. Accessed April 2004.

Douglas, J.D., ed. *The New Bible Dictionary.* Grand Rapids: Eerdmans, 1962.

Dubovsky, S. "DHEA May Be an Antidepressant—but Not a Cognitive Enhancer." *Journal Watch Psychiatry* 5, no. 9 (September 1999): 68.

_____. "Herbal Treatments Can Act Like Medications." *Journal Watch Psychiatry* 7, no. 3 (March 2001): 28.

Dubovsky, Steven. "Fish-Oil Supplements for Depression?" *Journal Watch Psychiatry* 9, no. 1 (January 2003), 2.

Dubovsky, Steven L. *Clinical Psychiatry.* Washington, D.C.: American Psychiatric Press, 1988.

Duke, James A. *The Green Pharmacy.* Emmaus, Pa.: Rodale Press, 1997.

_____. *The Green Pharmacy Herbal Handbook: Your Comprehensive Reference to the Best Herbs for Healing.* Emmaus, Pa.: Rodale Press, 2000.

Eisenberg, David M., Roger B. Davis, Susan L. Ettner, Scott Appel, Sonja Wilkey, Maria Van Rompay, and Ronald C. Kessler. "Trends in Alternative Medicine Use in the United States, 1990–1997." *JAMA* 280, no. 18: 1569–75.

Elkins, Rita. *Chinese Red Yeast Rice.* Pleasant Grove, Utah: Woodland Publishing, 1998.

_____. *SAMe.* Pleasant Grove, Utah: Woodland Publishing, 1999.

_____. *Stevia: Nature's Sweetener.* Pleasant Grove, Utah: Woodland Publishing, 1997.

Ellicott, Charles John, ed. *Ellicott's Commentary on the Whole Bible.* Grand Rapids: Zondervan, 1981.

Ellicott, Charles John. *Ellicott's Bible Commentary in One Volume.* Grand Rapids: Zondervan, 1971.

Ewald, Gregory A., and Clark R. McKenzie, eds. *The Washington Manual—Manual of Medical Therapeutics,* 28th ed. Boston: Little, Brown and Company, 1995.

Fadem, Barbara, and Steven Simring. *Psychiatry Recall.* Baltimore: Williams & Wilkins, 1997.

Fetrow, Charles W., and Juan R. Avila. *The Complete Guide to Herbal Medicines.* With a foreward by Simeon Margolis. New York: Simon & Schuster; Pocket Books, 2000.

First, Michael B., ed. *Diagnostic and Statistical Manual of Mental Disorders,* 4th ed. Washington, D.C.: American Psychiatric Association, 1994.

Flaherty, Joseph A., John M. Davis, and Philip G. Janicak, eds. *Psychiatry—Diagnosis and Treatment,* 2nd ed. Norwalk, Conn.: Appleton & Lange, 1993.

Forster, Francis M. *Clinical Neurology,* 3rd ed. St. Louis: The C. V. Mosby Company, 1973.

Gaebelein, Frank E., ed. *The Expositor's Bible Commentary.* Grand Rapids: Zondervan, 1981.

Geller, B. "Brain Changes in Adolescents with Early-Onset Schizophrenia." *Journal Watch Psychiatry* 7, no. 11 (November 2001): 87.

Gitlin, Michael J. *The Psychotherapist's Guide to Psychopharmacology,* 2nd ed. New York: The Free Press, 1996.

Goldberg, Burton, comp. *Alternative Medicine: The Definitive Guide.* Tiburon, Calif.: Future Medicine Publishing, Inc., 1999.

Goldberg, Burton, and the eds. of *Alternative Medicine Digest. Heart Disease, Stroke & High Blood Pressure.* Tiburon, Calif.: Future Medicine Publishing, 1998.

Goldberger, Leo, and Shlomo Breznitz, eds. *Handbook of Stress—Theoretical and Clinical Aspects.* New York: The Free Press, 1982.

Goldman, H. H., ed. *Review of General Psychiatry,* 2nd ed. Los Altos, Calif.: Lange Medical Publications, 1988.

Good, William V., and Jefferson E. Nelson. *Psychiatry Made Ridiculously Simple,* 2nd ed. Miami: MedMaster Inc., 1991.

Gottlieb, Bill. *Alternative Cures: The Most Effective Natural Home Remedies for 160 Health Problems.* Emmaus, Pa.: Rodale Books, 2000.

Gottlieb, Bill, ed. *New Choices in Natural Healing: Over 1,800 of the Best Self-Help Remedies from the World of Alternative Medicine.* Emmaus, Pa.: Rodale Press, Inc., 1995.

Grinspoon, Lester, ed. "Alzheimer's Disease: The Search for Causes and Treatments—Part II." *The Harvard Mental Health Letter* 15, no. 3 (September 1998): 1–5.

_____. "DHEA for Depression." *The Harvard Mental Health Letter* 16, no. 3 (September 1999): 7.

_____. "How Does Melatonin Affect Sleep?" *The Harvard Mental Health Letter* 12, no. 12 (June 1996): 8.

_____. "Inositol for OCD." *The Harvard Mental Health Letter* 13, no. 6 (December 1996): 7.

_____. "Schizophrenia and the Brain—Part I." *The Harvard Mental Health Letter* 15, no. 11 (May 1999).

_____. "What Is a Nocebo?" *The Harvard Mental Health Letter* 14, no. 1 (July 1997): 8.

_____. "Who Seeks Alternative Treatment?" *The Harvard Mental Health Letter* 16, no. 7 (January 2000): 7.

Hahn, Rhoda K., Christopher Reist, and Lawrence J. Albers. *Psychiatry 2003–2004 Edition.* Laguna Hills, Calif.: Current Clinical Strategies Publishing, 2003.

Haist, Steven A., John B. Robbins, and Leonard G. Gomella. *Internal Medicine On Call.* Norwalk, Conn.: Appleton & Lange, 1991.

Harrison, R. K. *Leviticus, An Introduction and Commentary.* Downers Grove: InterVarsity Press, 1980.

Heinerman, John. *The Power of Healing Herbs.* Boca Raton, Fla.: Globe Communications Corp., 1999.

Henderson, Donald R., and Deborah Mitchell. *Colostrum: Nature's Healing Miracle.* Sedona, Ariz.: CNR Publications, 2000.

Henry, Matthew and Thomas Scott. *Commentary on the Holy Bible.* Nashville: Thomas Nelson, 1979.

Hettinger, Mary Ellen. *Home Remedies from the Bible.* Boca Raton, Fla.: Globe Communications Corp., 1999.

Heymsfield, Steven B., David B. Allison, Joseph R. Vasselli, Angelo Pietrobelli, Debra Greenfield, and Christopher Nunez. "*Garcinia cambogia* (Hydroxycitric Acid) as a Potential Antiobesity Agent." *JAMA* 280, no. 18 (11 November 1998): 1596–1600.

Hollander, Eric, and Cheryl M. Wong. *Contemporary Diagnosis and Management of Common Psychiatric Disorders.* Newtown, Pa.: Handbooks in Health Care Co., 2000.

Hughes, Mark. *Herbalife Catalog.* Toronto: Gero Vita Laboratories, 2001.

Hyman, Steven E., George W. Arana, and Jerrold F. Rosenbaum. *Handbook of Psychiatric Drug Therapy,* 3rd ed. Boston: Little, Brown & Company, 1995.

Jacob, Leonard S. *Pharmacology,* 4th ed. Baltimore: Williams & Wilkins, 1996.

Janicak, Philip G. *Handbook of Psychopharmacotherapy.* Baltimore: Lippincott Williams & Wilkins, 1999.

Jarman, B. "Blood Levels of Vitamin C Associated with Lower Mortality." *Journal Watch* 21, no. 7 (1 April 2001): 54.

_____. "Glucosamine for Osteoarthritis." *Journal Watch* 21, no. 6 (15 March 2001): 47.

Jellin, J. M., P. J. Gregory, F. Batz, K. Hutchins et al. *Pharmacist's Letter/Prescriber's Letter Natural Medicines Comprehensive Database,* 6th ed. Stockton, Calif.: Therapeutic Research Faculty, 2004.

Kaplan, Harold I., and Benjamin J. Sadock. *Comprehensive Textbook of Psychiatry,* 7th ed. Vol. 1 and 2. Baltimore: Lippincott, Williams & Wilkins, 2000.

Kaufman, David Myland. *Clinical Neurology for Psychiatrists,* 3rd ed. Philadelphia: W. B. Saunders Company, 1990.

Keck, Paul, and Susan McElroy. *Overview of CNS Disorders 2001.* New York: McMahon Publishing Group, 2000.

Kirchheimer, Sid. *The Doctors Book of Home Remedies II.* New York: Bantam Books, 1995.

Klatz, Ronald, and Robert Goldman. *Fight Aging!* Boca Raton, Fla.: Globe Communications Corp., 1999.

Komaroff, Anthony L. "Endogenous Opioids Mediate the Placebo Response after Exposure to Painful Stimuli." *Journal Watch* 22, no. 7 (1 April 2002): 56.

_____. "One Mechanism for the Cardioprotective Effect of Red Wine." *Journal Watch* 22, no. 3 (1 February 2002): 21.

_____. "Vitamins: Disappointment and Hope." *Journal Watch* 24, no. 1 (1 January 2004): 7.

Kovach, Sue. *Super Herbs.* Boca Raton, Fla.: American Media Mini Mags Inc., 2001.

Lam, Y. W. Francis. "Efficacy and Safety of Herbal Products as Psychotherapeutic Agents." *Psychopharmacology Update,* November 2000, 1–4.

Lee, T. H. "Folate, Vitamin B$_6$ Intake Associated with Reduced Coronary Risk." *Journal Watch* 18, no. 5 (1998): 38.

_____. "More Evidence for Role in Inflammation in Atherosclerosis." *Journal Watch* 18, no. 5 (1998): 37.

Leonard, Brian E. *Fundamentals of Psychopharmacology,* 2nd ed. Chichester, England: Wiley, 1997.

Lewis, Melvin, ed. *Child and Adolescent Psychiatry, A Comprehensive Textbook.* Baltimore: Williams & Wilkins, 1991.

Ley, Beth M. *Castor Oil: Its Healing Properties.* Temecula, Calif.: BL Publications, 1989.

Lezak, Muriel Deutsch. *Neuropsychological Assessment,* 3rd ed. Oxford: Oxford University Press, 1995.

Long, Donlin M. *Contemporary Diagnosis and Management of Pain,* 2nd ed. Newtown, Pa.: Handbooks in Health Care Co., 2000.

Lullmann, Heinz, Klaus Mohr, Albrecht Ziegler, and Detfel Bieger. *Color Atlas of Pharmacology.* New York: Thieme Medical Publishers Inc., 1993.

Mabbett, Phyllis D. *Instant Nursing Assessment: Mental Health.* Albany, N.Y.: Delmar Publishers, 1996.

Marieb, Elaine N. *Human Anatomy and Physiology,* 2nd ed. Redwood City, Calif.: The Benjamin/Cummings Publishing Company, Inc., 1992.

Marscot, Mary Lynn, ed. *Curing Everyday Ailments the Natural Way.* Pleasantville, N.Y.: The Reader's Digest Association Inc., 2000.

Marton, K. I. "Gingko Biloba for Tinnitus? Try Something Else." *Journal Watch* 21, no. 5 (1 March 2001): 39.

_____. "Initiating ACE Inhibitors for CHF: Safe in the Primary Care Setting." *Journal Watch* 21, no. 1 (1 January 2001): 3.

_____. "Vitex Agnus Castus Fruit Extract for PMS." *Journal Watch* 21, no. 5 (1 March 2001): 38–39.

Matturri, Gina. "News Roundup." *NeuroPsychiatry Reviews* 3, no. 8 (September 2002): 2, 4–5.

Miller, James, and Nathan Fountain. *Neurology Recall.* Baltimore: Williams & Wilkins, 1997.

Miller, Michael Craig, ed. "Disappointing St. John's Wort." *The Harvard Mental Health Letter* 18, no. 2 (August 2001): 8.

_____. "GHB: Its Use and Misuse." *The Harvard Mental Health Letter* 17, no. 9 (March 2001): 7–8.

_____. "SAMe for Depression." *The Harvard Mental Health Letter* 17, no. 7 (January 2001): 4–5.

_____. "What Are the Uses and Dangers of Kava?" *The Harvard Mental Health Letter* 17, no. 5 (November 2000): 8.

_____. "Wine Drinking and Health." *The Harvard Mental Health Letter* 18, no. 9 (March 2002): 8.

Mindell, Earl. *Earl Mindell's New Herb Bible.* New York: Simon & Schuster, 1992, 2000; Fireside Books, 2002.

Minirth, Frank. *In Pursuit of Happiness: Choices That Can Change Your Life.* Grand Rapids, Mich.: Fleming H. Revell, 2004.

Morelli, Vincent, and Roger J. Zoorob. "Alternative Therapies: Congestive Heart Failure and Hypercholesterolemia." *American Family Physician* 62, no. 6 (15 September 2000): 1325–30.

_____. "Alternative Therapies: Part I. Depression, Diabetes, Obesity." *American Family Physician* 62, no. 5 (1 September 2000): 1051–58.

Morgan, Clifford T., Richard A. King, John R. Weisz, and John Schopler. *Introduction to Psychology,* 7th ed. Columbus, Ohio: McGraw-Hill, 1986.

Murray, Michael. *The Healing Power of Herbs: The Enlightened Person's Guide to the Wonders of Medicinal Plants,* 2nd ed. Roseville, Calif.: Prima Publishing, 1995.

Muskin, Philip R., ed. *Complementary and Alternative Medicine and Psychiatry.* Vol. 19. Washington, D.C.: American Psychiatric Press Inc., 2000.

Nemeroff, Charles B., and Thomas W. Uhde, ed. *Depression and Anxiety.* Vol. 12. New York: Wiley-Liss, 2000.

Newmark, Thomas M., and Paul Schulick. *Beyond Aspirin.* Prescott, Ariz.: Hohm Press, 2000.

Nicholi, Armand M., Jr., ed. *The New Harvard Guide to Psychiatry.* Cambridge, Mass.: The Belknap Press of Harvard University Press, 1988.

Nowak, G., M. Siwek, D. Dudek, A. Zieba et al. "Effect of Zinc Supplementation on Antidepressant Therapy in Unipolar Depression: A Preliminary Placebo-controlled Study." *Polish Journal of Pharmacology* 2003; 55 (November-December): 1143–47. Quoted in Kate Casana et al., eds. *Psychiatry Drug Alerts* XVIII, no. 3 (March 2004): 17–18.

Olson, William H., Roger A. Brumback, Iyer Vasudeva, and Generoso Gascon. *Handbook of Symptom-Oriented Neurology.* St. Louis: Mosby, 1994.

Ornstein, Robert, and Richard F. Thompson. *The Amazing Brain.* Boston: Houghton Mifflin Company, 1984.

Passwater, Richard A. *Lipoic Acid: The Metabolic Antioxidant.* New Canaan, Conn.: Keats Publishing, Inc., 1995.

Passwater, Richard A., and James South. *5-HTP: The Natural Serotonin Solution.* New Canaan, Conn.: Keats Publishing, Inc., 1998.

"PC Spes." *The Medical Letter* 43 (February 2001): 15–16.

*The PDR Family Guide to Natural Medicines & Healing Therapies.* New York: Three Rivers Press, 1999.

*PDR for Herbal Medicines.* Montvale, N.J.: Medical Economics Company, 1998.

"PMS Treated with Agnus Castus Fruit Extract." *Psychopharmacology Update* 12, no. 3 (March 2001): 4.

Preston, John, and James Johnson. *Clinical Psychopharmacology Made Ridiculously Simple.* Miami: MedMaster, Inc., 1993.

*Psychopharmacology Update 1997.* Houston: Department of Psychiatry, Baylor College of Medicine, 1997.

*Psychopharmacology Update 1998.* Houston: Department of Psychiatry, Baylor College of Medicine, 1998.

*Psychopharmacology Update 1999.* Houston: Department of Psychiatry, Baylor College of Medicine, 1999.

*Psychopharmacology Update Conference.* Department of Psychiatry, Baylor College of Medicine. Houston, Texas. 2000.

*Psychopharmacology Update Conference.* Department of Psychiatry, Baylor College of Medicine. Houston, Texas. 2001.

*Psychopharmacology Update Conference.* Department of Psychiatry, Baylor College of Medicine. Houston, Texas. 2002.

*Psychopharmacology Update Conference.* Department of Psychiatry, Baylor College of Medicine. Houston, Texas. 2004.

Ramachandran, Anand. *Pharmacology Recall.* Baltimore: Lippincott Williams & Wilkins, 2000.

Restak, Richard M. *The Modular Brain.* New York: Charles Scribner's Sons, 1994.

Ritchason, Jack. *The Little Herb Encyclopedia,* 3rd ed. Pleasant Grove, Utah: Woodland Health Books, 1995.

Ross, Gary, and David Steinman. *Cure Indigestion, Heartburn, Cholesterol, Triglyceride and Liver Problems with Artichoke Extract.* Topanga, Calif.: Freedom Press, 1999.

Roy-Byrne, Peter. "Antidepressant Effects of SAMe, Redux." *Journal Watch Psychiatry* 9, no. 1 (January 2003): 2.

Rutter, Michael, Eric Taylor, and Lionel Hersov, eds. *Child and Adolescent Psychiatry, Modern Approaches.* Oxford: Blackwell Scientific Publications, 1994.

Ryrie, Charles Caldwell, ed. *The Ryrie Study Bible, King James Version.* Chicago: Moody Press, 1978.

_____. *The Ryrie Study Bible, New American Standard Version.* Chicago: Moody Press, 1976.

_____. *The Ryrie Study Bible, New International Version.* Chicago: Moody Press, 1986.

St. Charles, Annell. *Integrated Nutrition.* Nashville: ES Enterprises, 2000.

"St. John's Wort." *Medical Letter* 39. (November 1997): 107–8.

"St. John's Wort." *Psychopharmacology Update* 12 (2001): 7.

Sadock, Benjamin J., and Virginia A. Sadock, eds. *Kaplan & Sadock's Comprehensive Textbook of Psychiatry,* 7th ed. Vol. 1. Philadelphia: Lippincott Williams & Wilkins, 2000.

_____. *Kaplan & Sadock's Comprehensive Textbook of Psychiatry,* 7th ed. Vol. 2. Philadelphia: Lippincott Williams & Wilkins, 2000.

_____. *Kaplan & Sadock's Pocket Handbook of Clinical Psychiatry,* 3rd ed. Philadelphia: Lippincott Williams & Wilkins, 2001.

_____. *Kaplan & Sadock's Pocket Handbook of Psychiatric Drug Treatment,* 3rd ed. Philadelphia: Lippincott Williams & Wilkins, 2001.

Sahley, Billie Jay. *GABA: The Anxiety Amino Acid.* San Antonio, Tex.: Pain & Stress Publications, 2001.

Saklad, Stephen. *The Psychopharmacology Desktop Reference.* Providence: Manisses Communications Group Inc., 2000.

"SAM-e: A 1950's Discovery Reappears to Treat Mild to Moderate Depression." *Psychopharmacology Update* 10, no. 6 (June 1999): 1, 6.

"SAMe for Depression." *Medical Letter* 41, no. 1065 (5 November 1999): 107–8.

Schatzberg, Alan F., and Charles DeBattista. *The Black Book of Psychotropic Dosing and Monitoring 2002.* New York: MBL Communications, Inc., 2002.

Schatzberg, Alan F., Jonathan O. Cole, and Charles DeBattista. *Manual of Clinical Psychopharmacology,* 4th edition. Washington, D.C.: American Psychiatric Publishing, Inc., 2003.

Schillenberg, R. "Chasteberry, Vitex." *Psychopharmacology Update* 12 (2001): 4.

_____. "Vitex Agnus Castus Fruit Extract for PMS." *Journal Watch Psychiatry* 21 (2001): 38–39.

Schwenk, T. L. "Androstenedione Supplements Not Helpful, Maybe Harmful." *Journal Watch* 21, no. 4 (1 January 2001): 2–3.

Scofield, C. I., ed. *The New Scofield Study Bible.* Nashville: Thomas Nelson, 1982.

Scully, James H. *The National Medical Series for Independent Study: Psychiatry,* 3rd ed. Baltimore: Williams & Wilkins, 1996.

Shaner, Roderick. *Psychiatry—Board Review Series.* Baltimore: Williams & Wilkins, 1997.

Shipman, James T., Jerry L. Adams, and Jerry D. Wilson. *An Introduction to Physical Science,* 5th ed. Lexington, Mass.: D.C. Health and Company, 1987.

Siegel, Mo, and Nancy Burke. *Celestial Seasonings Herbs for Health and Happiness: All You Need to Know.* Alexandria, Va.: Time Life Inc., 1999.

Silver, Larry B. *Attention-Deficit Hyperactivity Disorder, A Clinical Guide to Diagnosis and Treatment.* Washington, D.C.: American Psychiatric Press, 1992.

Silverman, Harold M., Joseph Romano, and Gary Elmer. *The Vitamin Book,* revised ed. New York: Bantam Books, 1999.

Simon, D. K. "Is Creatine Protective in Neurodegenerative Disease?" *Journal Watch Neurology* 3, no. 9 (September 2001): 67.

Simpson, John F., and Kenneth R. Magee. *Clinical Evaluation of the Nervous System.* Boston: Little, Brown and Company, 1973.

Skidmore-Roth, Linda. *Mosby's Handbook of Herbs & Natural Supplements*. St. Louis: Mosby, Inc., 2001.

Slaga, Thomas J, and Judi Quilici-Timmcke. *D-Glucarate: A Nutrient Against Cancer*. Los Angeles: Keats Publishing, 1999.

Smith, James, and M. Smith. "Herbal Toxicity." *Directions in Psychiatry* 19 (1999): 363–73.

Smith, Jerome H., ed. *The New Treasury of Scripture Knowledge*. Nashville: Thomas Nelson, 1992.

Solomon, Neil. *Tahitian Noni Juice: How Much, How Often, for What*. Vineyard, Utah: Direct Source Publishing, 2000.

Stahl, Stephen M. *Essential Psychopharmacology: Neuroscientific Basis and Practical Applications*, 2nd ed. Cambridge: Cambridge University Press, 2000.

Stern, Theodore A., and John B. Herman, eds. *Psychiatry: Update and Board Preparation*. New York: McGraw-Hill, 2000.

Stong, Colby. "Does Drinking Wine Help Keep Dementia Away?" *NeuroPsychiatry Reviews* 4, no. 1 (February 2003): 1, 21.

Studdert, David M., David M. Eisenberg, Frances H. Miller, Daniel A. Curto, Ted J. Kaptchuk, and Troyen A. Brennen. "Medical Malpractice Implications of Alternative Medicine." *JAMA* 280, no. 18 (11 November 1998): 1610–19.

Tierney, Lawrence M., Jr., Stephen J. McPhee, and Maxine A. Papdakis. *2003 Current Medical Diagnosis and Treatment*, 42nd ed. New York: Lange Medical Books/McGraw-Hill, 2003.

Tierra, Michael, and John Lust. *The Natural Remedy Bible: Revised and Updated*. New York: Simon & Schuster, 1990; Pocket Books, 2003.

Tomb, David A. *Psychiatry, House Officer Series*, 5th ed. Baltimore: Williams & Wilkins, 1995.

Tortora, Gerard J., and Sandra Reynolds Grabowski. *Principles of Anatomy and Physiology*, 8th ed. New York: Harper Collins, 1996.

"Troubling News on Kava—Plus a Look at Herbals in Drinks." *The Brown University Child and Adolescent Psychopharmacology Update* 4, no. 3 (March 2002): 1, 5–7.

Tucker, G. "Another Dietary Supplement, Another Drug of Abuse." *Journal Watch Psychiatry* 7, no. 3 (March 2001): 22–23.

———. "Endocrine Effects of Antiepileptic Drugs in Men." *Journal Watch Psychiatry* 7, no. 3 (March 2001): 23.

Tyler, Varro E. "Herb Nerve." *Prevention*, January 2001, 95–97.

Ulett, George Andrew. "A Rational Approach to Alternative Medicine." *Directions in Psychiatry* 19, Part 1, Lesson 4 (1999): 53–65.

Unger, Merril F. *Unger's Bible Handbook*. Chicago: Moody Press, 1967.

"Update on Memantine—New Drug for Alzheimer's Still Being Studied." *The Brown University Geriatric Psychopharmacology Update* 6, no. 10 (October 2002): 1, 6–8.

Vance, Mary Lee. "Can Growth Hormone Prevent Aging?" *The New England Journal of Medicine* 348, no. 9 (27 February 2003): 779–80.

Vine, W. E. *An Expository Dictionary of New Testament Words*. Old Tappan, N.J.: Fleming H. Revell Co., 1966.

Vine, W. E., Merrill F. Unger, and William White Jr. *Vine's Complete Expository Dictionary of Old and New Testament Words*. Nashville: Thomas Nelson, 1985.

"Vitamin C May Interfere with Chemotherapy." *The Integrative Medicine Consult* 1, no. 17 (1 December 1999), 160.

"Vitamin Supplements." *Medical Letter* 40 (July 1998): 75–77.

Walvoord, John F. and Roy B. Zuck. *The Bible Knowledge Commentary: New Testament Edition*. Wheaton: Victor Books, 1983.

Wasson, John B., Timothy Walsh, Richard Tompkins, Harold Sox, Jr., and Robert Pantell. *The Common Symptom Guide*, 2nd ed. New York: McGraw-Hill Book Company, 1984.

Watson, Elizabeth. *Vitamin and Mineral Bible*. Lantona: MicroMags, 1997.

Weber, Wim. "Gingko Not Effective for Memory Loss in Elderly." *The Lancet* 356 (October 2000): 1333.

Weil, Andrew. *Natural Health, Natural Medicine*. New York: Houghton Mifflin, 1998.

Weiner, Howard L., and Lawrence P. Levitt. *Neurology*, 5th ed. Baltimore: Williams & Wilkins, 1995.

Weiner, William J., and Christopher G. Goetz. *Neurology for the Non-Neurologist,* 3rd ed. Philadelphia: J. B. Lippincott Company, 1994.

Whitaker, Julian. *27 Most Overlooked Natural Remedies and Cures.* Potomac, Md.: Phillips International Inc., 1999.

_____. *Anti-Aging Miracles: Your Guide to Health Longevity.* Potomac, Md.: Phillips International Inc., 2000.

_____. *Breathtaking Sex at Any Age.* Potomac, Md.: Phillips International Inc., 2000.

_____. *Healthy Alternatives to the 100 Most Commonly Prescribed Drugs.* Potomac, Md.: Phillips International Inc., 1999.

_____. "Healthy Directions: Performance Vitamins That Heal." *Whitaker Wellness Institute Guide to Nutrients.* Summer 2001.

_____. *Miraculous Pain Relief.* Potomac, Md.: Phillips International Inc., 2000.

_____. *New Treatment for Prostate Problems.* Potomac, Md.: Phillips International Inc., 2000.

_____. *No Willpower Weight Loss System.* Potomac, Md.: Phillips International Inc., 2000.

_____. *Reverse Your Heart Disease Naturally.* Potomac, Md.: Phillips International Inc., 1999.

_____. "Seven New Breakthrough Cures." *Whitaker Wellness Journal.* Potomac, Md.: Phillips Publishing, 1998.

_____. *Slash Your Risk of Cancer.* Potomac, Md.: Phillips International Inc., 2000.

_____. *Today's Safest Hormone Replacement Therapies for Women.* Potomac, Md.: Phillips International Inc., 2000.

_____. *What I Would Do If I Had Cancer.* Potomac, Md.: Phillips International Inc., 1999.

Williams, David. "A New and Improved Way to Get Total Heart Support." *Mountain Home.* January 2001.

Wilson, Shannon, Stang. *"Nurses Drug Guide 2005."* Pearson Education Inc., 2005.

_____. "Some Day All Doctors Will Prescribe These Cures." *Alternative Health Journal.* Summer 2001.

Yager, Joel. "Can Omega-3 Fatty Acids Help to Treat Schizophrenia?" *Journal Watch Psychiatry* 8, no. 11 (November 2002): 90.

Youngblood, Ronald F., ed. *Nelson's New Illustrated Bible Dictionary.* Nashville: Thomas Nelson, 1995.

Yudofsky, Stuart C., and Robert E. Hales. *The American Psychiatric Press Textbook of Neuropsychiatry,* 3rd ed. Washington, D.C.: American Psychiatric Association, 1997.

Zhdanova, I., R. Wurtman, and C. H. Green. "How Does Melatonin Affect Sleep?" *Harvard Mental Health Letter* 12 (1996): 8.

"Zinc for the Common Cold." *Medical Letter* 39 (January 1997): 9–10.

"Zinc Has Little—If Any—Effect on Colds." *Journal Watch* 21 (January 2001): 10.

Zink, Therese, and Jodi Chaffin. "Herbal 'Health' Products: What Family Physicians Need to Know." *American Family Physician* 58, no. 5 (1 October 1998): 1133–40.

Zuger, A. "Zinc Has Little—If Any—Effect on Colds." *Journal Watch* 21, no. 1 (1 January 2001): 10.

Zvosec, D. L. et al. "Another Dietary Supplement, Another Drug of Abuse." *Journal Watch Psychiatry* 7 (2001): 22–23.

# About the Authors

**Dr. Frank B. Minirth** is a diplomate of the American Board of Psychiatry and Neurology, a diplomate of the American Board of Forensic Medicine, and certified by the American Society of Clinical Psychopharmacology. Holding doctorate degrees in medicine and theology, he has been in private practice in the Dallas area since 1975. He holds degrees from Arkansas State University; Arkansas School of Medicine; Dallas Theological Seminary, where he is an adjunct professor; and Christian Bible College.

Dr. Minirth is president of the Minirth Clinic, P.A., in Richardson, Texas. He is a consultant for the Minirth Christian Group at Green Oaks Behavioral Healthcare Services in Dallas, Texas; the Minirth Christian Services at Millwood Hospital in Arlington, Texas; the Minirth Christian Program at Fort Lauderdale Hospital in Fort Lauderdale, Florida; the Minirth Christian Program at Summit Hospital in Summit, New Jersey; the Minirth Program at Cedars on the Brazos in Glen Rose, Texas; and Big Creek Ranch in Harriet, Arkansas. He is heard weekly both locally and nationally on radio.

Dr. Minirth has authored or coauthored over sixty books, many of which have been translated into foreign languages. Best sellers include *Happiness Is a Choice, Love Is a Choice,* and *100 Ways to Overcome Depression.* He has more than four million books in print.

He and his wife of thirty-six years, Mary Alice, have five daughters.

For more information on the Minirth Clinic call 1-888-646-4784, or visit the Web site at www.minirthclinic.com.

**Dr. Virginia Neal** is an experienced clinician in pediatrics, psychology, and psychiatry. In her early career she worked both in neonatal and pediatric intensive care as well as general pediatrics. She served on a helicopter rescue team during the 1970s for Harbor General Hospital, a teaching hospital for UCLA. Other teaching experiences include instructing UCLA medical students on the *Initial Examination of the Newborn and Gestational Age Assessment of the Premature Infant.* In addition, she has taught intensive care nurses about resuscitation of critically ill infants. She has initiated and participated in research projects including recent studies on resistant depression, mood stabilization, encopresis in children, and treatment of aggression in adults and children.

Dr. Neal received her RN training at Los Angeles Harbor College of Nursing, attended UCLA for her nurse practitioner training, and received a master's degree from California School of Professional Psychology and Texas A&M University in Clinical Psychopharmacology. Dr. Neal also has a BS, an MA, and a PhD in psychology from Texas Women's University.

Dr. Neal is a licensed psychologist in Texas and currently works in the combined role as psychologist and nurse practitioner.

**Dr. Alan Hopewell** received his PhD in psychology from North Texas State University. He holds a master of science degree in clinical psychopharmacology from the California School of Professional Psychology. He was the first Texan to be board certified by examination in clinical neuropsychology. He is licensed as a prescribing psychologist in New Mexico. He is past president of the Texas Psychological Association. He is fluent in English, German, and Spanish.

**Dr. John Claude Krusz** received his PhD in neuropharmacology from State University of New York, Downstate Medical Center in 1975, and his medical degree from State University of New York at Buffalo School of Medicine in 1983.

Dr. Krusz is a diplomate of the American Board of Neurology and Psychiatry and the American Board of Forensic Examiners. He is board certified in Pain Management, EEG, and Quantitative Electroencephalography. He is the vice president of the American Board of Electroencephalography and Neurophysiology. Dr. Krusz currently serves on the editorial board of the American Academy of Pain Management and is an adjunct faculty member in the Department of Psychology at Southern Methodist University. He has been involved in extensive research in the area of headache and pain disorders.

Dr. Krusz is in private practice in neurology in Dallas, Texas, and serves as the head of his multidisciplinary clinic Anodyne Headache and Pain Care.